GO WITH YOUR FLOW

Dear reader,

Please remember that this book is an educational tool designed to help you better understand your body and advocate for your health. Therefore, it is not intended to diagnose, treat, cure or prevent any disease, and nor is it intended to be used as a replacement for diagnostic evaluation or medical treatment from a licensed healthcare provider. Please always consult with your own doctor before implementing any health-related strategies that you read about in this book, or anywhere else.

In health,

Dr. Alexandra MacKillop, DC

GO WITH YOUR FLOW

A Revolutionary Guide to Better Periods, Balanced Hormones, and a Cycle That Works for You

Dr. Alexandra MacKillop, DC

BLOOMSBURY ACADEMIC
NEW YORK • LONDON • OXFORD • NEW DELHI • SYDNEY

BLOOMSBURY ACADEMIC
Bloomsbury Publishing Inc, 1385 Broadway, New York, NY 10018, USA
Bloomsbury Publishing Plc, 50 Bedford Square, London, WC1B 3DP, UK
Bloomsbury Publishing Ireland, 29 Earlsfort Terrace, Dublin 2, D02 AY28, Ireland

BLOOMSBURY, BLOOMSBURY ACADEMIC and the Diana logo are trademarks of Bloomsbury Publishing Plc

First published in the United States of America 2025

Copyright © Alexandra MacKillop, 2025

All rights reserved. No part of this publication may be: i) reproduced or transmitted in any form, electronic or mechanical, including photocopying, recording or by means of any information storage or retrieval system without prior permission in writing from the publishers; or ii) used or reproduced in any way for the training, development or operation of artificial intelligence (AI) technologies, including generative AI technologies. The rights holders expressly reserve this publication from the text and data mining exception as per Article 4(3) of the Digital Single Market Directive (EU) 2019/790.

Bloomsbury Publishing Inc does not have any control over, or responsibility for, any third-party websites referred to or in this book. All internet addresses given in this book were correct at the time of going to press. The author and publisher regret any inconvenience caused if addresses have changed or sites have ceased to exist, but can accept no responsibility for any such changes.

Library of Congress Cataloging-in-Publication Data Available

ISBN: PB: 979-8-8818-0417-6
ePDF: 979-8-7651-6519-5
eBook: 979-8-8818-0418-3

Typeset by Deanta Global Publishing Services, Chennai, India
Printed and bound in the United States of America

For product safety related questions contact productsafety@bloomsbury.com.

To find out more about our authors and books visit www.bloomsbury.com and sign up for our newsletters.

To my daughter.
And to my sister, my nieces, my friends; to my patients, and to women everywhere.
You are fearfully and wonderfully made.
And to my son, you too are made in His image.

CONTENTS

Foreword by Dr. Felice Gersh		ix
1	Why Knowledge Matters	1
2	To Fertility and Beyond	17
3	Structure Determines Function	31
4	How Your Hormones Work	49
5	Um, Is This Normal?	59
6	Building a Balanced Foundation	71
7	Really Getting to Know Yourself	109
8	Harness Your Hormones	129
9	Birth Control: Know Your Options	143
10	Fertility and Family Planning	169
11	Treatment: Making Your Cycle Work for You	187
Closing Thoughts		235
Acknowledgments		237

Appendix: Hormone Imbalances	239
Notes	249
Bibliography	281
Index	307
About the Author	317

FOREWORD

When I first learned about this book on periods and hormonal contraception, I instantly agreed to write its preface. This is a topic very dear to me and one I cover frequently when I speak on podcasts and health summits, and on the many webinars and lectures I deliver. I repetitively say that whether one decides to conceive or not should be one's own private decision, but that regardless of whether one procreates or not, it should be acknowledged that the prime directive of life is the creation of new life. Everything in the female body evolved for optimal reproductive success, a process requiring that every organ system optimally function. Fertility and pregnancy necessitate a healthy cardiovascular system, neurological system, musculoskeletal system, and immune system, as well as an optimal genitourinary system. Essential to the healthy function of every organ system is optimal ovarian hormone production of estradiol, the estrogen that ovaries make, and progesterone—the ovarian hormones of the menstrual cycle. Of course, other hormones play a role in successful reproduction, but these ovarian hormones are foundational. I have come to no longer call them sex hormones. Instead, I call them "life hormones." Estrogen, as estradiol, is the master of metabolic homeostasis, the hormone that creates harmony throughout the body, optimizing energy production and utilization and orchestrating a synchrony of function among all the organ systems to facilitate successful reproduction and ideal health.

Successful reproduction requires that every organ system operates with excellent health, in a beautiful synchrony with the other organ systems. To achieve that end, there are receptors present in every organ for estradiol and progesterone, and optimal levels and rhythms of those hormones are essential for the organs to operate at peak function. These amazing ovarian hormones, and their lunar rhythm, should not be lightly tossed aside in favor of the chemical hormonal mimics found in hormonal contraceptive pills, rings, and patches, which are recognized officially as endocrine disruptors. Such chemicals were designed specifically to prevent pregnancies by interfering with normal ovarian function, and they have a variety of undesirable impacts on health. Clearly, optimal female health necessitates normal ovarian function and production of ovarian hormones.

There are undeniably benefits to the use of such hormonal contraceptives. Pregnancies can successfully be prevented, an extremely important benefit. Menstrual cramps can be reduced, along with heavy bleeding. Sometimes premenstrual syndrome (PMS) is helped. But there are other, more natural ways to address these problems, if one is willing to investigate the problem and then do all that is necessary to improve the period problem. Optimal health requires the individual to do the work to achieve it.

Periods have taken a bad rap for decades, labeled the "curse" when I was an adolescent, and imbued with negativity. Instead, the menstrual cycle should be recognized and appreciated as a beautiful cycle of health and vitality of women. Celebrating the beautiful rhythms of the female body should occur with the first menstrual cycle and continue for the duration of reproductive life. When problems occur with the menstrual cycles, ideally, the root cause of the problem should be found and remedied in the most natural ways possible, to support optimal hormonal production and function, rather than replacing human hormones with chemical mimics, delivered in an unphysiological manner. Changing how one views periods is foundational to female self-love.

But unwanted pregnancies must be prevented and, admittedly, healthy young females can readily conceive. When contraception is needed, utilizing methods that do not modify the production and rhythms of the female ovarian hormones are preferred, if possible. Utilizing two barrier methods together can provide a high level of protection from undesired pregnancy, in highly motivated individuals. My hope is that all sexually active individuals act responsibly.

I applaud the readers of this book for showing high levels of motivation to understand their bodies and their beautiful life hormones, and because they are clearly acting responsibly by wanting to better understand the options available for contraception and what it means to their bodies to use hormonal contraception. I congratulate you on your decision to learn about hormones, cycles, and contraception. Whatever decisions you make are yours alone. But to make any decision wisely requires a deep understanding of the situation and of all options available. Hopefully, once you've read this book, you'll be optimally equipped with the foundational knowledge needed to make the best decisions for you.

Dr. Felice Gersh, MD, OB/GYN

1

WHY KNOWLEDGE MATTERS

If you are a woman and have periods, you've probably wondered at times if your experience is normal; and when you have these questions, who do you ask for help? Most of us turn to other trusted women in our lives—mothers, sisters, and best friends. But in a society where the subject of menstruation is still somehow taboo in many contexts, even this may feel intimidating and awkward. Ideally, we would feel comfortable enough to ask our doctors about our period concerns too. But unfortunately, many women don't feel comfortable or confident enough to bring their concerns to their physicians, who are sometimes too quick to dismiss them or offer prescriptions that weren't wanted in the first place. So, instead of being able to understand their bodies and make empowered decisions about how to best care for themselves, women assume that what they're experiencing is normal and never get the health care they deserve. If that's you, you're reading the right book.

As a woman, you deserve to know how your body works and what it means when things aren't functioning quite as they should. This knowledge gives you the power to be fully in charge of your own body, equipped to make decisions that support your health, in alignment with your values. It's your right to be the one in charge of this arena and to know what's going on with your hormones so that you can feel your very best. In this book, you'll find answers to all your hormone-related questions and, at the same time, receive the education you deserve but never got in sex education—"sex ed"—as a teenager. You'll learn what's normal and what's not and how to fix it without having to take birth control (and without the side effects that usually accompany it). You'll learn how to embrace your body, harness its hormonal power, and set its systems back into balance with full confidence. While our societal systems still have a long way to go with regards to female reproductive care, this book will bridge the gap for you and other women until that day comes.

A BROKEN SYSTEM

Thanks to cultural movements over the past few hundred years that have pushed for health freedoms, we've made significant progress in the area of female wellness. However, we still have a lot of work to do. Here's why: one of the most commonly prescribed drugs for the treatment of women's health, contraception, and fertility is the birth control pill. While family planning has benefited women and the societies in which we live in tremendous ways, the pill itself simply isn't a great solution for fertility and hormone problems. That's because the whole point of it is to *prevent* fertility and *override* hormones! That's not to mention that even when used as a contraceptive, the birth control pill still comes with side effects and risks, and most of the time when it is prescribed, doctors don't inform women of their alternative options. But other options—arguably better options—do exist, both for contraception and to fix period problems.

As a form of birth control, oral contraceptives (i.e., "birth control pills") seem simple and straightforward: pick a time of day to pop it in your mouth and you can have a painless, predictable period without the risk of pregnancy. Even better, choose the right pill and you can eliminate periods once and for all! But nothing is ever that simple. The pill comes with serious safety concerns, including blood clots, cancer risks, and fertility problems for women who want to pursue pregnancy at a later time. It also increases the risk of mental and emotional disorders such as anxiety and depression and disrupts the important, often spiritual connection between our minds and our bodies. That's because its action as a contraceptive is only possible because of the fact that it completely shuts down our reproductive systems, parts of our bodies that were put in place for good reason.

Contrary to popular belief, our periods have a purpose beyond procreation. They aren't just an inconvenience, a side effect, or background noise, so to speak. They play a vital role in our well-being, and we feel better when we are having healthy, natural periods than when we aren't. As if feeling our best isn't enough of a reason, the case for natural cycles doesn't stop there. While the main point of menstrual and ovulatory rhythms from an evolutionary perspective is to reproduce and further the human species, that's only a single piece of the puzzle. Our reproductive function is also intricately interwoven with every other system of our bodies. The hormonal communication between our brains and ovaries that prompts monthly bleeding is also responsible for coordinating our metabolism, mood, thyroid function, stress responses, and more. Nearly every cell in our bodies has sex hormone receptors, which means that the forces that drive our menstrual cycles also touch on every other aspect of our health. As we'll discuss in more detail throughout this book, the influence of our periods doesn't even stop within the confines of our own bodies. Our hormonal cycles also have intricate connections with the earth, with the seasons, and even with other people. Periods aren't just about creating new life, they're a foundational element of female livelihood as a whole.

As will become abundantly clear throughout this book, our health system falls short in addressing women's health. Parsing out our medical care model into a system-by-system approach loses sight of the integrative nature of our bodies, which explains the unfortunate ubiquity of hormonal contraceptives. That being said, there is no shame in using the birth control pill or in making any other decision for your health that you want to make. The problem instead comes from not knowing what's available to you and, therefore, not having the opportunity to make an informed choice with full knowledge of all the risks, benefits, and alternatives. I too have used birth control pills to try to "fix" my period, and that experience along with my training in women's health has highlighted to me that it really hurts women when they don't know what all their options are. My hope for those of you reading this book is that you would be empowered with the knowledge you need to make your own best decisions. If that includes hormonal contraceptives, that's great! But if you're looking instead to identify the root cause of your symptoms, balance your hormones, and utilize other, non-pharmacological, strategies, keep reading because you'll find all of that and more in the coming chapters.

HOW I MADE THE DECISION TO START USING THE PILL

Like I just mentioned, I too have taken the pill before, and it didn't do for me what I was hoping it would. Here's my story—maybe you can relate:

I made my first gynecologist appointment when I was eighteen. The problem that prompted me to see the doctor wasn't really anything new. In fact, I already had my own suspicions of why my period was missing—restrictive dieting and my intense exercise schedule had lowered my body fat enough to suppress my cycle. But despite putting on weight and cutting back on my workouts, my period was still MIA. Over the previous five years of a rocky relationship with dieting and exercise, I'd noticed a pattern with my periods: Aunt Flo would disappear during marathon training, or if my calorie counting caused the scale to drop below a certain number. Then, in the offseason, or if I relaxed some of my food rules a little bit, she would return for a few months at a time. Then, I'd start a new diet or training schedule, and we'd take another break from each other. It was a different kind of cycle for me, with less bleeding but a similar degree of predictability.

Except, that's not what was happening this time around. It was December, and my last period had been the previous February. My cycle had disappeared for the same reason it always had during my triathlon training in the spring, but it hadn't returned once there was less exercise and more food in the picture. Though I was no stranger to bouts of intermittent *amenorrhea*, the technical term for a missing period, I figured my cycle would have returned already. The doctor said she would have assumed the same, and she ushered me out of her office with a prescription for birth control pills in my hand. "Take this," she said. "It'll kick-start your period."

I waited a few weeks before taking my first pill, even though I'd filled the prescription that same day. Reading the pamphlet on the inside of the box made me nervous, though. Next to the instructions, with details about how to use the calendar of pills, the importance of taking the medication at the same time each day, and the note about making sure the blister packs weren't prematurely punctured, was a text box with a harsh, bold headline: "WARNINGS. Myocardial infarction. Thromboembolism. Cerebrovascular diseases. Carcinoma of the reproductive organs and breasts. Hepatic Neoplasia. Ocular Lesions. Gallbladder Disease. Carbohydrate and lipid metabolic effects. Elevated blood pressure. Headache. Bleeding Irregularities"—the list went on and on.[1] Why had I never heard of these risks before? Why hadn't my doctor brought them up to me? Were these real risks, or were they merely associated with the use of the pill rather than caused by it? (You know, correlation versus causation and all that other statistics jargon.) I decided to reach out to a friend of mine who'd shared with me that she also was taking the pill for menstrual problems, though her predominant symptom was extreme pain—*dysmenorrhea*—rather than an altogether missing cycle. Her dad was a doctor, so I brought up my concerns with him, too. He assured me that the risks were very rare. "They're only a concern," he said, "For people who are already unhealthy." *But was I healthy?* I wasn't so sure, anymore. After all, a major system of my body was malfunctioning. If the aspect of physiology that defined my womanhood was missing, could I truly say I was a fit and well female? And if I wasn't, were those risks truly negligible for me?

I ultimately decided to take the pill after mulling over the issue a little more on my own. I figured that the doctor must have thought the benefits outweighed the risks if she wrote me the prescription in the first place. Plus, I'd heard of other women taking birth control to kick-start their reluctant cycles, and surely it must be safe if it was so common. So, I swallowed the first pink pill and sure enough, twenty-four days later, I rejoined the club of "healthy, menstruating women"—or so I thought.

After a few months on the pill, I left for a hiking trip and accidentally left my pill package at home. When I returned from the vacation, I picked back up with number twenty (after tossing out the previous five pills, which I was supposed to have already taken) expecting to see my period come on schedule. But when that day came and went, and my period was nowhere in sight, I was confused. True, my doctor had told me that it would affect the contraceptive function of the pill if I deviated from the predictable schedule. But she never said that skipping a few days would make my period disappear. She'd actually told me the opposite—that the pill would restart my body's natural periods. *Unless*, I thought, *the pill wasn't actually kick-starting my cycle like it was supposed to.*

What my doctor didn't tell me, and what I didn't find out until months after discontinuing Yaz, was that the breakthrough bleed I experienced during the four days of placebo pills wasn't a real period. Sure, I used tampons and avoided light-colored pants for a few days every few weeks, but that monthly bleed was very different from a true, fertile period. In order to have a real menstrual cycle, I needed to ovulate—something I wasn't doing before the pill or during my use of it, and something that still wasn't happening even after I chose not to refill my prescription. For me, the persistent absence of my cycle was the first red flag that birth control pills weren't everything they were advertised to be.

A few months later, I made an appointment with an integrative physician. My still-missing cycle wasn't the only issue I wanted to bring up with her, but I was sure to mention it along with my other symptoms, such as weight gain, dry skin, and tummy troubles. When my lab results came back, she told me I had hypothalamic amenorrhea and secondary hypothyroidism caused by a combination of stress (thanks, college) and my long history with disordered eating. She explained that I had gained weight partly because I needed to (which my body knew, even if I refused to admit it) and partly because my thyroid was under-functioning. The low levels of thyroid hormone also explained the constipation, the fatigue, the puffiness in my face, and the dizziness I felt when standing up too quickly. "Of course, the pill didn't fix the amenorrhea," she noted, "Because it didn't address the root cause. It was just a Band-Aid over a wound that still hasn't healed." I'm so grateful for that doctor because she helped me realize what I really needed to do in order to get my health back. After just a few months of changing my eating habits, addressing my stress levels, and taking my prescribed supplements, my natural period returned—no drugs required.

This experience opened my eyes to the incredible wisdom and power of my body. Even though I wasn't taking care of myself as I should have been, my body had its own self-protection mechanisms built in. To prevent the loss of valuable biological resources such as nutrients and blood that takes place throughout a menstrual cycle, my body naturally shut down my reproductive functions in response to the food deprivation and chronic stress I was going through. My body also knew that pregnancy at that time, should it occur, would be dangerous to both me and the baby on account of my under-functioning thyroid. So, it sent my reproductive system into protection mode, preventing the possibility of a pregnancy that could potentially be fatal to both parties involved. The significant risks of not menstruating, which we'll explore in more detail later, were less than the risks of potentially needing to grow an entire new human when the original one—me—didn't even have what she needed to be well. Recognizing this sense of innate intelligence that my body had, all on its own, clued me in to the fact that the health of my menstrual cycle could tell me a lot about other areas of my well-being, such as my thyroid function, my nutrition patterns, and more. In awe of the amazing creation that was my physiology, I vowed never to return to the pill and instead let my body do what it was designed to do.

HOW I REALIZED THAT BIRTH CONTROL PILLS AREN'T ALWAYS OUR OWN DECISION

A few years later, I made an appointment with a family practice doctor in my college town for a physical before traveling internationally. The doctor wrote me a prescription for Cipro so I wouldn't be in a pinch if I contracted a UTI and Loperamide in case of food poisoning. "Are you still taking birth control?" He asked, "Because I can write you a refill, so you have enough while you're on your trip." When I shared that I'd discontinued Yaz, I was surprised when he told me he thought that was a bad idea. "Unplanned pregnancy is the worst thing that could happen to your career.

It doesn't matter that you say you're not sexually active right now. You can have the purest of intentions, but you never *really* know what you're going to end up doing." He pushed and pushed despite me declining his offer, and even wrote me a prescription anyway, against my wishes. "In case you change your mind," he said.

I was beyond annoyed by the time I left the appointment, so much so that I nearly threw away the other prescriptions he wrote, too. (I still wish I had, since I never ended up needing them anyway.) *Who did he think he was, telling me that I couldn't trust myself or the choices I'd made with my sexuality? Who gave him permission to (try to) dictate my values, my education, and whether or not I wanted to have children and when? In what world did he think it was okay to make the decision* for me *about whether or not I wanted to use birth control pills*? Until then, I hadn't really considered much in terms of female reproductive rights, as it had never seemed relevant to my life. But once the seed was planted, I couldn't stop thinking about it.

From that moment, the phrase "birth control" became a trigger for me. It caught my attention even if the conversation in which it came up was one that I was merely overhearing, rather than participating in. It was like my ears were programmed to pick up the phrase, and whenever I heard it, my brain waves short-circuited to the place where emotions like anger and indignation were stored. After my frustrating experience with the family practice doctor, the context for conversations surrounding birth control that I was exposed to also seemed to grow increasingly negative. For example, a family friend told me that when she was prescribed the pill for hormonal imbalances, her symptoms not only failed to improve, but actually worsened. Another friend shared with me that the pill triggered the worst bout of depression and anxiety she'd ever dealt with. Her first panic attack, she said, came just a week after starting the pill even though her anxiety had been well controlled for months.

The narratives only worsened as time went on. In graduate school, a classmate of mine was hospitalized for bilateral pulmonary embolisms. The blood clots in both of her lungs that nearly killed her were caused by the synthetic estrogen compounds in the birth control pills she was taking. Around the same time, another friend's sister fell into a coma following an embolism caused by birth control that traveled to her brain. Hearing those stories brought me back to the moments of deliberation before I'd first started taking Yaz. The potential risks and complications listed in the Food and Drug Administration (FDA) insert of my prescription box flashed in the back of my mind: *Myocardial infarction. Thromboembolism. Cerebrovascular disease.* "Minimal risk of adverse events" doesn't seem quite so minimal anymore when you actually meet someone who falls into that 1 percent. It seemed even more significant when I became a doctor myself and started treating my own patients, including more of that supposedly miniscule percentage of women who are harmed from taking oral contraceptives. In my intern year alone, I met three more patients who had developed blood clots as a consequence of taking birth control, as well as two women who had experienced uterine perforation from their intrauterine devices (IUDs). That was all on top of the double-digit number of patient accounts of becoming pregnant even while on the pill. The additional stories of such events occurring in the lives of my patients, friends, and family members seemed never ending.

But high-risk contraceptives aren't the only issue we're facing in the realm of women's health care, though they are indeed problematic. In addition to scary complications like blood clots and organ rupture, countless women experience side effects from hormonal contraceptive use that are even worse than the symptoms that drove them to use it in the first place. Many of my patients seek my help with problems like irregular bleeding, debilitating pain, PMS, weight changes, and acne after already seeing their gynecologists. They, too, were given prescriptions for birth control, not as a contraceptive but as a "treatment." However, they found the pill so intolerable that, like me, they discontinued use after just a few months. Unwilling to try another brand of synthetic hormone, these patients were left without any other options in the traditional medical paradigm, which is how they ended up seeking help through functional medicine.

Meeting these women and hearing their stories changed me. Not only has my work as a functional medicine doctor and acupuncturist expanded my understanding of just how much harm is caused by birth control drugs but it's opened my eyes to the epidemic lack of informed consent. Patients aren't aware of what could happen to them as a result of using hormonal contraceptives. Now, when I hear stories or read articles about complications and side effects, the faces of real-life women come to my mind. It's no longer just a scientific discussion of statistics and risk factors for me; it's a matter of my patients' lives and livelihoods, people whom I care deeply for and have a responsibility to protect from a medical standpoint. But I know that the problem stretches far beyond the four walls of my office. The lack of education in the realm of reproductive health affects every woman. It affects me, and it affects you. It affects our mothers, our sisters, our daughters, and our friends. It even affects men, because each of us—every human being on this planet—is only here because of the full functioning of a woman's reproductive system. The status quo of our medical system and its infringements on the reproductive rights of women is a critical issue that can no longer be ignored.

The problem with our medical system's current approach to women's health doesn't end with birth control pills, however. Really, the biggest problem we face is the fact that doctors feel the need to prescribe them at all. I truly believe that health care providers, even the one who bullied me about my own contraceptive preferences, usually have good intentions. They want to help their patients, but they aren't always equipped to do so in the best possible way. Most physicians prescribe birth control for women's health concerns because it's what they learned to do. We desperately need this to change. In addition to offering safe and effective treatment options, health care providers have a responsibility to help patients to not only heal but also to thrive. If all women knew that other treatment options are available, and if we all understood more about our own bodies and how they function, we'd have much less need for interventions like the birth control pill. In women's reproductive health, this means having more than just a tolerable cycle but, rather, a painless, peaceful, and—dare I say it—enjoyable one as well.

In addition to helping you understand the risks of birth control and the alternative methods you can use to manage your reproductive health, I want you to be able to experience how truly enjoyable a hormonally balanced cycle can be. PMS symptoms like a low mood, cramping, or breast tenderness don't need to be your usual anymore. In fact, I would even argue that they shouldn't be. When you know how to work with your body and interpret the signals it is giving you, you are empowered to make changes that allow your hormones to naturally fall back into balance. Most of the time, all your body needs is a little TLC, and knowing the next right step to take makes a world of difference.

Sisters, that's exactly the reason I wrote this book. I want to provide you with the information you need to advocate for and protect your personal health so you can feel your very best. It is my goal to educate and empower you to see your body as an ally rather than a burden because once you realize that it really is on your side, you can more easily cultivate the vibrant, fulfilling life you deserve. At the same time, I hope to ignite a passion in you for learning about your own body and inspire you to keep exploring your fertility even outside the binding of these pages. Sure, some of what you read in this book might seem like old news—things you already know. Some of the information might even confirm long-standing suspicions you had about your health that were never acknowledged by your doctor. But other things might altogether surprise you, and I hope that the astonishment motivates you to keep digging to see what else you can find out about yourself.

The process of writing this book opened the door to conversations with the women in my life that might ordinarily be reserved for patients within the private, protected setting of my office. But once my friends and family members learned that I was writing a book about periods *of all things*, they started bombarding me with all the questions they'd wondered about for years with regards their own bodies, but they never knew where to turn for answers. One of my best girlfriends even followed up her questions with, "You're a doctor, so that's why I'm telling you this." *Right*, I thought, *that, and you never actually brought it up with your own doctor!* Ladies, you deserve to have your questions answered, and my hope is that this book will inspire you to bring up these topics with your health care team. But don't let it stop there—keep the dialogue going with your friends, mothers, sisters, and daughters. Let's start a revolution and change not only our personal conversations but the cultural ones as well.

SEX ED NEEDS A MAKEOVER

I can only speak from personal experience in this case, but the sexual education I received when I was growing up came mainly from my friends and classmates who, like me, had no clue what was going on with their bodies. All of us were trying to figure out how to cope with what was happening to us while, at the same time, maintaining at least the bare minimum level of coolness. For most of us, this meant averting our eyes and making fun of the teacher whenever topics like *Reproduction* or *Sexual Intercourse* came up in class. As if the educational videos and awkward slide shows weren't bad enough already, few of us actually paid any attention at all.

My first introduction to fertility came from a book I found on our family's bookshelf titled *How Babies Are Made*. From what I remember, it involved cartoonish illustrations of puppies, kittens, *chickens* of all things, and, finally, a man and a woman with brief explanations of how 1 + 1 eventually equals 3. I remember being simultaneously horrified and intrigued by the sentence, "In the beginning, you were smaller than the size of a pencil dot." Fast-forward to fourth grade when my teacher announced that we would be dividing into two groups—according to gender—to discuss *puberty*. I remember lots of whispering and uncomfortable shuffling as the girls in my class corralled into a neighboring classroom. A teacher I didn't recognize explained to us the following key points:

- "Sometime in the next one to five years, you will get your period. You'll have it every month until you don't anymore."
- "No, it won't hurt. But you might have a stomachache."
- "Here's some deodorant."

Once again, I remember experiencing conflicting feelings of curiosity and disgust as a word that used to hold no significance beyond a small, round punctuation mark became suddenly taboo. When discussing the subject quietly among ourselves, my best friend and I came up with a code word for periods—the *apple*. I can't decide if it was the way my teacher talked about it that day, or how my classmates responded, or the fact that the whole subject was "hush hush" in general, but my earliest memories of conversations surrounding periods and female reproductive health were laced with silence and shame.

Not much changed in high school, when the birds-and-the-bees conversation took on a new life and my health teachers started setting the stage for birth control. My own health teacher was next to famous for his "triple protection plan," which involved not only the recommendation that girls use birth control pills but that couples employ both the use of condoms *and* the withdrawal method. Of course, safe sex is important, but the safest sex is the kind that involves both parties' full awareness of the functioning of their bodies. Because sex, like periods, is still a taboo topic, health education classes often serve as the only guaranteed time for adolescents to learn about their own reproductive health in a safe space. But these educational opportunities are disastrously limited to fearmongering lectures about the horrors of sexually transmitted infections (STIs) and teenage pregnancy. In sex ed classes, as they're currently run, there is no discussion of what's normal with a menstrual cycle, how abnormalities can affect a woman's life, or what can be done to support the natural, healthy function of her body. Instead, students are ushered out of the classroom and into adulthood, left to wonder about their reproductive symptoms until they become overwhelming enough to seek advice from a health care provider who simply recommends birth control pills. (That is, if the woman isn't already taking them.)

INFORMATION IS THE PATH TO EMPOWERMENT

"When you know better, do better." Maya Angelou is credited with these powerful words, inspiring women away from the shame of regret and into a stance of hopefulness and action. But when we read between the lines a little bit (I know, I know, we usually shouldn't do that) we can see the important undertones that give substance to the quote: when presented with full knowledge of our circumstances, many of us would choose differently. We would choose to learn what is and isn't normal from a young age, to learn how to advocate for ourselves, and be the ones in charge of making decisions about our bodies. All the while, we would choose to do so while equipped with full knowledge of all of our options. This is the whole premise of informed consent in medicine; we can't safely make decisions about our health and what happens to us—something that is our right—when we don't fully understand the risks, benefits, and alternatives to a given intervention. When we don't know something, it's not our fault. But it also means that the power to make that decision never truly belonged to us.

So many of my patients come to me as adults dealing with period problems that started when they were teenagers because nobody ever told them that what they were experiencing wasn't normal. Still others started taking the pill per the advice of their physician due to menstrual irregularities only to come off it and find their cycle even more irregular than it was prior to starting. Others are surprised that they have no cycle at all or, perhaps, have new symptoms of "premenstrual syndrome" that they'd never previously experienced, such as cramps, heavy bleeding, acne, or headaches. The result of such a lack of information is the antithesis of female empowerment. When I work with patients who have been wronged by the medical model in this way, they are shocked to learn just how much they had allowed someone else to steer the wheel of their health, sometimes in ways contrary to what they would have chosen had they truly been allowed the informed consent they were entitled to. You don't have to sit back and accept the role of passenger in your own life.

In fact, countless studies have shown that individuals who take an active role in their well-being are happier,[2] healthier, and tend to live longer than their more passive counterparts, sometimes more than a decade longer.[3] Advocating for yourself and becoming an ally with your body really does allow you to not only survive but also to thrive—periods included! I won't lie, periods in general are not particularly fun. Even if they are completely painless (as they should be), they are still time-consuming, inconvenient, and seem to have a vendetta against white jeans. Many of us feel that our lives would be better if we didn't have to deal with menstruation at all. But I think that when things go right, they can really be considered an ally, and I hope that after reading this book, you will too. Instead of a burden and a hindrance, science and history show that our periods—and our bodies—are a good thing. Our natural physiology is an asset, and we're better off when we embrace and honor it.

A CHANGE IN PERSPECTIVE

If that sounds insane to you, I get it. I felt that way too for many years. But as I slowly learned more about the female body and all its intricacies, the more I realized how powerful and important our menstrual cycles are. Once I understood that my period didn't have to hinder my lifestyle and goals but, instead, could enhance them, everything changed for the better. That is exactly what I'll be teaching you about in the coming chapters. But in order to truly be able to receive and process the information held in the remaining pages of this book, we're going to have to shift our perspective away from the desire to control and subdue our bodies and instead start seeing them as our allies, as something to be honored.

Because of the way our culture teaches us to think of our bodies, it's easy to feel like they are working against us rather than being members of the same team. So often, it seems like Aunt Flo arrives on exactly the wrong day, that nights of insomnia always strike right before a big event (or when our young children actually happen to sleep), or that our bodies are trying to oppose all of our diet and fitness goals. (Have you ever felt like you gain weight just by *looking* at pizza?) But many of these seemingly inconvenient occurrences are merely symptoms of a deeper problem with our health, signals that our bodies are giving to let us know that something is amiss. In fact, some of these symptoms actually create a protective effect for our health, shielding us from the full brunt of the forces underlying our problems. Many of us dismiss these symptoms, seeing them as an inconvenience, but if we slow down and tune in to our bodies instead, we'll save ourselves a whole lot of grief and frustration in the long run.

Menstruation is a key example of this. We often see our periods as limiting. Men don't have to "overcome these inconveniences," we argue, so women shouldn't have to, either. Even commercials for feminine protection products market themselves as a "solution" or "cure" for periods, allowing women to do exactly what they want to do, regardless of what's going on with their bodies. But ignoring our periods isn't as easy as putting in a tampon and getting back on the tennis court. Anyone who has had a period knows that certain activities seem much more appealing than others during that time of the month. But rather than a limitation or a problem to be overcome, our periods, and our other bodily processes, serve to enhance our vitality and well-being. The signals our bodies give us are valuable tools, giving us information about how we should live so that we can take the best possible care of ourselves. When we ignore those signals about what we truly *need* in order to do what we *want*, we paradoxically end up worse for wear. True freedom is not found in transcending the reality of our bodies and succumbing to the pressures and expectations of a society that antagonizes normal, natural hormonal fluctuations but, rather, in having permission to live life according to our natural design.

SOME NOTES ABOUT HOW THIS BOOK IS ORGANIZED

As we get started, be aware that there are several themes interwoven throughout this book. First and foremost: knowledge is power. It's a serious disadvantage to be able to climb a mountain, program a computer, change the oil in a car, cook a gourmet meal, or perform any of the other incredible tasks that your female body can perform if you don't actually know how it works. I want you to become an advocate for yourself so that you never have to question if you would've done things differently had you known you had other options. Next, we'll dive into the science. In our discussions of anatomy and physiology, you'll learn what is and isn't normal in terms of your female body's structure and function, and how to use changes in your menstrual cycle as a sounding board for whether or not other systems in your body are healthy too. In other words, we'll be talking about your fertility. Spoiler alert: it has to do with way more than your ability to get pregnant or your lack thereof. Finally, we'll get practical. I will teach you how to track your cycle and hormone levels without ever having to undergo invasive fertility testing. You can do this easily at home with your own two hands (and a thermometer, if you have one). You'll also learn how to align your lifestyle with your body's inborn, natural hormonal fluctuations so that you can feel your very best. Finally, in chapters 10 and 11, we'll talk about your options for family planning and truly fixing your period without a birth control prescription, if that's what you prefer to do. And if you still want to use the pill? Do it—judgment free! My heart's desire is for you to make that choice while armed with the full knowledge of its risks, benefits, and alternatives. That's informed consent, and it's every woman's birthright.

SOME NOTES ABOUT MY BACKGROUND

If you're going to be taking my advice, which I hope you do, I feel it's important for you to know the woman behind the pages. I'm Alexandra MacKillop, a functional medicine doctor with, as you probably have already picked up on, a fiery passion for women's health and fertility. I see patients both online and in person at an integrative clinic near Chicago and write a blog through which I share articles about the same sorts of topics you'll find in this book. Prior to entering the world of functional medicine, I ran a nutrition business where I helped women break up with dieting and learn how to eat their favorite foods without feeling guilty. You'll therefore also find themes about gentle nutrition and making peace with your natural body size in this book.

I earned my bachelor's degree in food science at Purdue University in West Lafayette, where I then completed graduate coursework in clinical nutrition and public health. When I returned to Chicago, I did so in pursuit of my doctoral degree in chiropractic medicine at the National University of Health Sciences, where I also completed advanced training in functional medicine with an emphasis on endocrine disorders and fertility. I am also a wife, mother, and sister and a cheerleader for all other women who want to take their health back into their own hands so they can make decisions for themselves about how they want to care for their bodies.

If that describes you, let's get started!

2

TO FERTILITY AND BEYOND

How do you know that you're alive? That may seem like a strange question because it has an obvious answer. I imagine that you're probably thinking something along the lines of, *Well, I'm here reading this book, so clearly, I'm alive.* Right—you're breathing, your heart is beating, your skin is warm to the touch, and blood is flowing through all your vessels. Health care providers use these indicators of life, appropriately dubbed "vital signs," to assess whether someone is alive. But, merely living isn't necessarily the gold standard. There's a difference between the state of being alive and the state of thriving.

So, here's another question: How do you know that you're thriving? In contrast to the first, painfully obvious question, this one may challenge us a little more. On an emotional level, giving an answer is highly subjective. *Am I fulfilling my purpose in life?* But from a biological standpoint, things are much more straightforward. The dictionary definition states that something is thriving if it is growing and developing well or vigorously. In essence, the question of physical thriving ultimately depends on fertility. *Do we have the ability to grow and develop, to create new life?* Whether or not we feel emotionally, spiritually, or financially ready to have a child isn't the question but, rather, if we have a high enough level of health that we could if we wanted to. We use this language with animals too—we say a certain species is thriving if it is rapidly multiplying and the offspring stay alive long enough to reproduce and care well for their young. For this reason, many experts refer to fertility signs in women as vital signs themselves. Linguistically speaking, this makes a lot of sense given that the word *vitality* is defined as "the power giving continuance of life, present in all living things."

Of course, we don't want to get too caught up in semantics because plenty of alive and thriving individuals are no longer fertile. But in general, fertility signs translate to well-being. Fertility isn't just about pregnancy or the lack thereof, it's about your body's functions, abilities, and health status as a whole. As women, this means that changes to or abnormalities with your periods tell you a lot about your health, and you don't necessarily need to visit a medical clinic to get that vital information about yourself.

YOUR PERIOD, A HEALTH-O-METER

Periods make us pay attention. Try as we may, we can't ignore our periods; they have a very obvious way of making themselves known and reminding us of our fertility. From the very first time that Aunt Flo arrives, we become attuned to her cyclic presence in our lives. We maintain a general knowledge of when she comes and how long she stays around. We take note of her appearance as well, filing away notes about color, flow, clots, and more in the back corners of our minds. Although we may not be aware of our analysis of such information in the moment, we always notice enough to be able to recognize when something atypical happens. If we experience mid-cycle spotting when we usually don't, we notice. If we normally see bright red bleeding with a thin texture, symptoms like clots or dark discolorations catch our attention. When a period comes early or late or altogether fails to show up, if we notice a heavier or lighter-than-usual flow, and most certainly if we experience atypical pain—whether breast pain, headaches, or cramping—we notice.

Variations in our cycle almost always signal a change in the status of our health. While the changes themselves might seem benign or maybe even preferable (who wouldn't like to skip or delay dealing with a period now and then?) there's always an underlying physiological reason for that change, and it ultimately reflects the status of another system of our bodies. Sometimes we write off these changes because they're so common among women that we don't think they're important, such as a period coming late because of stress. But despite being "normal," meaning that they happen frequently among women as a whole, these changes aren't insignificant. A delayed cycle due to stress should be a red flag. It's not "no big deal," it's a sign that our stress levels have heightened enough to harm us physically. You should also keep in mind that if something affects your periods, it affects every other system of your body too. Using the example of stress, it may not seem like an issue for Aunt Flo to delay a few days. But it is definitely a big deal for stress hormones to be running high. Not only do these chemicals affect the regulation of our reproductive hormones (and hence, the timing of our periods) but they also affect levels of inflammation, risk of cardiovascular disease, metabolic maintenance, and blood sugar control, as well as just about every other aspect of our health. If our bodies pump the brakes on fertility, it means they'll slow down other systems too.

However, stress hormones aren't the only driver of change in reproductive function. Anything that affects our health and vitality also impacts fertility. This applies both in the short term, such as with a cycle or two that's delayed, but also in the long term, creating the risk of chronic reproductive health problems. Let's take a closer look at some of the most common health conditions affecting women in the United States and the impacts they have on the menstrual cycle.

Illnesses, Infections, and the Immune System

Perhaps you've noticed that your annual winter cold throws off your cycle for a month or two. If you catch the flu, for example, your body knows it's not a good time to conceive and carry a pregnancy, so it reduces your reproductive function until your immune system has cleared out the invaders. This was apparent to many menstruating women amid the COVID-19 pandemic when COVID infections and even the COVID vaccinations caused periods for many to be delayed or altogether skipped, sometimes for several cycles in a row.[1] Bacteria and viruses pose a risk to developing fetuses, so it's a good idea for your body to self-regulate in this way. But the germs themselves aren't the only reason that your body chooses to reduce fertility during periods of illness, and reduced fertility isn't the only effect that illnesses and infections have on the reproductive system.

The body's immune system fights off foreign invaders, accomplishing this in a couple of different ways. One example is through fever. Increasing the resting temperature of the body prevents bacteria and other pathogens from growing and reproducing. Every organism thrives at its own unique temperature, so changing the environment to a less-than-ideal temperature (or, rather, greater-than-ideal temperature) greatly impacts whether or not that bug will survive. The same holds true for human cells, which is why fevers concern us so much during pregnancy: they can damage a developing baby. Our bodies, wise in their own right, want to protect us from invaders as much as they also want to protect pregnancies. So, if we start to get sick and the immune system cranks up the temperature as the best next step, the body will also send signals to the reproductive organs to prevent ovulation.[2] Anovulation may result in very short cycles or very long cycles depending on other aspects of the woman's health.

INFLAMMATION

Another way that the immune system attacks germs is by secreting a cascade of chemicals called *prostaglandins* that create inflammation. We generally think of inflammation as a bad thing because chronic exposure to it wreaks havoc on our health, but the upside of inflammation is that it affects the health of bacteria and viruses too. This makes it difficult for them to survive. These inflammatory chemicals break down the cell walls of bacteria and disrupt the genetic material of viruses. However, the inflammation also has a secondary effect of causing discomfort for our own bodies, too. Sickness makes us feel run down, achy, swollen, and sore because of our own immune system's inflammatory activity, mediated through chemicals called prostaglandins. As a consequence of these prostaglandins, things that ordinarily hurt only a little bit end up hurting even worse. While periods normally bring the sensation of mild tenderness and pelvic fullness, the additional prostaglandins released due to illness makes that discomfort downright painful. This is one reason that the first period after a bout of sickness may be accompanied by more severe cramping than usual, and why chronic inflammatory conditions such as endometriosis often make periods outright unbearable.

CHRONIC INFECTIONS

Some illnesses and infections directly impact fertility and conception too. Many bacterial and viral infections pose a direct threat to pregnancy in all stages, but this is especially true in the early days when cell division and fetal development occur at maximum speed. These include foodborne illnesses like listeriosis, a disease caused by the bacteria *Listeria monocytogenes*, which naturally occurs in soil but can contaminate protein-rich foods like meat and cheese. Unfortunately, some bacterial and viral infections also may become chronic, meaning they last for months or years, which poses a challenge to women planning to conceive even months or years down the line. Most notably, *Borrelia burgdorferi* (the tick-borne bacteria responsible for causing Lyme disease) and Epstein-Barr virus (the culprit behind mononucleosis) both potentially cause chronic disease with secondary effects of pregnancy loss or infertility. This is partly because the immune cells responsible for killing these infectious agents can also end up inadvertently destroying fetal tissue too. In the case of chronic infections, some women experience loss of their menstrual cycles, or periods accompanied by more painful cramping.

AUTOIMMUNITY

With problems like Lyme disease or other infections, the culprit is the virus or bacteria responsible for the illness. However, in some cases the immune system reacts without a reasonable cause and starts destroying the body's own tissue, mistaking itself for a pathogen. We refer to this self-reactivity as autoimmunity, and autoimmune diseases significantly affect the menstrual cycle and subsequent fertility. Many autoimmune diseases also tend to occur more frequently in women compared to men, especially Hashimoto's disease, rheumatoid arthritis, lupus, and multiple sclerosis.[3] Menstrual changes commonly occur with autoimmune diseases, with impacts on flow, frequency, and premenstrual symptoms. While we don't have a predictable pattern for how a period will change with any particular autoimmune disease, for many women they cause lighter periods, mid-cycle bleeding, heavy cramping, and irregular or absent cycles. It's therefore important to recognize that persistent changes in the menstrual cycle, such as bleeding between cycles or the absence of periods for several months, could be due to an autoimmune disorder. Unlike a short-term, acute infection, however, menstrual changes due to autoimmune diseases tend to stick around for several months or years. Fortunately, once we identify and address the autoimmune disorder, cycles return to normal.

ANEMIA OF CHRONIC DISEASE

Anemia is another common concern in menstruating women. The term "anemia" broadly refers to a lack of quality red blood cells, the most common cause being iron deficiency. In this condition, a person's diet lacks sufficient iron to make red blood cells. When a woman loses blood each month, red blood cell numbers and iron levels both drop. It's always important to understand the root cause behind a problem such as anemia, because it can come from many places. In cases where menstruation leads to anemia without a concomitant concern like an extremely heavy flow (a problem in and of itself), we always need to figure out the driving force behind the anemia. Autoimmune disorders notoriously cause a form of anemia related to inflammation. We refer to this as "anemia of chronic disease" and, clinically, it looks just like any other type of anemia. If a person's low-grade anemia results from an autoimmune disease, for example, monthly periods may put them over the edge to develop cyclically related iron deficiency anemia as well. While the problem appears to be monthly blood loss from periods, the problem actually stems from the underlying autoimmune disease.

GASTROINTESTINAL DISORDERS

Autoimmune diseases are just one reason for an underlying anemia in a patient. Gastrointestinal disorders that impact the body's ability to absorb iron and other necessary nutrients also play a role in development of anemia. Celiac disease is an autoimmune disease in which gluten consumption triggers the immune system to attack the small intestine. This leads to iron loss in two ways: first, because it compromises the body's ability to absorb iron in food and, second, because of the potential for gastrointestinal bleeding to occur as a complication of the autoimmune reaction. Blood loss from intestinal inflammation compounded by menstrual blood loss makes an existing anemia far worse.

Gastrointestinal (GI) disorders also often bring additional symptoms beyond anemias. Given the location of the gastrointestinal tract in the abdomen and pelvis, many times doctors miss GI disorders or inappropriately blame the symptoms on premenstrual syndrome (PMS). Celiac disease is a common example of this, with its accompanying cramping and diarrhea often attributed to other pelvic organs, such as the uterus. Although we often consider the amalgamation of symptoms constituting PMS "normal," please know that, if your symptoms negatively impact your quality of life, they aren't normal. Compounded by the fact that some changes in bowel motility do commonly accompany menstruation, it's all too easy to blame more severe gastrointestinal symptoms on periods. But periods shouldn't hurt!

MICROBIOME

One of the other key means by which gut health influences the menstrual cycle is through the human microbiome. While nobody would argue that killing a pathogen, such as the one responsible for strep throat, is a bad thing, note that millions, billions, and even trillions of other bacteria live in and on our bodies that play an essential role in our health. We collectively refer to these other, good bacteria as our microbiome. The microbiome plays innumerable roles in promoting and protecting health, but a few of the key areas in the context of reproductive health include maintenance of homeostasis in the immune system and nutrient absorption,[4] as well as regulation of sex hormone levels. We've already discussed many of the ways that the immune system affects the cycle, and, in a large capacity, the microbiome directly mediates this effect. The same is true of the relationship between nutrients and the menstrual cycle such as with iron absorption and anemias. The microbiome also mediates other nutrient deficiencies or excesses such as vitamin K, a vitamin involved in blood clotting. Vitamin K is produced in large part by our good gut bacteria,[5] and if we lack good bacteria in amount or variety, vitamin K deficiency results. Because vitamin K plays such an intricate role in the process of blood clotting, microbiological imbalances and subsequent vitamin K deficiencies potentially lead to extremely heavy menstrual bleeding.

Just like the microbiome affects nutrient absorption, it also participates in blood sugar regulation, detoxification, and even the metabolism of sex hormones. In the scientific community, we understand the gut microbiome to be "one of the principal regulators of circulating estrogen" and a major influence over the development of estrogen related diseases. One study detailing the estrogen-gut microbiome axis (another way of describing the relationship between two facets of the human body) noted that the effect of the gut microbiome on estrogen levels has been implicated in the development of "obesity, metabolic syndrome, cancer, endometrial hyperplasia, endometriosis, polycystic ovary syndrome, fertility, cardiovascular disease, and cognitive function."[6] Barring a major diagnosis such as the ones just listed, estrogen balance still manifests very clearly in the menstrual cycles of everyday women. Excesses of estrogen result in heavy cramping, heavy bleeding, large clots, swelling, and inflammation; likewise, estrogen deficiencies cause irregular cycles, light bleeding, or sometimes the absence of periods altogether. The microbiome's influence over sex hormone levels is just one of the innumerable ways that it impacts reproductive health.

Sex Hormone Imbalances

In our discussion of the microbiome, we touched on one mechanism of estrogen imbalance: a consequence of bacterial disruptions in the gastrointestinal tract. However, many other hormones besides estrogen play important roles in regulating reproductive health. We also need to pay close attention to progesterone, testosterone, and dehydroepiandrosterone, also known as DHEA. Typically, we think of these hormones as produced by the ovaries on a monthly cycle, regulated by input from the brain. We'll discuss some of the nuances of this finely controlled system later in this book, but for now we will make the generalization that the ovaries do what they do because the brain tells them to do so. When the brain sends signals to the ovaries throughout the month, the ovaries then respond by producing those four hormones—estrogen, progesterone, testosterone, and DHEA—at specific times and in specific amounts to accomplish the goal of releasing the egg, thickening the endometrial (uterine) lining, and then consequently shedding that lining through menstruation. But if something disrupts the levels of these hormones, period problems result. Here are a few of the most common imbalances.

ESTROGEN DOMINANCE

We use the phrase estrogen dominance when a woman's estrogen level is altogether too high, or high in relation to progesterone. Because estrogen levels fluctuate throughout the menstrual cycle, we classically measure them on the twenty-first day of the cycle when progesterone levels should also be highest. Then, we can clearly understand the relationship between those two hormones. However, high estrogen levels at any point of the cycle cause problems, and we would refer to this as an estrogen excess type of estrogen dominance. In terms of periods, high circulating estrogen levels classically lead to painful cramping and heavy bleeding with clots. We also assign an estrogen pattern to periods that come too frequently. However, when estrogen levels reach extremely high levels, they can also cause irregular, very light, or absent periods.

Estrogen also stimulates cells in breast tissue during pregnancy to prepare for lactation. This cellular stimulation also occurs at a low level each menstrual cycle whether pregnancy occurs or not, which often leads to mild breast swelling or sensitivity. However, when estrogen dominance occurs, a woman may experience significant swelling and tenderness in the premenstrual period. Long term, this also increases the risk of developing breast or uterine cancer.[7]

ESTROGEN DEFICIENCY

Low estrogen, or estrogen deficiency, is exactly what it sounds like: it occurs when the ovaries produce too little estrogen in a given cycle. While we most often think of this problem as occurring during the perimenopausal time when a woman's ovulation becomes less and less frequent, it also may occur in women who have not yet reached this season of life. Note that estrogen deficiency doesn't exist alone; progesterone deficiency almost always comes along with it. So, many of the problems associated with low estrogen go hand in hand with low progesterone, which we will talk about in the next section.

Women of reproductive age with low estrogen levels typically struggle with irregular or altogether absent periods. These periods, if they come at all, also tend to be very light and can be accompanied by hot flashes, insomnia, mood swings, low libido, and vaginal dryness. Many women also experience dry skin and an increased risk of developing urinary tract infections. Low and declining estrogen levels also notoriously contribute to menstrual headaches and migraines.

PROGESTERONE DEFICIENCY

As noted in the previous section, estrogen and progesterone tend to drop together. However, in the case of low hormone levels, we attribute some symptoms specifically to the low estrogen and some to the low progesterone. While some of the symptoms described previously such as low libido, hot flashes, and migraines also result from low progesterone, progesterone deficiency additionally causes spotting between periods, long but light periods, fertility problems like early miscarriage, or difficulty conceiving such as in the case of luteal phase defect.

Although progesterone typically runs low when estrogen does, it can also be low with normal or high estrogen levels. Progesterone deficiency is technically a form of estrogen dominance (because the estrogen levels are high in relation to progesterone levels), but it's important to understand this nuance because estrogen dominance due to excess estrogen differs from estrogen dominance due to insufficient progesterone. These two clinical pictures have different underlying causes, and we consequently treat them differently.

HIGH ANDROGENS

Just like we need estrogen and progesterone levels to be in the proper range to feel our best, we also need our testosterone and DHEA levels to be in the proper range. We use the term androgens to collectively refer to testosterone and DHEA. While in our culture, we classically talk about estrogen and progesterone as "female reproductive hormones" and chemicals like testosterone and DHEA as "male reproductive hormones," all people produce all four hormones. The difference is that men and women need different levels of those hormones in order to function optimally. As an example, high testosterone levels in men lead to better blood sugar control and reduced risk of obesity, whereas in women, they instead contribute to insulin resistance and increase the risk of weight gain, obesity, and developing diabetes.[8]

Elevated testosterone and DHEA levels in women also negatively affect reproductive function and the experience of menstruation. High androgen levels classically cause long cycles, meaning a large number of days between periods and irregular ovulation. Elevated androgen levels also drive up estrogen levels in women, so heavy bleeding, pain, and clotting also commonly accompany periods in women dealing with high androgens. Because these hormones also contribute to irregular or absent ovulation, many women with high androgens only menstruate a handful of times per year rather than according to the ideal monthly rhythm. High androgen levels in women also cause oily skin, cystic acne, hair growth on the face, chin, or abdomen (known as hirsutism), hair loss on the scalp, and contribute to difficulty conceiving and maintaining pregnancy.

LOW ANDROGENS

With everything in health, balance is key. While elevated androgen levels cause all the problems noted above and more, low androgen levels also create problems. Low androgen levels in women contribute to depression, low libido, fatigue, loss of muscle mass, lower resting metabolic rate, and more. Low androgen levels tend to accompany low estrogen and low progesterone levels, so the trifecta of these deficiencies leads to light bleeding, irregular menses, and fertility problems. One of the most common times that we see these three levels low together is in perimenopause, a historically very overlooked season of female reproductive health.

You might have noticed that many of the period problems associated with hormonal imbalances overlap with each other. Patterns of course exist, but it's really impossible to know exactly which types of imbalances a patient has just by looking at their symptoms. That being said, any of the problems listed above whether they be periods that come too often or not frequently enough, whether they are heavy or light, whether they are too long or short, signal a problem in the body that needs to be investigated further. Lab testing comes into play here, not just for reproductive hormones but for other aspects of health as well. For more information about lab tests and how to advocate for appropriate testing in a physician's office, see the "testing" section at the end of this book.

Stress, Allostatic Load, Thyroid Function, and Sex Hormones

Reproductive hormones don't exist in isolation. As we discussed at the beginning of this chapter, everything from the gut microbiome to the immune system impacts reproductive hormone levels and subsequent menstruation. However, stress hormones and thyroid hormones connect so closely with reproductive hormone function that the medical literature often groups them together as: the hypothalamic-pituitary-adrenal-thyroid-gonadal-axis, or HPATG axis for short. Therefore, when we encounter clinical problems like menstrual cycle irregularities, or symptoms of hormone imbalances, we never merely look at estrogen or measure testosterone levels. We need to evaluate reproductive hormones together with adrenal and thyroid hormones.

In short, the term "HPATG axis" describes the fact that the thyroid, ovaries, and adrenal glands (responsible for producing stress hormones such as cortisol) all talk to each other, with the brain at the center, moderating the whole conversation. More specifically, two parts of the brain called the hypothalamus and the pituitary gland send signals to the thyroid, ovaries, and adrenal glands to tell them whether or not to increase or decrease production of hormones. When they do, those hormones then interact with each other to fine-tune bodily systems like menstruation. That's why times of stress cause a woman's period to come late or be altogether missed, and why an underactive thyroid contributes to light or irregular periods in addition to the other symptoms that hypothyroidism is known for causing, like weight gain or hair loss. (This is yet another reason that the hormonal picture is so nuanced, because hair loss, for example, may result from elevated androgens, low estrogen, hypothyroidism, or excess cortisol.

Then again, the root cause may stem from a completely separate issue, like nutrient deficiencies!)

THYROID IMBALANCES

As we've already discussed, menstrual problems arise from many different places and the thyroid is no exception. However, we must also address a few other key areas when considering thyroid function and its impact on fertility. An underactive thyroid, known as hypothyroidism, classically slows down the body's functions, creating symptoms like constipation, dry skin, hair loss, weight gain, low body temperature, depression, and more. It also consequently decreases fertility, leading to irregular or missing periods and difficulty conceiving. Hypothyroidism may produce either really heavy or really light periods.

On the flip side, we associate an overactive thyroid, known as hyperthyroidism, with excess activity in the body—things like increased heart rate, nervousness or anxiety, high blood pressure, weight loss, diarrhea, increased sweating, elevated body temperature, and racing thoughts. Like an underactive thyroid, overactivity of the thyroid affects periods by making them lighter, irregular, or altogether absent.

STRESS

Periods of high stress result in increased production of stress hormones, which through the various communication pathways noted above create changes to the menstrual cycle. This stress comes in many forms. While we classically think of stress as a psychological phenomenon, which it absolutely can be, it may also result from physical stress like running a marathon, nutritional stress like insufficient calorie intake, lack of sleep, illness or injury, a shift in circadian rhythm resulting from travel or jet lag, depression or anxiety, certain medications or drug use, and more. The increased cortisol production that accompanies stress notoriously causes irregular periods, skipped ovulation, and painful cramping. This occurs because cortisol acts like a brake pedal on the brain's signaling pathways to all the organs on the HPATG axis. When the brain experiences stress, it goes into conservation mode, slowing the body's use of resources by reducing metabolic rate via the thyroid and eliminating nonessential functions, like fertility. High cortisol levels also create inflammation which, if you remember from our discussion about the immune system, makes everything hurt worse than it already does. So, stress can also show up in the menstrual cycle as painful cramping, tender breasts, headaches, and so much more.

At the end of the day, all the systems of our bodies interrelate with one another. Because of this, problems with our immune function, gut and microbiome, stress response, thyroid function, and more all show up in our periods. But we can get the help we need when we pay attention, and we know what we're looking for because our bodies clue us in to these problems early on through changes to our periods. But if we instead assume that being a woman means we must put up with feeling crummy every month, our health will deteriorate until we can't ignore the symptoms anymore. At that point, treatment becomes much more difficult. So, here's my charge to you: commit to getting to know your body and how it functions so you can face problems head-on—all things the coming chapters will help you with!

3

STRUCTURE DETERMINES FUNCTION

Our collective understanding of the natural world expands exponentially every day. The earliest records of anatomical science date back to the ancient Egyptians, who identified that blood flows out from the heart and noted that the skull is made up of several individual bones rather than just one.[1] They deserve a lot of credit for these discoveries considering the lack of modern medical technology at that time. Their early anatomy efforts weren't without error, though. Around 800 BC, Euro-Asian medical practitioners believed that semen was produced by a man's whole body rather than from a single organ,[2] and the study of women's health was no better: Claudius Galen, a Greco-Roman physician, surgeon, philosopher, and early anatomist, influenced much of the prevailing medical thought and theory at the time. One noteworthy conclusion he made was that that females are the anatomical equivalents of men, only the inside-out version: "all the parts, then, that men have, women have too, the difference between them lying in only one thing, namely that in women the parts are within, whereas in men they are outside."[3] Fortunately, we have come a long way from that level of anatomical ignorance, though most women don't have access to the detailed truth if they haven't attended medical school themselves. This, sisters, is a problem.

We've already spent a couple of chapters discussing how expanded knowledge of the way our bodies work empowers us to make truly informed choices as we manage our health. We've discussed the problem—lack of education—in detail, and now it's time to solve it. It's time to stop relying on watered-down or misinformed explanations of our biology or—worse—deferring to others instead of pursuing that knowledge for ourselves. We have a right to understand how our bodies work and to live into the fact that our female bodies aren't just the inside-out version of our fathers, brothers, and husbands. In order to do this, though, we first need to understand the parts we have, what they do, and how they all work together. In other words, structure determines function. In medical schools, anatomy and physiology are taught first, before anything else. That's because we first need to know what's normal before we can appropriately identify what's not, and what that means. We'll be following the same pattern in this chapter, examining the ins and outs of a healthy female body in detail followed by a discussion of how those specially designed pieces work synergistically together. Later, we will expound on that foundational knowledge to pave a path forward for addressing problems as they arise when normal anatomy and physiology go haywire.

STRUCTURE (ANATOMY)

A little disclaimer as we get started here: if you hated science in high school or very intentionally did not take a biology class in college, don't worry. This won't be the same textbook exposition that made you bored, or anxious, or maybe a little nauseated back then. Think of it instead like having taken one of those "Get to know yourself" quizzes online and now you get to read the results. Only, instead of revealing your identity as a member of Gryffindor House or Bamm-Bamm Rubble from the Flintstones, you are . . . *a woman*, and here's the updated, grown-up version of "The Talk." For best results, I recommend using a mirror as your study partner so you not only understand what this book says about female anatomy but also about your own unique body as its proud owner.

External Genital Anatomy

Growing up, most of us were well versed in the fact that boys have penises and girls have vaginas—only, the conversation stopped there. Truth be told, there's a lot more involved in female reproductive anatomy than just the vagina. In fact, the vagina doesn't even fall into the category of "external genitalia" at all. Rather, the area that most people refer to as a "vagina" is actually called the vulva, the term we use for the female genitals located on the outside of the body. This includes the mons pubis, labia majora (outer lips), and labia minora (inner lips), clitoris, vestibular bulbs, vulva vestibule, Bartholin's glands, Skene's glands, urethra, and vaginal opening,[4] all pictured in figure 3.1.

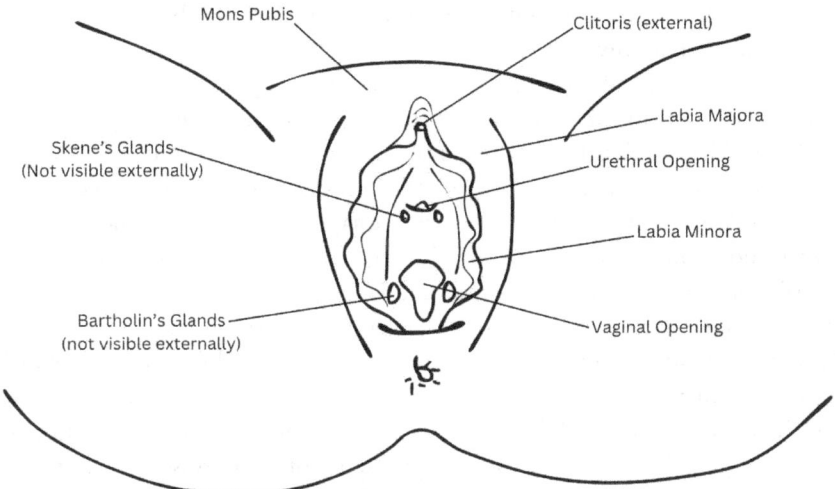

Figure 3.1 Female External Genital Anatomy

The mons pubis is an area of fatty tissue above the pubic bone, a central anterior point of the pelvis. Pubic hair normally covers this area in women who don't shave or wax. The mons pubis protects the pubic bone from impact or injury and also contains oil glands that release pheromones. Pheromones are a type of special scent released by various glands of the body. Carefully controlled by fluctuating levels of reproductive hormones, these chemical messengers travel through the air to influence mood and sexuality. The composition and level of these pheromones change throughout the menstrual cycle, which explains why you may notice a different smell at different times of the month.[5]

Most of us think of body odor as something to avoid, but pheromones usually aren't something we're consciously aware of. Yet, they have the power to influence both sexual attraction and mate selection. Taking the birth control pill actually changes the level and composition of pheromones, and some scientists believe that this change even influences what humans find attractive in a mate. In her article "A Scientific Basis for Human Vitae and Natural Law," physician Angela Lanfranchi, MD, FACS, concludes: "The role these changes have caused in attractiveness and selection of mate by both males and females in preferences concerning major histocompatibility genes is examined. These changes have also resulted in societal changes in sexual behavior and family structure and have led to increased violence against women."[6] For small chemicals that we can't see or even really smell, those effects are huge, stretching far beyond a simple discussion of anatomy.

Below the mons pubis, we find the labia majora and labia minora, named as such from the Latin words for "large lips" and "small lips." These are easily identified as the long folds of skin and tissue stretching from the mons pubis down to the perineum (the muscular transition between the vulva and the anus). Structurally, the labia majora and minora serve to cover and protect the area within, but they also play an interesting additional role. Underneath the skin of the labia reside important pelvic floor muscles called the *ischiocavernosus*, *bulbospongiosus*, and *corpus spongiosum*, also known as "vestibular bulbs." These muscles swell with blood during sexual arousal, similar to a male erection, and contribute to sexual pleasure. They also help stabilize the pelvis during movements like running and jumping, and through other experiences of increased abdominal pressure, like sneezing, coughing, and laughing. These superficial muscles also connect to the deeper muscles of the pelvic floor that are responsible for urinary and fecal continence, stability of the hips and abdomen, and suspension of organs in the pelvic cavity. (When pelvic organs don't stay put, we call that "prolapse," but we'll save that discussion for another time.) These muscles are among those strengthened during pelvic floor physical therapy exercises known as "Kegels," which I recommend for every postpartum and perimenopausal woman. Muscles that are too tight also cause problems such as with pain during intercourse, worsened menstrual cramps, and constipation. Pelvic floor therapy helps with these issues too.

Corpus cavernosum refers to another type of erectile tissue in females, more commonly known as the clitoris. Located below the mons pubis, just below the point where the right and left labia minor diverge, sits the clitoris—as we typically think of it in vulvar anatomy. However, that protrusion of tissue actually only constitutes a small piece of a much larger whole. The clitoris itself consists of three parts, the body (hidden in the pelvis), the glans (the small piece located within the vulva), and the external protective hood. Despite what the medical community believed for centuries, the clitoris is much larger than the small glans appears from the outside. Approximately 90 percent of the corpus cavernosum tissue resides within the pelvic cavity. At up to nine centimeters in diameter, it contains an estimated eight thousand nerve endings,[7] which explains the extreme sensitivity of that area of the body. However, this not-so-small detail wasn't recognized by the larger medical community until 2005 when the Australian urologist Helen O'Connell utilized a combination of magnetic resonance imaging (MRI) and cadaveric examination to dissect the whole truth.[8] Ironically, the clitoris had a name before we ever discovered the majority of its structure. *Clitoris* comes from the Greek word *Kleitoris*, which we translate to mean "little hill." Talk about medical misinformation!

The geographic term "vulva vestibule" refers to the area and structures found between the left and right labia minora. In other words, "the vulva vestibule" collectively involves all the other anatomical structures of the vulva that aren't visible outside of the labia. This area includes both the urethra (the opening for urine to pass) and the opening to the vagina, with the urethra located beneath the glans clitoris and the vaginal opening located below that. The vulvar vestibule also contains two types of glands: Bartholin's and Skene's. Bartholin's glands are located near the vaginal opening and release a lubricating substance that protects the vulvar and vaginal tissues from infection and friction, such as that caused by sexual intercourse or rapid movement like running. Hormones influence the activity of these glands, with phases of low estrogen such as during breastfeeding or menopause notoriously causing vaginal dryness.

Similar to Bartholin's glands, we find the Skene's glands just outside the urethral opening, which secrete an antimicrobial lubricant to protect the urethra from inflammation and infection. Atrophy of these glands due to low estrogen partially contributes to the increased likelihood of urinary tract infections after menopause.[9] Some medical writers theorize that Skene's glands are the external, female equivalent of the internal male prostate. However, I beg to differ; unlike the prostate, women have *two* Skene's glands, and the lubricant released plays no role in transporting sperm (which is the main function of a male's prostate and is more closely mimicked by the lubricant that Bartholin's glands and the cervix itself secrete). Let this be another resounding reminder to Mr. Caludius Galen and his fans that women are not inside-out men and are, instead, their own uniquely beautiful creation.

Breast Anatomy

While we may not typically think of breasts as genital organs, they are considered as such in women. That's because we can't separate the main function of our reproductive system, procreation, from our need to continue nourishing and growing the baby after birth. Even if a woman never has children or if she chooses not to breastfeed, we still expect breasts to function in accordance with certain characteristics, with medically normal and medically abnormal ways that they can behave.

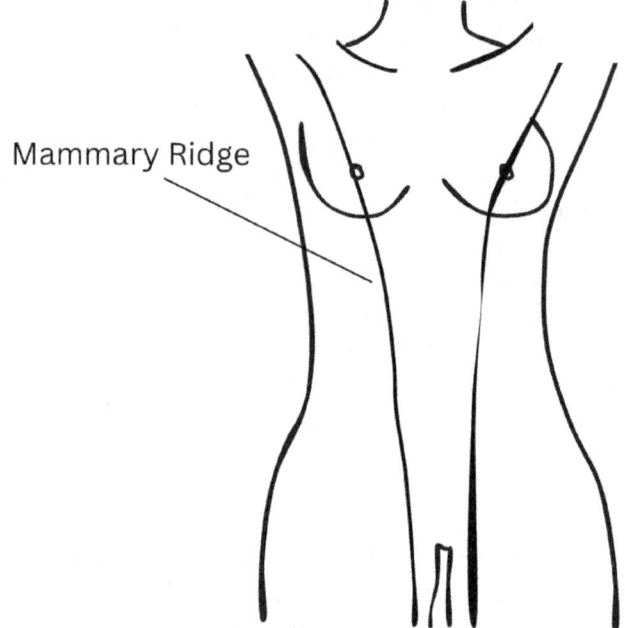

Figure 3.2 Mammary Ridge

Starting with the basics, most women have two breasts. This number can of course change because of surgery, as a partial mastectomy (removal of one breast but not the other) is a common part of treatment for breast cancer. However, both men and women can also be born with polythelia, the term for extra breast tissue. We most commonly see this as supernumerary/accessory or "extra" nipples. A review of breast anatomy published by the National Institute of Health estimates that as many as 4 percent of people have a supernumerary nipple,[10] which means that you probably know somebody who has one, or perhaps you have one yourself. Because polythelia doesn't always involve any extra visible tissue beyond the nipple, many people don't realize they have them at all and instead mistake them for moles or skin tags. Many women end up noticing them for the first time during pregnancy, when they start to grow and change like other breast tissue due to increasing hormone levels.

These supernumerary nipples occur along a pathway of the body called the mammary ridge, or mammary milk line. We typically think of breast location as mid-chest, just below the armpits on each side; however, variation in placement follows this mammary ridge pathway (see figure 3.2), which can span from the shoulders down to the pelvis on each side. This is similar to how other mammals have several nipples on each side, following a curved or linear path stretching down from the chest and abdomen toward the pelvis. Just as no two women have breasts located in exactly the same place, there can also be variations in location and other characteristics on the same person between the left and right sides. Sometimes this variation reaches an entire cup size or more! Size disparity of this nature typically results from variations in levels of glandular (milk-producing) tissue (see figure 3.3), though women may also notice asymmetries from structural changes to the spine, like kyphosis and scoliosis (curvatures in the spine) or pectus deformities (changes in the shape of the rib cage and sternum).

Breast tissue overlies the pectoralis muscle on the chest, beginning with a deep layer of tissue called fascia, which separates the breast tissue from the muscle beneath it. Think about fascia like a type of superthin tendon, or maybe a very thick sort of skin. Fascia connects and separates major muscle groups all throughout the body. Beneath the breasts, it exists as a thin layer that covers the entire pectoralis muscle, which is why it's named "pectoral fascia." This fascia then branches out into very thin ligaments called the suspensory ligaments of the breast, which help keep the breasts elevated or "suspended" on the chest. It probably doesn't come as a shock to know that breasts are not meant to just hang there in the air, though sometimes we treat them that way. Movement should naturally occur in and throughout the breast that maintains tension and strength of the suspensory ligaments

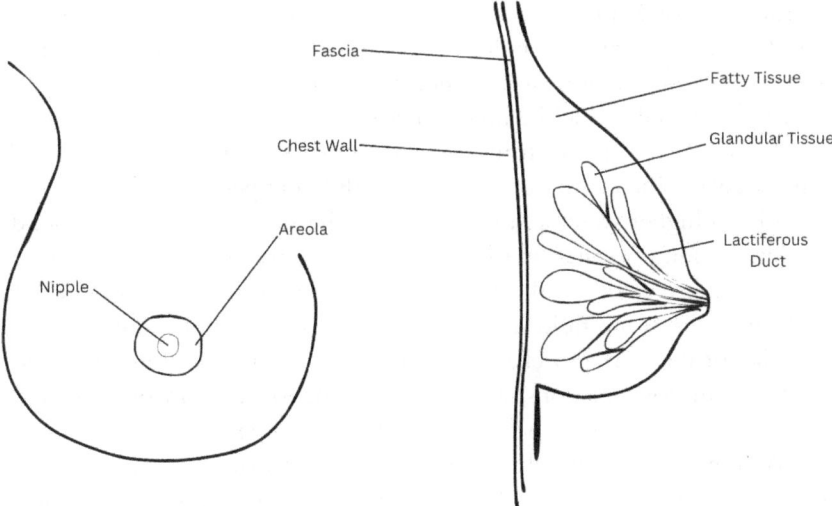

Figure 3.3 Breast Anatomy

to keep breasts from sinking down too much. Paradoxically, offering too much external support such as through overuse of bras may actually lead to saggier breasts over time! Breast movement is also important because it contributes to the flow of lymph (a type of liquid that helps clear away toxins) and stimulates cellular activity. In fact, biomechanist and movement advocate Katy Bowman notes that restricting breast movement too much also increases risk of developing breast cancers and other disorders of the breast in addition to provoking structural changes.[11] So, even though the breasts themselves don't have their own muscles as we classically think about them, their location allows them to benefit from the movement of the muscles below. It's a smart design if you think about it!

The fatty tissue of the breasts themselves serves to protect and support the active glandular tissue within. This glandular tissue is comprised of "modified" sweat glands that have been biologically reprogrammed to produce milk. This milk then drains into lactiferous ducts that converge at the nipple to express during breastfeeding or pumping. The amount of fat in relation to glandular tissue varies from woman to woman, and changes throughout different hormonal states such as pregnancy, postpartum, or menopause. During periods of low estrogen such as menopause, the breasts undergo a hormonal reconstruction in which the level of glandular tissue decreases and fat levels of the breast increase. So, even if you find yourself large-breasted or small-breasted now, that may change over time.

Just like breasts come in different shapes and sizes, nipples are all different too. For a long time, scientists calculated that the nipple needed to protrude at least 7 millimeters for breastfeeding to be successful; however, that idea has been long since disproven.[12] Even women with inverted nipples can successfully breastfeed—and, yes, nipples can be long, short, flat, and even inverted and all be physiologically normal. Keep in mind as well that the nipple is different from the circle of darkened skin that surrounds it, the areola, which varies in diameter for different people. In women, the areola has a higher water and lipid level on the surface than the surrounding skin, making it softer and less likely to become dried out.[13] There are even specialized glands in the areola called Montgomery's tubercles, which produce a lubricating fluid to protect the skin from chafing. Interestingly, the color of the skin also changes over time, darkening during pregnancy due to hormonal variations, a process thought to occur in order to help babies reach their target when initiating breastfeeding.

A thin layer of muscle lies beneath the areolar skin that classically contracts and relaxes as part of breastfeeding but also responds to temperature variations. When nipples are exposed to cold, they sometimes become enlarged or "erect." Many online blogs and forums suggest that this occurs as part of the pilomotor complex, the process responsible for causing goosebumps around hair follicles when we catch a chill. However, the specialized skin of the areola and nipple doesn't have any hair follicles normally, and the change in nipple status actually comes from the activity of two special muscles, called the muscle of Sappey and muscle of Meyerholz. So, there's your next fun fact for bar trivia![14]

Breast anatomy isn't all just fun facts, however. I've included it in this discussion because premenstrual problems like breast tenderness have a hormonal root cause, and those hormones directly influence the structure of breast tissue. It's important to understand that breasts aren't solely comprised of fatty tissue, and that their important structure and function exists even outside of nursing a baby. The ability to recognize health problems requires knowledge of normal anatomy, which holds true even outside of premenstrual syndrome (PMS). Just like with the other external female genital anatomy, you should take the time to familiarize yourself with your own equipment—not just textbook diagrams. Yes, breasts come in all different shapes and sizes, but if your own breasts start to change shape or size, you need to be able to recognize if that's normal or not. This is why medical providers recommend women complete frequent breast self-exams as an early detection tool for problems like cysts, fibrosis, and even cancer. If you've never performed a breast self-exam before or need a refresher, check out the following:

BREAST SELF-EXAM

Breast self-exams should be performed every month. To perform one on yourself, start by standing upright in front of a mirror with your arms by your sides. Look for visual changes in the contour or shape of your breasts, color changes, dimpling, swelling, or other changes or irregularities around the breast and nipple. Take another look while raising both arms up above your head.

Next, raise one arm above your head and use the middle three fingers of the opposite hand to systematically apply increased levels of pressure, checking for lumps, knots, thickening, or changes in texture throughout the entire breast area stretching from your collarbone (clavicle) down to your rib cage. Be sure to check the sides, near and including your armpit as well. Gently pinch the nipple to check for abnormal discharge, too. Then, repeat the process on the other side.

Internal Genital Anatomy

Now, let's circle back to our discussion about the vagina. We've already clarified that excluding breasts, we refer to a woman's external genital anatomy as her vulva, but we also can't forget about the vagina and everything else inside the body. The external opening to the vagina is located within the vulva, but the vagina itself is an internal organ. Other internal genital organs include the cervix, uterus, fallopian tubes, and ovaries.

Although most pictures demarcate the vagina as a hollow tube, it's actually not hollow at all. Rather, the walls of the vagina normally touch each other unless they're being stretched apart. This helps protect the delicate lining of the vaginal canal and maintains the appropriate moisture, acidity, and other conditions to prevent infection and inflammation. The vagina primarily serves as a pathway connecting the uterus to the outside of the body.

We typically think of the uterus as the main female pelvic organ. For such an important anatomical structure, it's actually quite small—only about two inches by three inches in a nonpregnant female. Smooth muscle primarily makes up the uterus, a type of muscle tissue that we don't have autonomous control over the way that we do with our arms and legs. However, the uterus doesn't have a mind of its own altogether; our brains control uterine contraction and relaxation through a series of hormonal signals. The uterus also normally tilts a little bit forward—we use the term "anteverted"—and bands of tissue called "round ligaments" hold it in place. Sometimes these ligaments can be very tight—too tight—causing pain during pregnancy, the postpartum period, or even around menstruation. While many period problems are caused by hormonal imbalances, not all of them are. Sometimes it's truly a structural problem like too-tight round ligaments or inflammation of nearby structures such as the digestive tract, that bump into the uterus and cause pain. Structure determines function as well as *mal*function.

As pictured in figure 3.4, the uterus itself consists of two layers, the endometrium and the myometrium. The muscular portion, or myometrium, contracts during menstruation and childbirth, and we use the term "endometrium" to refer to the inner lining that thickens and sheds each month with menstruation. With disorders like endometriosis, this inner lining spills over from inside the uterus to outside, forming on other structures in the pelvic cavity like the intestines and ovaries. Naturally, this causes a lot of pain and inflammation. The endometrial lining also causes problems

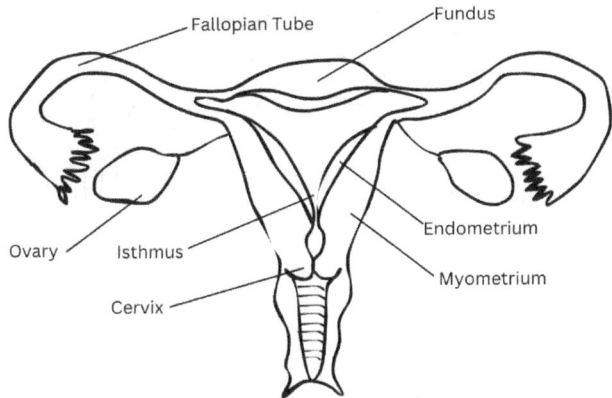

Figure 3.4 Female Internal Genital Anatomy

if it grows too far within the uterus itself, pushing into the muscular walls of the uterus, a condition we refer to as adenomyosis.

In addition to the endometrium's potential to cause pain throughout the cycle, the muscular walls of the uterus themselves can also develop problems such as when they form growths called fibroids. These are benign tumors, so they aren't cancerous, but they often cause pain or heavy bleeding and may even result in an enlarged uterus. Although problems like endometriosis, adenomyosis, and fibroids involve a change in the structure of the uterus, these structural changes are also subject to hormonal influence. All three are considered estrogen-dominant conditions, and endometriosis is also understood to have an autoimmune component. Structure determines function but, sometimes, function of other systems determines the structure of our reproductive organs.

In addition to its two layers, the uterus also has four geographical parts that make it up, which include the fundus, body, isthmus, and cervix. Most of the action takes place in the largest part of the uterus, called the body; the cervix is the opening that sits at the top of the vaginal canal; and the fundus constitutes the top "wall" of the uterus. We refer to the narrow bottom portion of the uterus leading down to the cervix as the "isthmus." For most women, the uterus has a pear shape. However, some women have what's called a bicornuate uterus (see figure 3.5), which is heart shaped. If the middle, muscular portion of the uterine fundus extends all the way down to the isthmus and divides the uterus into two parts, we use the term "septate uterus." Women with a bicornuate or septate uterus usually can conceive normally, barring other concomitant conditions, but the structure of the uterus may complicate pregnancy and delivery.

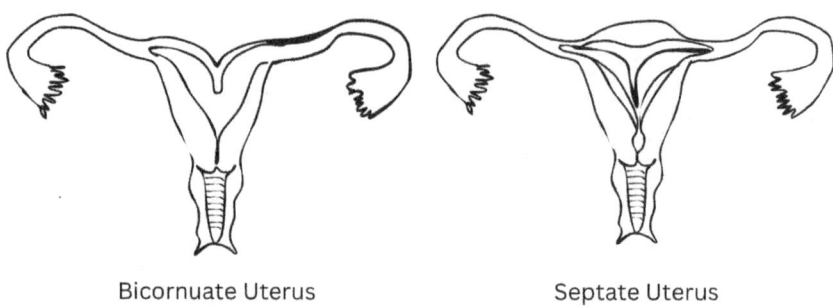

Bicornuate Uterus   Septate Uterus

Figure 3.5 Select Uterine Anomalies

Think of the cervix as a muscular doorway into the uterus allowing sperm in, washing bacteria away, and pushing menstrual blood out. Additionally, the cervix produces a type of fluid that changes in consistency to either help or hinder sperm from passing through depending on the phase of the cycle. It also protects the uterus from infection by washing away bacteria or plugging the entrance to the uterus and preventing infectious organisms from entering. During pregnancy, a thick band of cervical fluid develops, called the mucus plug, which blocks anything from entering the uterus and potentially hurting the baby by causing a uterine infection. Although many companies produce special vaginal cleansers or "douche" kits, there's no need to do anything special to maintain vaginal health apart from showering regularly. In fact, inserting any liquids into the vagina disrupts the delicate microbial balance and washes away this carefully produced cervical fluid, increasing the likelihood of developing yeast or bacterial infections. Chronic infections may lead to pelvic inflammatory disease, a condition associated with both infertility and increased risk of cancer. The vagina already has everything it needs to stay healthy as long as we don't meddle with it.

The opening to the cervix is small and round in a woman who has never been pregnant but becomes stretched and elongated after dilating to allow for delivery of a baby. The opening of the cervix and its texture also change throughout the cycle: opening and closing, shortening and lengthening, and becoming firm or soft. You can determine what your own cervix feels like by inserting one or two clean fingers (with trimmed nails) into your vagina until you reach the smooth, rounded cervix. Completing this self-assessment, known as "cervical checking," regularly provides you with valuable information about your fertility, which we will discuss in more detail later in this book.

The cervix sits at the top of the vagina and protrudes down into it. This forms two pockets which we refer to as the "anterior fornix" and "posterior fornix" of the vagina, located in front of and behind the cervix, respectively. When using a tampon, the correct location for insertion is the posterior fornix, and incorrect insertion may result in irritation of the vagina or worsened menstrual cramping. When a tampon resides in the posterior fornix, it's located high up in the vaginal canal, behind the cervix. However, if part of the tampon sits underneath the cervix itself, contraction of the uterus during menstruation bumps the cervix into the tampon, causing pain. Picture this as the difference between punching the air versus punching a wall. Ouch!

On the sides of the uterus, we find the fallopian tubes and ovaries, small glands about the size and shape of an almond, which house and release eggs throughout a woman's life through a process known as ovulation. The ovaries also release hormones and communicate with the brain, uterus, and other organs about various reproductive processes. At birth, a woman already has all the eggs she ever will already present in her ovaries, however only a tiny fraction of these millions of eggs will ever mature and release into the fallopian tubes. Healthy ovaries, despite their status as small, internal organs, can usually be felt externally during a physical exam. Ovaries with cysts on them will feel larger and asymmetrical, which can offer clues when investigating the cause for a woman's pelvic or menstrual pain. Various ligaments hold the ovaries in place to keep them close to the fallopian tubes when they release their eggs.

During the process of ovulation, the brain sends signals to the ovaries to begin maturing eggs. Yes, you read that correctly, *plural: eggs*. During each cycle, as many as one thousand eggs begin to change and progress but not all of them survive. Among the ones that do, only a couple (though usually only one) mature enough in any given cycle to be released through ovulation. It takes anywhere from 90 to 120 days for an egg to reach full maturity. In women with polycystic ovarian syndrome (PCOS), many more of these eggs reach maturity at any given time, forming what appear to be cysts and making the ovaries appear bumpy—hence the term "polycystic." (*Poly* means "many," and *cystic* refers to the bumpy cyst-like structures seen on ultrasound.) Women with PCOS are also more likely to release multiple mature eggs in any given cycle, increasing the likelihood of conceiving fraternal twins.

Once the ovary releases the egg or eggs, they travel to the fallopian tubes, where fertilization occurs if a healthy sperm is ready and waiting. The hollow fallopian tubes are about eleven or twelve centimeters in length, with an interior space of less than one millimeter in diameter. The fallopian tubes have an arc shape, with the top of the arc known as the ampulla, where fertilization most often occurs. If a woman has unprotected sex in the days leading up to ovulation, the sperm swim through the cervical fluid, up through the uterus and into the fallopian tube where they join with the egg shortly after its release and form an embryo—the earliest stage of an unborn baby. The embryo takes eight to ten days to travel through the fallopian tube and implant, most typically, in the uterine body's endometrial lining.[15] Amazingly, just a few days after leaving the fallopian tube itself, the early form of fallopian tubes begin developing within the embryo if it happens to be a female.[16] This astounding level of early development shows the importance of physical structure in terms of what it means to be a woman.

REMOTE REPRODUCTIVE ORGANS

The modern medical model classically separates bodily systems according to medical specialties: gastrointestinal doctors for digestive problems, neurologists for nerve problems, and so on and so forth. In many cases, this can be a very good thing because if you have a heart problem, you're better off working with a specialist who sees cardiac patients all day every day rather than another type of provider who only encounters a patient with a heart problem once every three months. The downside of this model, though, is that it doesn't take into account that those various bodily systems are very delicately interwoven; it's nearly impossible to understand what's going on with a woman's heart or nerves or ovaries without also considering the other systems of her body.

From a textbook perspective, the only true organs of the female reproductive system are the ones we've already discussed: the vulva, breasts, vagina, uterus, cervix, ovaries, and fallopian tubes. However, looking at these organs from a functional viewpoint, we really can't separate their activity from that of the other systems of the body—most notably, the brain, thyroid, and adrenal glands. Because the structure of an organ or system determines its function, we therefore also have to consider the remote influence of these other organs' functions and how they relate to the genital organs. We'll dive into the details of how, exactly, these organs interrelate in the next chapter (physiology) but for now we want to cover the structural basics. We need to learn about these glands because their activity influences period health, too, and may actually be directly responsible for some of our period-related symptoms.

As pictured in figure 3.6, you can find your own thyroid gland on the front side of your neck, just below a piece of firm cartilage tissue called the thyroid cartilage, which elevates and drops when you swallow. In men, we sometimes casually refer to this structure as the Adam's apple and women have one too, only smaller. The middle portion of the thyroid—called the isthmus—sits about one finger's length below the thyroid cartilage, with two lobes of tissue (the right lobe and left lobe) located on either side. The thyroid doesn't normally protrude from the neck enough to be seen past the other muscles and cartilage of the neck. However, there are some cases when the thyroid can become swollen, form nodules, or change texture and consequently become enlarged enough to see. Iodine deficiency causes goiter, a profound swelling of thyroid tissue that makes the lower portion of a person's neck bulge outward, usually permanently. Infection or inflammation of the thyroid, such as in the case of the autoimmune thyroid disease Hashimoto's, can also cause temporary swelling, pain, or a change in texture that we call *bogginess*. Cysts and nodules also may form in the thyroid as a result of injury, autoimmune activity, or infections, and are a common source of asymmetry between the right and left lobes. While some thyroid nodules can be cancerous, an estimated 95 percent are benign.[17]

Our thyroid plays an important role in regulating the various metabolic systems of the body. This metabolic function includes the way we burn or store calories and regulation of heart rate, blood pressure, muscle contraction, speed of digestion, brain development, and maintenance of

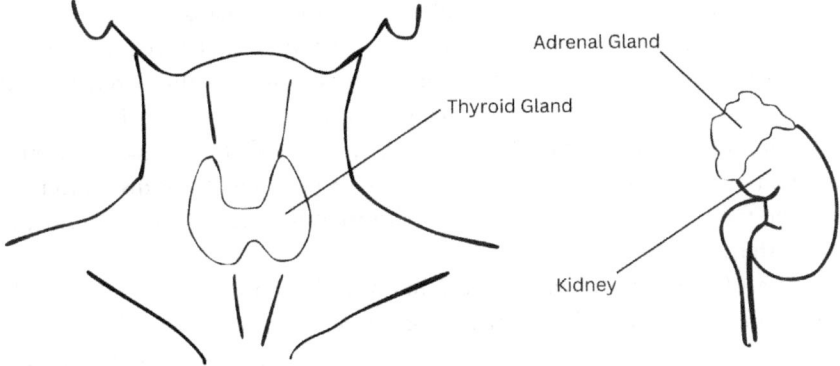

Figure 3.6 Thyroid Gland and Adrenal Gland

bone density. Structural problems with the thyroid such as goiter, swelling, nodules, or cysts can affect the thyroid's ability to carry out these functions. The thyroid carries out its functions in the body via two main hormones—triiodothyronine (T3) and tetraiodothyronine (T4)—and we'll discuss what these hormones do in the next section. For now, however, it's important to know that T3 and T4 are structurally very similar: they are each made up of protein molecules connected to three or four atoms of iodine, respectively. About 80 percent of the body's thyroid hormone comes in the form of T4, which can be converted to T3 by removing one atom of iodine. This is why iodine is so crucial for thyroid function, as it plays a key structural role in thyroid hormones!

The way T3 and T4 do their job of talking to cells also depends on function. Like other hormones, thyroid hormones bind to cell receptors that are specially shaped protein locations on the exterior of the cell. Think about these cell receptors as keyholes on a car. T3 and T4 (and other hormones) are like keys, which fit into the keyhole to turn and start the engine. Most of the thyroid hormone in the body travels to cells through the bloodstream by riding on proteins called thyroglobulins, which are like city buses that carry the hormones to their cellular destinations. We can measure levels of thyroid hormones, cortisol, and sex hormones in both their bound or unbound states, referring to whether they are attached to the globulins or free in the bloodstream where they can do their jobs.

The adrenal glands sit on top of the kidneys (see figure 3.6) and produce hormones responsible for regulating the body's fight-or-flight response. Unlike the thyroid gland, we can't feel our adrenal glands from outside our body, so it's more difficult to identify structural problems with them. Fortunately, structural problems with the adrenal glands such as cancer are very rare. Instead, most problems with the adrenal glands result from abnormal functioning—that is, the release of abnormal levels of adrenal hormones. Like the thyroid, the hormones secreted by the adrenal gland influence metabolism, salt and water (electrolyte) balance, levels of reproductive hormones, and the immune system. The effects of these hormones are widespread and extremely nuanced, so for the sake of this discussion we will be focusing on just a few of those hormones: cortisol and dehydroepiandrosterone (DHEA).

Last but not least, we have the brain. It's almost laughable to include the brain last on the list because it is the central regulator of absolutely everything that happens in the body. However, it makes a good segue for talking about physiology, which we'll turn to next. The brain is made up of nearly innumerable different structures, and they are so detailed that a person could earn a PhD in any one of them. Our goal here isn't to dissect every neuronal connection in the brain but, rather, to understand that the brain talks to the reproductive organs (as well as the thyroid and adrenal glands, who all in turn "talk back" to the brain). The main structures involved in sending messages to the ovaries, adrenal glands, and thyroid are called the hypothalamus and the pituitary glands. These tiny structures in the brain kick-start all the other hormonal systems. They're like the spark and the fuel that get the fire burning in the first place. First, the hypothalamus sends its signal to the pituitary gland, then the pituitary sends its signal out to the adrenal glands, thyroid, or ovaries (also known as *gonads*—from the Latin root "to give birth"). Remember the HPATG axis we talked about earlier? Well, here you go. The hypothalamic-pituitary-adrenal-thyroid-gonadal axis: the triangular interrelationship of the different hormonal systems with your brain smack-dab in the center.

That's the structure, so now let's uncover how it all works together.

4

HOW YOUR HORMONES WORK

Talking about hormones can get really confusing really fast, so in this chapter we will do our best to take something abstract (as in, we can't even see hormones with the naked eye) and make it accessible to you to think and talk about freely. Like our anatomy conversation, we need to understand how our hormones are supposed to work before we can even broach the subject of what can go wrong with them. To keep it simple, we'll simplify our terminology because, let's be honest, hypothalamic-pituitary-adrenal-thyroid-gonadal axis is just way too long to say. So we'll refer to it as the HPATG axis from here on out.

Let's circle back to the brain. Even though we discussed it *last* in the anatomy chapter, everything really begins up there. To recount the basics, the hypothalamus tells the pituitary gland what to do, and the pituitary gland then tells everything else what to do. Note that these are reciprocal interactions, meaning that the organs receiving signals from the brain (adrenal, thyroid, and gonads/ovaries) also send signals back to it—we call these feedback loops—as well as to each other. It's like a big, three-way conversation, depicted with a triangle in figure 4.1. So, if you have a thyroid problem, for example, your brain talks to your thyroid and then your thyroid talks back to your brain, which then corresponds with your adrenal glands and ovaries, causing a slowed metabolism and infertility. So now, you would clinically appear to have an adrenal problem and a fertility problem when in actuality the whole thing stems from your thyroid going awry in the first place. Let's flesh out how, exactly, all of this happens.

Really, it all boils down to hormones. We've used the word "hormone" a thousand times already at this point and have even specifically named some of them (estrogen, progesterone, etc.). But let's make sure

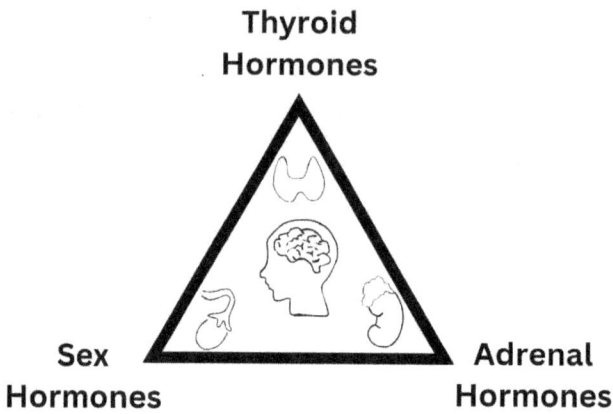

Figure 4.1 Interrelationships Among Thyroid, Adrenal and Sex Hormones

we lay the groundwork with a good, old-fashioned definition. Hormones are molecules that exist in the body for the purpose of communication. This signaling occurs when one organ or organ system releases a chemical messenger—called a hormone—into the bloodstream so it can travel to another part of the body, located somewhere else. Think of it like sending a letter via snail mail from one part of the country to another; you can't see with your own eyes what's happening on the other coast, but you can receive letters in the mail from your friends telling you about it. This messaging service gives all the organs in the body awareness of the goings-on elsewhere and allows them to communicate with each other. It also allows the brain ultimate control of what happens with metabolism, fertility, and more (whether or not we are even consciously aware of it). When a hormone "talks to" another organ, it does so by binding to a location on that cell's membrane (outer structure) and triggering a series of chemical reactions that then cause the receiving organ to do something else. Think about this like a key fitting into a car ignition, which revs the engine. But rather than taking a drive, on a cellular level, the triggered activity involves something like increasing or decreasing activity (like heart rate), increasing or decreasing a chemical (such as blood sugar), or by stimulating that organ to then produce hormones itself. The brain monitors all of this by perceiving these hormone levels in the blood (like you would monitor the dashboard of your car) and deciding whether or not to send more signals to further increase that process, or fewer signals to decrease that process. We call this surveillance activity by the brain over other remote bodily systems "feedback loops," and these feedback loops allow all the other activities of the HPATG axis to take place.

Although all the pieces of the HPATG axis interconnect with each other, we often separate them into three separate axes in the scientific community in order to communicate more easily. These divisions include the hypothalamic-pituitary-gonadal axis (or HPG axis), the hypothalamic-pituitary-adrenal axis (HPA axis), and hypothalamic-pituitary-thyroid axis (HPT) axis. All of these divisions of the HPATG axis are important, and we can't experience fully functional fertility without them all working properly. However, we just won't have enough pages in this book to give the HPA and HPT axes the attention they deserve, so we will instead focus the bulk of our attention on the HPG axis in this chapter. However, it's important to remember the adrenal glands and thyroid in our discussions of physiology because they do influence fertility, and we must also consider them when troubleshooting period problems.

HYPOTHALAMIC-PITUITARY-GONADAL AXIS

Like we already mentioned, the HPATG axis starts in the brain, most specifically the hypothalamus, which sends a signal to the pituitary gland through a hormone called gonadotropin-releasing hormone or GnRH. The pituitary then sends its own signal out to the ovaries. Things get interesting here. The pituitary uses two different hormones to communicate with the ovaries for two different purposes: follicle-stimulating hormone (FSH) and luteinizing hormone (LH); but unlike GnRH, these hormonal signals don't produce instantaneous results. When the hypothalamus talks to the pituitary, it instantly responds. The ovarian reproductive cycle, on the other hand, takes twenty-eight days on average to reach completion (or however long a given women's menstrual cycle lasts). Once the ovaries receive their pituitary signal, they produce hormones that travel through the bloodstream and affect nearly every other cell in the body to varying degrees throughout the month. These hormones, of course, include estrogen, progesterone, testosterone, and DHEA.

The menstrual cycle really is all about the ovaries and what they do. Paradoxically, though, the uterus and its monthly bleed typically get all the hormonal credit. After all, that's how we quite visually see the effects of our HPATG hormonal signaling: as monthly blood loss. But it's the ovaries that make our reproductive hormones, and so that's where we need to focus our attention when it comes to understanding how our cycles work on a chemical level.

OVULATION: THE BIG "O"

With menstrual cycles, we typically think of periods or the actual bleeding as the main event. However, we need to shift that perspective and start thinking about ovulation as the most important aspect of the fertility cycle. That's because fertility ultimately derives from ovulation—the release of an egg—not the bleeding. We can experience bleeding in many different forms, including from our uterus, without being fertile (able to conceive and carry a pregnancy) at all. It's absolutely possible to have monthly bleeding without ovulation, and unfortunately pretty common as well. (Abnormal menstrual bleeding might even be one of the reasons you are reading this book!) But without ovulation, we can't conceive, and if we haven't transitioned to menopause yet, we can't truly call ourselves healthy and fertile either. If a given menstrual bleed doesn't involve ovulation, it's not really considered a period at all and is simply an episode of bleeding. So, when we talk about fertility, or having healthy periods, we need to keep ovulation as our focus.

The menstrual cycle exists in four phases beginning with bleeding, followed by the follicular phase that gears the body up for ovulation. The third phase is ovulation itself, and the final phase, the luteal phase, involves everything the ovary and uterus do after ovulation to prepare for a possible pregnancy (or to clean up shop if pregnancy doesn't occur).

THE CYCLE STORY

Think back to when you first learned about periods. What do you remember? For most of us, explanations about menstruation went something like this: "Once a month, a woman has a period that lasts for a few days and then a few weeks later it happens again. This repeats until menopause when it stops." That might be just enough to shut down a conversation with a confused elementary schooler and move to a less taboo topic, but it's not enough for a grown up, ovulating, self-directing woman who wants to reclaim her feminine power and actually take charge of her fertility. So, rather than water it down to two categories, bleeding and not bleeding, in this section we're going to talk through everything that happens in the four full phases of the menstrual cycle, day by day. Then we'll talk through it all over again with all the hormonal details back in the conversation. Keep in mind throughout this discussion that a twenty-eight-day cycle isn't standard, it's simply average, and referring to it this way makes it easier to divide the cycle into predictable phases for the sake of explanation. However, the length of cycles varies, and the optimal length is actually a little longer, around thirty or thirty-one days.[1]

Let's start with the ovulatory phase: ovulation occurs an average of two weeks before a period begins. With a textbook twenty-eight-day cycle, we therefore refer to ovulation as occurring on day fourteen. In response to signaling from the hypothalamus, the pituitary gland sends a strong signal to the ovaries, where many immature eggs called *follicles* had been maturing over the course of several months. When the pituitary gives word, the most advanced and mature follicle breaks open, releasing an egg which then starts its journey through the fallopian tube. In most cases, only one ovary releases an egg in any given cycle, with the body alternating sides from month to month. After the follicle releases the egg, it transforms into a specialized cyst called the corpus luteum, which is where the luteal phase gets its name. The egg then travels through the fallopian tube toward the uterus and, if it encounters a sperm, will become fertilized and likely implant in the uterine lining. If the egg doesn't encounter sperm, or if the embryo formed by an egg that's found her mate is not viable, it will disappear by twenty-four to forty-eight hours after ovulation.

In the luteal phase, the corpus luteum produces progesterone and a special form of estrogen over the course of eight to twelve days to fine-tune the uterine lining in the case of possible fertilization and pregnancy. This helps the endometrium to strengthen its blood supply to nourish a possible baby and produces a mucous layer to trap and embed the embryo as it enters the inside of the uterus. If pregnancy doesn't take place, the corpus luteum breaks down and stops producing these hormones, leading to a sudden, steep drop-off of hormone levels. It is this hormonal drop-off, over the course of a few additional days, which allows bleeding to occur.

During the menstrual phase, the inner endometrial layer of the uterus breaks down. At this point, the tissue contains prostaglandins, cellular debris, and waste products, as well as special chemicals to prevent clot formation. During the menstrual phase, the prostaglandins irritate the uterine wall and stimulate contraction, which pushes the endometrial blood, waste, and cellular debris out through the cervix. At this time, reproductive hormone levels drop to their absolute lowest. Once bleeding finishes, hormone levels slowly begin to rise again, and the body gears up for the next ovulation.

This next phase, the follicular phase, involves all the hormonal changes required to prepare the uterus and ovary for the next egg release. During this phase, the endometrial lining of the uterus regrows rapidly. In response to signaling from the brain, immature follicles begin to develop on the ovaries, and these follicles communicate with each other to favor the development of one, main follicle—the one that will eventually release an egg. The other, partially developed follicles will resume their growth in subsequent menstrual cycles.

Hormonal signaling allows all of these structural changes to happen throughout the four phases of the menstrual cycle. (Refer to figure 4.2 for a visual representation of how these hormonal changes translate to the physical development of uterine tissue throughout the cycle.) We typically describe estrogen as the main hormone at work during the follicular phase. The brain hormone FSH tells the ovaries to start the follicle (egg) maturation process and, in doing so, those follicles produce increasing amounts of estrogen. The estrogen produced in this phase interacts with the uterus to increase the thickness of the endometrial layer and stimulates the growth of new arteries to enrich the blood supply. Estrogen also interacts with the

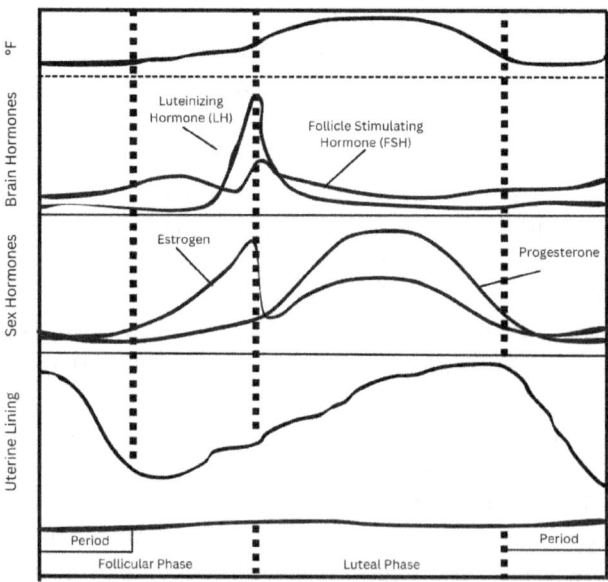

Figure 4.2 Cyclic Fluctuations in Sex Hormones, Brain Hormones, Body Temperature and Thickness of the Endometrium

cervix, allowing it to retract and open, softening as it produces a watery cervical mucus to support sperm motility and allow their passage from the vagina into the uterus and fallopian tubes where fertilization occurs.

As these estrogen levels rise, the hypothalamus receives this feedback signal and responds by telling the pituitary to produce large amounts of LH, a phenomenon referred to as the "LH surge."[2] This sudden spike in LH causes the now mature follicle to break open and actually release the egg through ovulation. The sharp rise in LH also stimulates the ovary to produce androgens—testosterone and DHEA—which typically convert into estrogen within the cells of the ovary itself as well as in fat cells throughout the body.

Once the follicle breaks open, it no longer is able to produce estrogen, resulting in a sudden drop-off of blood levels. The corpus luteum then forms where the follicle once existed. As we discussed earlier, the corpus luteum is a special gland formed by the ruptured follicle that produces primarily progesterone. Low-level, continued release of LH is how the brain communicates with the ovaries during the luteal phase. This LH is what stimulates the corpus luteum to produce progesterone as well as some additional (albeit lower levels of) estrogen. Progesterone plays the important role of preventing the endometrial lining from becoming too thick (and consequently preventing periods from becoming too heavy). Progesterone also helps the blood lining mature, storing energy to potentially feed a growing embryo and refining the arteries within in case they need to help sustain a new pregnancy. The cervix also responds to progesterone, changing in texture to become firmer and closed, as the egg by this point has either already been fertilized or has dissolved. The consistency of the cervical mucus changes in response to progesterone, becoming thicker and less elastic, as there is no longer any reason for sperm to enter the uterus.

As these progesterone levels rise, they signal to the hypothalamus in two ways. For one, progesterone stimulates the thyroid to increase body heat production. (We measure this as an increase in basal body temperature, which we will discuss more in a few chapters.) It also creates a negative feedback loop along the HPATG axis. When the hypothalamus perceives a sufficient progesterone level, it reduces signaling to the corpus luteum and, consequently, the progesterone and estrogen levels begin to fall. If, however, an embryo implants in the uterine lining, early pregnancy hormones override the negative feedback loop and allow those progesterone and estrogen levels to remain elevated in support of the pregnancy until the placenta forms and takes over. As progesterone levels drop in the absence of pregnancy, the endometrial layer sheds.[3] This is menstruation, occurring when reproductive hormone levels reach their absolute lowest. Then, everything starts all over again!

Occasionally, a woman might naturally experience an anovulatory cycle, meaning that she experiences bleeding, but ovulation does not occur. In these cases, an egg/follicle complex fails to completely mature due to inadequate hormone signaling, whether from low estrogen levels, low LH/FSH, or low receptivity of the ovary to these hormonal signals as may occur in polycystic ovarian syndrome (PCOS). Estrogen allows the endometrial layer of the uterus to form, but absence of progesterone results in a typically thicker albeit chemically different uterine lining.[4] Anovulatory cycles are infertile cycles because pregnancy is not possible. These constitute the type of "periods" that occur when hormonal contraceptives function correctly.

BEHIND THE SCENES OF "PERIODS" ON THE PILL

Another important difference between the monthly bleeds seen when using the pill and natural periods, apart from the lack of ovulation, is the difference in the hormonal picture. As we already outlined, hormonal activity normally ebbs and flows throughout the cycle with dramatic highs and lows, all carefully and magnificently orchestrated by the web of signaling from the brain and body. Estrogen has its time to shine just before ovulation, and progesterone steps into the spotlight during the luteal phase. Neither of these hormones is typically high all the time or low all the time. But with birth control, it's a different story. When you swallow your little pink combination pill, hormone levels rise pretty quickly once the active component starts to absorb and travel through the bloodstream. Then, throughout the day, the liver and gastrointestinal system clear away that hormone, only for the whole process to repeat the next day, and the next, until you reach the placebo part of your pack. (Never mind that the drugs in birth control pills aren't chemically the same as estradiol and progesterone, so they don't interact with our cells exactly the same way.) Because of this, the pattern we see throughout the month on a hormonal scale also looks a lot different between women who use the pill and those who don't.

Take a look at figure 4.3; as you can see, the hormonal fluctuations seen with the pill cycle daily, until they don't anymore, with dramatic peaks in the morning and valleys in the evening. This makes every day of a pill cycle sort of "averaged" or modulated compared to cycles without it, which is why many women notice changes in energy, drive, motivation, mood, and other experiences of life when using hormonal contraceptives.

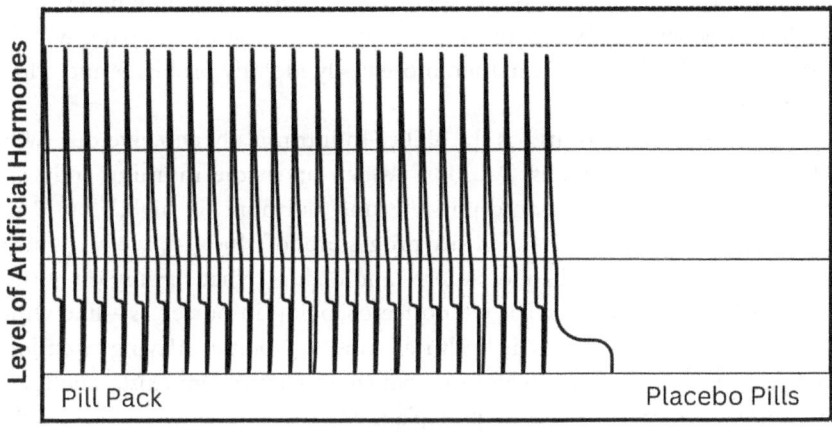

Figure 4.3 Cyclic Fluctuations in Sex Hormones When Using Hormonal Contraceptives

We will discuss more about how to harness the power of those hormonal fluctuations throughout the month later, but for now the main takeaway is that the web of hormones in fertile cycles differs pretty dramatically from what happens when you take the pill, and that difference touches on all the other aspects of the HPATG axis, too. Studies show that hormonal birth control suppresses the body's ability to regulate cortisol release in response to stress[5] and they reduce activity of thyroid hormones too.[6] (Note that other types of hormone imbalances can also induce these effects, they aren't just brought on by contraceptive use.) But as Sarah Hill, PhD, a researcher who has dedicated her career to studying the psychological effects of the birth control pill writes, "We should all be alarmed by the fact that the stress hormone profiles of women who are on the birth control pill look more like those belonging to trauma victims than they do like those belonging to otherwise healthy young women."[7] Yikes!

PHYSIOLOGY, IN A NUTSHELL

If it's even possible to summarize the widespread web of fertility, the main takeaway is this: our hormones communicate with each other, primarily through feedback loops with our brain, which in turn carefully control variations in these hormone levels throughout the month and throughout our lives. Of course, because the effects of our hormones stretch so far and wide, and because there is so much normal variation over time in terms of our hormone levels, it's easy for things to go awry. But by knowing what's normal and what isn't, we can then more easily identify problems and what they mean.

Of course, none of us has the ability to intrinsically perceive our own relative levels of hormones. We don't wake up in the morning and say, "Hmm, I think my gonadotropin-releasing hormone is high," or "My DHEA feels out of balance with my progesterone." Instead, we recognize our body's own structures and patterns and deduce what's going on at the hormonal level based on what we notice changing in ourselves—like with our menstrual cycles and their health-alerting capabilities. Paying attention to deviations from normal helps us recognize *that* a problem exists, and then our knowledge of hormones helps explain *why* that problem exists. It's only once we understand the problem that we then can fix it. That will come. But for now, let's take a look at what's normal on a symptomatic level: *your* periods and how *you* experience them.

5

UM, IS THIS NORMAL?

Have you ever wondered if something going on with your body is normal, but you've been too embarrassed to ask? Not knowing something like this really amps up stress levels. This is especially true if you don't have the tools to do something about it, or don't feel comfortable with the tools available to you—situations this book is designed to change. Not to mention, the unknown can just outright scare us sometimes. Or maybe, as we commonly see with period problems, it's not a question of fear, but rather of annoyance, discomfort, or something getting in the way of how you want to live your life. For example, many health care providers say PMS is normal, cramps are normal, breast tenderness is normal. "Most people experience these things," they say, "But if it's really bad or it bothers you that much, you can take the pill." But what if you don't want to take the pill? Or what if you aren't so sure you believe that what you're experiencing is healthy? Just because it's seemingly normal doesn't mean it's optimal, and it most certainly doesn't mean that you have to continue to experience it.

On the other hand, sometimes an experience in your body may seem atypical but still falls into the category of "healthy"; it's not normal per se, but it's still okay or even good. For example, we often talk about a twenty-eight-day menstrual cycle as normal but it isn't necessarily. In fact, "normal" cycles can last several days more or less than that. In this chapter, we'll take a deep dive into how we quantify *healthy and normal* so that you can decide for yourself if what you experience on a monthly basis—your "normal"—is how you want to keep living, or if you'd like to make a change. At the end of the day, you are the one who gets to choose how to manage your health and if or when you'd like to do things differently.

THE NORM

By now, you're basically an expert. You know the anatomy, you know the hormones, and next we'll break down the normal data in a quantitative and qualitative way. The characteristics of what does and does not constitute a "normal" period are summarized in table 5.1, and we'll flush out the details of each section in this chapter. Compare it to your own experience: are you comfortable with the differences you find?

Frequency and Cycle Length

We define cycle length as the number of days between the first day of your period and the first day of your next period. As an example, if your period comes on September 1 and again on October 1, that cycle is thirty days. One of the most important markers of a "normal" cycle is whether or not your periods follow a regular interval, meaning they tend to come each time after about the same number of days in between. The law of averages only applies to cycle length if they are predictable in this way: a woman may have an "average" thirty-day cycle if her period comes every thirty days, but also if she has a twenty-one-day cycle followed by a thirty-nine-day cycle. We therefore define normal frequency as a cycle length that stays about the same from month to month, with only a few days of wiggle room.

Different resources describe a "normal" cycle length differently. For example, the Mayo Clinic describes a normal cycle as twenty-one to thirty-five days,[1] the *Merck Manual*, a leading medical education company, gives a twenty-four-to-thirty-eight-day range[2] and the National Library of Medicine estimates that between twenty-six and thirty-five days is normal.[3] So, where does all the discrepancy come from? In reality, it's because different sources use different measuring sticks. Some sources calculate based on averages among all women, and others calculate based on fertile women, meaning women who are likely to conceive in any given cycle based on ovulation rates. But at the end of the day, a woman with a period problem such as a short cycle, long cycle, or a diagnosed disorder like endometriosis still may conceive just as easily as a woman who more closely matches the average.

A large study reviewing outcomes in reproductive technology noted that most fertile cycles resulting in successful conception last between thirty and thirty-one days.[4] Another study of approximately 1.5 million women using a common period-tracking app noted that 80 percent of women aged

Table 5.1 Normal Period Characteristics

Cycle Length	Period Length	Color	Texture	Flow	Cramps or Pain	Discharge	Mood Changes
Cycle Day 1 defined as first day of spotting or menses followed by at least 3 consecutive days of full bleeding	Defined as the number of days of bleeding including post-menses spotting and the first day (if applicable) of premenstrual spotting that immediately precedes full bleeding	Defined according to the days of full bleeding, excluding days of spotting		36.5 mL to 72.5 mL cumulatively over the course of the period	Mild swelling or tenderness of pelvis is normal	White, yellowish, or clear fluid that varies in quantity throughout the cycle is normal	Mild transitions from high-energy to more subdued are normal
30 days ± 3 days	4 to 5 days, with all bleeding and spotting resolved in < 8 days	Bright or deep red	Similar to a watery mucus, without clots	Approximately 9 to 18 fully saturated "regular" tampons or pads (4 mL each)	Severe or widespread pain, enough to take medicine, is not normal	Green, dark yellow, gray, pink, or brown is not normal	Depression, anxiety, lethargy, and irritability are not normal

eighteen to twenty-nine have a median cycle length between approximately twenty-eight and thirty-three days, though that range moves to between twenty-seven and thirty-two days for the thirty to thirty-four age group. So, while we don't have a clear-cut range for what's considered normal, irregular cycles or a cycle length that deviates more than two-to-three days on either side of the thirty-to-thirty-one-day window in combination with other sub-optimal symptoms clues you in about something amiss. Keep in mind that menstrual cycles do tend to become slightly shorter with age. For women aged thirty-five to thirty-nine, 80 percent have a median cycle length of between twenty-six and thirty-one days, and the forty-plus age group has a median cycle length of between twenty-four and thirty days.[5] This mirrors the decline in fertility we see after age thirty-five in combination with the data that most fertile cycles hover around the thirty-to-thirty-one day range.

Period Length

Tracking cycle length and regularity depends on the definition used for the first day of a period, or cycle day one. Stated simply, the first day of your menstrual cycle is the first day of your period. But what if you have spotting on and off for a few days before the bleeding really picks up? What about spotting afterward, do those count as period days too?

Spotting and actual menstrual bleeding are not the same thing. Spotting includes light-pink or light-brown-tinged vaginal discharge that may appear mid-cycle, or at the start or end of a period. We'll discuss more about when spotting is or isn't normal in a bit, but typically we don't include days of spotting in the count. Instead, the first day of your cycle, or CD1 refers to the first day of full, red bleeding. That being said, an algorithm commonly used in research studies to define onset of menses, developed by Paige Perry Hornsby, includes premenstrual spotting in the cycle count so long as it does not exceed one day and that it is followed consecutively by at least three days of full bleeding.[6]

The normal number of days of bleeding also differs among resources and ranges anywhere from two to ten days. However, cycles with fewer than four days of bleeding result in pregnancy less frequently whereas those with more than five days have a reduced risk of miscarriage, with a range of four-to-five days considered most likely to result in successful conception.[7] By the logic of optimizing fertility outcomes, periods lasting four or five days, coming every thirty (plus or minus three days) are optimal.

Spotting

Apart from the conditions listed in the previous section in which a single day of spotting immediately precedes at least three consecutive days of fully bleeding, we do not consider premenstrual spotting optimal. Another exception is when very light bleeding occurs at the end of a menstrual cycle which may result from bleeding trailing off or old blood in the uterine isthmus and vaginal canal that washes away more slowly over time, mixing with cervical fluid to appear light brown or pink-tinged. However, the International Federation of Gynecology and Obstetrics (FIGO) Menstrual Disorders Committee (MDC) outlines in its parameters that even this light bleeding or spotting at the end of a cycle must conclude within eight days to be considered normal.[8] Authors of a study published in the *American Journal of Endocrinology* regarding menstrual bleeding patterns note that irregular patterns of bleeding and spotting, including midcycle bleeding "may be indicative of endocrine dysfunction and uterine abnormalities, and such patterns have been associated with infertility, breast and ovarian cancers, type 2 diabetes and cardiovascular disease." They also note that variations in bleeding patterns result from hormonal imbalances, given that endometrial growth and shedding are under hormonal control.[9] Numerous research studies have also concluded that spotting of two days or more strongly correlates with endometriosis, particularly when lab work also demonstrates elevated TSH.[10] We also see premenstrual spotting more commonly with hypothyroidism, estrogen dominance patterns, and structural problems with the uterus like polyps or fibroids.

Color

Menstrual blood comes in a variety of colors but bright and dark red are the only ones considered normal apart from pink or brown spotting at the very beginning or end of a period.[11] Pink menstrual blood during the bulk of a period often signifies a deficiency of the uterine lining, whether from an estrogen deficiency, inflammation, or decrease in red blood cell count such as what we see with anemia. This type of bleeding correlates with increased risk of miscarriage.[12] Gray or orange bleeding likely relates to an infection (make an appointment with your doctor), though spotting at the end of a period involving a mixture of old and new blood may sometimes appear orange. Relatively uncommon, black blood typically results from very old menstrual blood that was once red, then brown, and finally turned black. Because most blood typically exits the vagina before achieving this color change, black blood may signal something blocking the cervix or vagina.[13] Keep in mind that old blood on a pad or tampon may appear black if the pad hasn't been changed quickly enough, so change your products at least every three or four hours.

From the perspective of Traditional Chinese Medicine (TCM), deviation in the color of menstrual blood often points to imbalances elsewhere in the body with other certain associated patterns and risk factors. From this perspective, pale pink bleeding often relates to nutritional insufficiency and difficulty getting enough food energy. Menstrual bloating, fatigue, and as noted earlier, fertility problems often accompany a pattern like this. Likewise, Traditional Chinese Medicine associates a darker shade—a deep red color—as abnormal if a thick texture accompanies it. We associate this with inflammation in the body. A dark purplish color with clots is also seen as pathological, relating to poor detoxification. Finally, TCM describes dark brown colored blood with clotting as resulting from poor blood flow, or "blood stagnation."[14]

Texture

Menstrual tissue is made up of more than just blood, so it's different from the red beads that form on your skin after a papercut, or what fills the collection tube during a blood draw. The material passed during a period also includes vaginal and uterine mucus, old cells that need to be cleansed from the uterus as well as stem cells.[15] Because of this, the consistency of menstrual blood more typically resembles a watery but viscous mucus rather than a thin liquid. Variations in texture often reflect hormonal imbalances, such as with thyroid disorders, sex hormone imbalances, and related disorders like endometriosis and PCOS. Clots often accompany heavy menstrual bleeding, and they are considered abnormal if larger than 1 centimeter.[16] With heavy menstrual bleeding, the tissue pools in the uterus before being expelled and coagulates, which manifests as passing clots when the tissue leaves the body. These clots may increase pain and cramping, and from a Traditional Chinese Medicine perspective, they relate to increased risk of miscarriage.[17]

Decidual casts, also known as membranous dysmenorrhea, is another textural change we can see with the menstrual cycle. This involves shedding the uterine lining all at once, in one piece or a few pieces, rather than slowly shedding over the course of several days. The tissue often appears bloody, but doesn't have the same liquid, red appearance as a typical bleed. Rather, the tissue is thick, firm, and sometimes actually uterus-shaped, as the entire three-dimensional lining sloughs off in a single piece. Understandably, the appearance and passing of a decidual cast might alarm you, however they aren't themselves dangerous unless accompanied by heavy bleeding. Hormone imbalances are associated with deciduous casts, particularly those induced by progestin-only contraceptives or irregular use of the birth control pill.[18]

Flow

Although it often seems like more, an average, medium-flow period only involves the loss of around sixty milliliters (mL) of blood, about the equivalent of two to three tablespoons.[19] Because menstrual flow typically varies throughout the cycle, and because menstrual products vary in composition and size, we don't classify bleeding according to a daily or hourly basis but rather according to the total blood volume lost throughout the course of a cycle. We define light periods as 36.5 mL or less, medium periods as between 36.5 mL and 72.5 mL, and heavy periods as greater than 72.5 mL total over the course of the entire period. We estimate this as between nine and eighteen fully saturated, regular-size pads or tampons over the course of the period, each amounting to about 4 mL. Light tampons or pads typically hold up to 3 mL and super tampons hold up to 12 mL. Similarly, we estimate that overnight pads hold up to 10 mL.[20] Because all women are different, "normal" spans a range of several ml. However, if you use more than eighteen or fewer than nine regular-sized pads or tampons in a four-to-five-day cycle, something is off with your hormones. How does your own flow compare to these measurements, summarized in table 5.2?

Table 5.2 How to Measure Menstrual Blood

Pads	Volume	Tampon	Type	Volume
0.25 Full	1 mL	0.25 Full	Light	0.25 mL
			Medium	0.5 mL
			Super	1 mL
0.5 Full	2 mL (Regular)	0.5 Full	Light	0.5 mL
	3 mL (Overnight)		Medium	1 mL
			Super	2 mL
0.75 Full	3 mL (Regular)	0.75 Full	Light	1 mL
	6 mL (Overnight)		Medium	1.5 mL
			Super	4 mL
Completely Full	4 mL (Regular)	Completely Full	Light	3 mL
	10 mL (Overnight)		Medium	4 mL
			Super	5 mL

Cramps and Pain

Simply put, cramps and pain during the menstrual cycle are not normal. That being said, we do normally expect some changes in inflammation to occur. At the end of the luteal phase, when progesterone production declines, it triggers an immune system surge and subsequent release of two types of pro-inflammatory chemicals called prostaglandins and cytokines which help break down the endometrial lining and trigger bleeding and uterine contraction.[21] This is just a "little bit" of inflammation and typically remains very localized to the uterus and related structures. It does, however, explain why the pelvic area often feels a little swollen or tender leading up to and during the first few days of menstruation. We should not expect excessive bloating, pain, or cramping though, and often these result from excess levels of inflammation in the body that compound the localized prostaglandin and cytokine activity. They may also point to a progesterone deficiency, as low progesterone allows this immune system reaction in the first place. Without enough progesterone, inflammation gets out of control. As a general rule of thumb, the normal inflammatory and immune changes we see around the onset of menstruation should not last more than a few days or cause you to do anything more than rest up a bit. If it's bad enough to take medicine or lands you in bed, doubled over with pain or fatigue, it's time to take a closer look at hormone balance and inflammation.

Discharge

Vaginal discharge or cervical mucus, like menstruation, also fluctuates according to hormones. The cervix produces this fluid to lubricate and protect the vagina, wash away bad bacteria or yeast, and if it's the right time of the month, aid sperm in traveling up through the uterus and into the fallopian tubes to help fertilize an egg.[22] Cervical fluid is difficult to differentiate from menstrual fluid when you're on your period, but after the bleeding stops, cervical mucus tends toward a dry or sticky texture, and may appear white or slightly yellowish. As estrogen rises throughout the follicular phase, it stimulates the cervix to swell with blood and produce a mucus that has an increasingly watery texture. As ovulation approaches, the fluid transitions to a creamy white consistency, followed by a clear and slippery texture, and culminating with a gelatinous clear or whitish stretchy fluid that resembles raw egg whites. This type of mucus signifies the greatest level of fertility and usually indicates that ovulation will occur in the next couple days. Following ovulation, the cervical fluid rapidly becomes drier with a more gluey consistency. Because hormonal contraceptives suppress the monthly variations in sex hormones, users of the pill see less cervical mucus production overall, while breastfeeding tends to increase the number of days of fertile mucus (watery or egg-white consistency) seen throughout the cycle.[23] Cervical irritation caused by IUD placement often stimulates a greater total volume of cervical fluid production but with less fertile quality.[24] Yellow, gray, or green cervical fluid is not normal, and usually signals an infection such as bacterial vaginosis or a sexually transmitted infection. White, clumpy discharge accompanied by itching, burning or redness may indicate a yeast infection, and pink or brown discharge apart from the immediate premenstrual or post-menses periods is considered irregular or mid-cycle bleeding and is also not normal. The normal characteristics of cervical discharge are summarized in table 5.3. Anything outside of these parameters should be evaluated by a health care provider for appropriate treatment and follow-up.

Mood Changes

If you flip back to the physiology chapter, you'll remember that reproductive hormone levels fluctuate dramatically throughout the menstrual cycle. This is normal and good. Because all of your body's cells, including your brain, have receptors for estrogen, progesterone, testosterone, and DHEA, it's normal to experience changes in your mood throughout the cycle—not just around your period. Estrogen is a very invigorating hormone, so many women experience more energy, increased libido and feel peppier and more upbeat when estrogen surges during the follicular phase. Progesterone makes you feel cool, calm, and collected, so you should expect to feel a little more relaxed, peaceful, and introverted during the second half of your cycle. As hormone levels drop off before your period, it's normal to feel a little tired—that's your body telling you to rest in anticipation of what's to come. That being said, it's *not* normal

Table 5.3 Cervical Mucus Throughout the Menstrual Cycle

Cycle Day	Amount	Consistency	Phase
1 to 7	None to Low	Not able to distinguish from menses	Menstruation
8 to 10	Medium	Milky, wet, whitish, or clear	Follicular
11 to Ovulation	High	Wet, clear, watery, slippery, and stretchy	Ovulation
Ovulation to 28	Medium	Thick and sticky	Luteal phase

to become depressed, anxious, irritable, or so drained of energy that you can't function in your daily life. If you experience these things, it almost guarantees a hormone imbalance, and the birth control pill won't fix it. In fact, women using the birth control pill are at a 130 percent higher risk of developing depression than women who don't.[25]

Breast Changes

Because of the influence of estrogen over breast tissue, which we do consider a genital organ, breasts normally change somewhat throughout the cycle. Remember from our discussion of anatomy that estrogen stimulates the glandular tissue in breasts to begin developing in case of a possible pregnancy. Therefore, it is normal and expected for breasts to become a little fuller and maybe a bit more sensitive just before ovulation and again mid-luteal phase when estrogen surges. However, this shouldn't affect your daily life too much, and you might not even notice it. Ovulation certainly shouldn't cause pain of any kind, including breast pain.

PMS Symptoms

The concept of premenstrual syndrome, or PMS, comes with quite a bit of controversy. The term first appeared in medical literature in 1931 and became a bigger part of the medical model in women's health around the 1960s through the work of British physician Katharina Dalton.[26] However, since the term's introduction into clinical conversations, it almost always leads to one of two outcomes: women being medicated or women being dismissed.

Have you ever yourself ignored your own symptoms because you assumed they were "normal PMS?" Well, PMS in general is not normal. The very word "syndrome" speaks to the fact that debilitating symptoms surrounding menstruation are a medical abnormality, and you shouldn't have to suffer through them. You're not "just hormonal" or "PMSing" or in any other way less-than because of your periods. You should think of your fertility as a superpower, not an Achilles' heel. So let's get to the bottom of it: if you can't function at your best before and during your period, your hormones need some help. However, let's not forget that the dimension added to the female experience of life on account of hormonal variations throughout the cycle does involve both some highs and lows. We will discuss the details of these changes, what they mean and how you can use them to your benefit in a few chapters. But for now, I want you to recognize that some degree of variation in your desire for sociability, how engaged or invigorated you feel, your interest in sex, your need for rest, and your appetite is to be expected. That being said, headaches, irritability, brain fog, bloating, heart palpitations, flu-like symptoms, digestive problems, insomnia or hypersomnia, pain, or pimples are not normal. They are not "just PMS" and you do not need to carry on experiencing them until you reach menopause.

Whether you experience long cycles with cramping and heavy bleeding, short cycles with light bleeding and clots, or debilitating PMS, you can get to a place where your periods are painless, predictable, and even become a positive force in your life. But in order to do that, even before we get into specifics like herbs for treatment or a method like cycle syncing, you need to lay some basic groundwork needed for a healthy foundation. Read on to make sure that you have what you need to set yourself up for period success.

6

BUILDING A BALANCED FOUNDATION

No pill can solve the problem of an unbalanced lifestyle, whether pharmaceutical, herbal, or otherwise. Just like the birth control pill doesn't fix the root cause of period problems, using herbal or any other type of medicine to address different facets of conditions like polycystic ovary syndrome (PCOS) or endometriosis really won't serve you in the long term if you don't have a foundation in place for an overall healthy life. For example, if your periods are missing because of hypothalamic-pituitary-adrenal (HPA) axis dysfunction, no supplement can bring it back if you don't eat enough. Likewise, insulin-sensitizing herbs won't completely solve PCOS if you don't exercise regularly, get enough sleep, or employ dietary strategies to support your blood sugar. While there's no such thing as a one-size-fits-all approach to health, and different strategies may be more or less appropriate for different women in the context of their individual lives, some universal principles apply to everyone. That's why this chapter is so important: these principles lay the groundwork for minimizing inflammation and supporting a hormonally balanced environment in your body so that you can maximize the effectiveness of other interventions and protect your overall well-being.

SLEEP

I like to start with sleep because it really epitomizes the fact that our bodies are governed, in part, by forces beyond us. We have no control over what happens in our bodies, the movements we make, or our brain activity while we sleep. Of course, our hearts beat, our hormones travel around in our bloodstream, and our brain regulates everything that goes on during awake times too. But it's hard not to become awed by the brilliance of it all when we think about how our bodies function completely on their own while sleeping. We wouldn't be able to have input even if we tried! That being said, we *can* influence our hormones and nervous system responses through the ways that we set ourselves up for sleep. Problems like insomnia or hypersomnolence stretch beyond the scope of this book, so instead I want to focus on how we can support our hormones through the aspects of sleep that do fall under our control.

When we sleep, our hormones undergo a "reset." In the medical literature, we use the term "diurnal" to refer to the fact that the body releases many of its hormones in a predictable daily rhythm, controlled by the brain, in response to the sleep-wake cycle. Research shows that thyroid-stimulating hormone (TSH),[1] cortisol,[2] luteinizing hormone (LH),[3] and estradiol[4] levels all reach their peak in the morning hours. This plays a biological role of kicking the body's systems into gear when metabolic activity is highest too. After all, it makes sense to engage in reproductive processes when the body is also consuming and digesting food, communing with other people, and otherwise moving through the world rather than resting, during which the priority is restoration and rejuvenation.

The American Academy of Sleep Medicine recommends that adults age eighteen and older sleep about seven to nine hours per night, noting that quality and pattern of sleep matter just as much as the number of hours of sleep.[5] This means that the body functions best when following a predictable, daily schedule for falling asleep and waking up, and that we pay attention to factors that may interrupt sleep and affect how deeply we sleep. Some of these factors may not be within our control, such as interrupted sleep by children, or for individuals who engage in shift work. However, as much as possible, it's important to try to wake up and go to sleep around the same time each day. If you experience difficulty sleeping, it may result from:

- unaddressed stress;
- stimulant use, such as caffeine, cold medications containing pseudoephedrine, or other drug use;
- exercising too close to bedtime;
- hormonal imbalances involving the thyroid, adrenal glands, or ovaries;
- blood sugar dysregulation, especially low blood sugar;[6]

- screen use: research shows that using screens in the evening, especially for more than two hours, increases the risk of insomnia and negatively impacts sleep quality;[7]
- certain nutrient deficiencies, such as vitamin D, magnesium, and omega-3 fatty acids; or
- mental health disorders.

You may find that your sleep quality improves if you minimize ambient light such as by using blackout curtains, reduce noise exposure from pets or traffic by using a fan or sound machine, and by keeping your bedroom a few degrees cooler than you keep your home during the day. It's also a good idea to follow a predictable bedtime routine, completing the same activities in the same order before bed. This cues the brain through pattern recognition that the time for sleep is coming.[8] While much of the research regarding bedtime routines and sleep quality involves children (for good reason, as parents have a vested interest in their children sleeping well) it also applies to adults. The human brain is as the human brain does.

Sleep medications pose a similar problem in the context of health that birth control pills do. They mask symptoms and can become dependency-forming, while the underlying cause remains unaddressed. If you establish good sleep hygiene as outlined above, correct any nutritional deficiencies, address stress in your life through psychotherapy, spirituality, meditation, or other practices, and still experience difficulty sleeping, please make an appointment with a sleep specialist.

Supplements to Support Sleep

- Phosphatidylserine plus omega-3 fatty acids
  - Dosage: 100 mg phosphatidylserine, 119 mg DHA, 79 mg EPA[9]
  - How it works: regulating cortisol release and regulating brain function[10]
- Magnesium glycinate
  - Dosage: 500 mg in the evening with food[11]
  - How it works: decreases evening cortisol and regulation of neurotransmitter synthesis[12]
- Ashwagandha
  - Dosage: 600 to 1,000 mg in the evening before bed[13]
  - How it works: supports the "rest and digest" parasympathetic division of the nervous system

- Melatonin
  - Melatonin is a hormone, not a "natural sleeping pill" as many companies market it. This chemical interacts with other hormones in the body and even acts on the ovaries. While melatonin use doesn't cause dependence, many people feel groggy in the morning after taking it and describe difficulty falling asleep after extended periods of using it as a sleep aid. For this reason, I recommend avoiding melatonin as a daily sleep support, reserving it for situations like jet lag or a period of significantly disrupted sleep, no more than 3 mg for seven days taken before bed.
  - Because of its hormonal and anti-inflammatory effects, melatonin offers many other benefits apart from sleep, when used strategically. These include PCOS, addiction,[14] and certain inflammatory disorders.[15] It also improves egg quality, especially in cases of age-related fertility decline.[16]

EXERCISE

There's a saying in the world of physical therapy that "movement is life." And I agree. All living things move, even when at rest. Cellular processes hum along while we sleep, and of course, our broader physical selves carry us through the movement of life during the day. We were made for movement, in many ways. Doctors recommend regular exercise because of its metabolic effects in preventing chronic lifestyle diseases, and it also profoundly influences hormones. Regular exercise:

- maintains blood sugar and insulin sensitivity;[17]
- regulates the stress response via the HPA axis;[18] and
- increases blood flow to the ovaries.[19]

The most important type of exercise is always the type you enjoy doing, because that's the type that will keep you coming back for more. We were not put on this earth to simply burn calories; rather, we want our movement to be productive and enjoyable. Don't feel pressured to follow an intense exercise regime such as the type often touted on social media. You don't even need to join a gym to get enough exercise to support your health. Brisk walking, at-home body weight exercise, and team sports all "count" as movement. That being said, I encourage you to also include a regular regime of stretching in your exercise routine. This oft-neglected area of movement protects our posture, prevents injury, and preserves mobility.

There's no simple rule for how much exercise you need. This varies from day to day, from person to person, and from season to season. Factors like injury, stress, childbirth, illness, and other demands of life all influence movement patterns. However, it's a good idea to aim to move your body in some way every day, even if that just means some simple stretching, an at-home yoga video, or a walk in fresh air. The Centers for Disease Control and Prevention (CDC) recommends that adults engage in 150 minutes per week of moderate-intensity physical activity, which amounts to about thirty minutes, five days per week.[20] Movement breaks are perhaps as important as formal exercise. Try to avoid sitting for more than two hours in the same position before getting up to take a break to walk and stretch. Doing so on an hourly basis is even better, and it gives your brain a break from whatever you were doing, too.

The 150-minute rule is a good minimum for forming the habit of exercise, but it's okay if your favorite fitness classes in combination with walking your dog exceed that. There really isn't a straightforward upper limit to what a person's body can handle before it becomes a form of stress—and yes, exercise can add stress to your life and harm your hormones if you push yourself too hard. There is such a thing as *too much* exercise. Out of balance with rest and nutrition, exercise adds stress to the body. If you feel completely exhausted from exercise rather than energized by it, or if soreness lasts more than twenty-four hours, you need to cut back.

Exercise also contributes to psychological stress if you feel dependent on exercise to control anxiety or to micromanage the size and shape of your body. If you notice a change in your sleep habits or periods following a new training schedule, I encourage you to cut back for a while until things regulate. Then, pay special attention to your built-in rest time and nutrition habits as you resume your training plan. Likewise, if you find that you feel stressed or anxious when you fail to keep up with a particular exercise plan, or if you worry about changes to your body that may occur as a result of skipping a workout, you might be suffering from an eating disorder, and I urge you to make an appointment with your doctor and a therapist to discuss this. Movement is a gift and a celebration of what your body can do, not a punishment for what you ate.

STRESS

Stress impacts fertility in virtually infinite ways. We touched on the details of how, exactly, stress impacts the hypothalamic-pituitary-adrenal-thyroid-gonadal (HPATG) axis back in the chapter about physiology. From stealing the building blocks to make progesterone, blocking estrogen production, shocking your metabolism into submission, and causing the pituitary to pump the brakes on it signaling output to the ovaries, thyroid, and adrenal glands, the body just can't catch a break when the brain perceives stress. That stress can come in many forms, not just the work demands or relationship conflicts that we typically blame for stress reactions in the body. We already touched on exercise, and we'll get to the nutrition piece. But illness, poor sleep, exposure to toxins in the environment, and an otherwise unbalanced lifestyle all also contribute to what we call "allostatic load," or stress on the body. Think about allostatic load like a bucket. It can be filled with many things, but once the level reaches the brim, just one more drop makes it spill over. That's when we see an impact on hormones and fertility and start to experience stress-related symptoms like hair loss, weight gain, and fatigue. When allostatic load exceeds what the brain and body can handle, we call it "HPA axis dysfunction," or as you may have heard it described, "adrenal fatigue."

In addition to the hair loss, weight gain, and fatigue mentioned earlier, HPA axis dysfunction also contributes to insomnia, decreased libido, blood pressure changes, cravings for salt or sugar, suppressed immunity, and brain fog. With your periods, it contributes to premenstrual syndrome (PMS) symptoms and irregular or missing periods, as well as increased bloating and cramping from the inflammation it causes. You should also know that using hormonal contraceptives such as the birth control pill contributes to HPA axis dysfunction.[21] The pill also reduces ovarian production of dehydroepiandrosterone (DHEA), which the adrenal glands also produce at meaningful levels. When the pill blocks the ovaries from making DHEA, and HPA axis dysfunction blunts adrenal production of it, the body no longer has any way of producing this valuable mood-regulating, energy-boosting, libido-driving hormone.[22] This again exemplifies how birth control doesn't fix health problems and, often, actually worsens the exact symptoms it is prescribed to "solve."

You've probably got the message by now that stress does nothing good for your body. So, how do you lay a foundation for health and wellness in the context of stress and allostatic load? Some of the not-so-simple processes have simple-sounding answers. If you are dealing with relationship problems, do some soul-searching, set boundaries, and maybe go to counseling. If you find yourself struggling to cope with the demands of your life, please see a therapist and get the help you need. Screen for underlying infections and imbalances in your body and treat them as needed. For everything else? Build in some strategies to support stress tolerance and recovery. Some of my favorite stress-mitigation and wellness techniques include:

- *Cultivating a spiritual practice*: Research shows that people who have robust spiritual practices cope with stress better, have fewer instances of mood disorders, and reduced risk of developing obesity and metabolic dysregulation.[23] Perform a quick Google search of religious and spiritual groups in your area such as churches or Bible studies and consider attending a meeting sometime in the next month. You also might consider checking out a book from a library to learn more about a spiritual topic that interests you.
- *Meditation and mindfulness*: Although meditation and mindfulness are often considered spiritual practices of their own right, they aren't exclusive to any one religious paradigm. Rather, the practice of meditation helps facilitate a reduced-stress psychological state, independent of environmental stressors. A large systematic review of 17,801 articles, a type of research study that factors in the findings of many individual scientific studies, reported that mindfulness strategies improved anxiety, depression, and pain reports in participants.[24] Getting started with meditation may seem confusing if you've never tried it before, so I like to share this quote from Jon Kabat-Zinn in his book *Wherever You Go, There You Are*: "Give yourself permission to allow this moment to be exactly as it is, and allow yourself to be exactly as you are." Consider using this quote as a journaling prompt.
- *4-7-8 breathing*: One of the most studied breathing techniques, 4-7-8 breathing has been demonstrated in the research to increase comfort, relaxation, pleasantness, vigor, and alertness, and to reduce symptoms of arousal, anxiety, depression, anger, and confusion.[25] This breathing technique, popularized by Dr. Andrew Weil, MD, effectively reduces stress at home or anywhere else. To perform it, intentionally override your existing breathing pattern to follow a cadence of four seconds inhaling, holding breath for seven seconds, followed by a slow release of breath over the course of eight seconds.
- *Ditch multitasking*: For many of us, multitasking is a superpower. Our households thrive on our ability to clean up, prepare dinner, make

sure everyone feels loved, and get work done, all while keeping the family schedule in mind. But this mad efficiency comes with a cost—our own well-being. Psychological research shows that we aren't really multitasking at all but, rather, rapidly switching back and forth between two thought processes or tasks. Doing so ultimately comes at the expense of accuracy, memory formation, and attention span,[26] with an overall increase in stress levels. It's like the difference between leisurely enjoying a cup of coffee and chugging an energy drink just for the caffeine jolt: one adds to your life, the other pulls you out of the present moment. I recommend making a list of the tasks (including mental tasks) that you want to accomplish in a given day, and checking them off one by one, rather than all ten at once. And, if possible, throw out the ones that maybe don't matter as much as your mental health does.

- *Clear your schedule*: Are you a "yes girl"?—meaning, do you agree to commitments, responsibilities, and invitations out of obligation? Passion projects, community groups, and initiatives you care about absolutely deserve a spot on your schedule, but perhaps not the ones you don't want to do, which add no value to you or your family, that you are simply reluctant to turn down on account of what others might think. It's much more difficult to enjoy the commitments already on your calendar if you don't make time to recharge afterward—something that's really hard to do when you've scheduled out every last minute of your day. Take a look at your planner and make a list of the things you've written down that ultimately detract from your quality of life rather than add to it. Practice how you might politely decline the next invitation so that you have more time to care for your health.
- *Get outside*: Nothing puts life's problems in perspective like a reminder of how very big the world is. Not only does the great outdoors put in perspective the piles of unfolded laundry or the mess of filing cabinet papers, but getting outside also puts some distance between us and the news, which hardly ever shares anything good, as well as the endless stream of notifications coming in through our phones. We see clear benefits of the natural world in the research, too: getting outside lowers markers of both physical and psychological stress. It's not just the change of scenery that benefits us, either, although visiting indoor recreation facilities does offer some relief too. However, research shows the greatest stress-reducing benefit when visiting natural environments compared to urban green spaces

or indoor locations (which offer the least benefit).[27] How much time should you stay out? We have clear data on that, too: the more the better. In a 2018 study published by the *Journal of Behavioral Medicine*, the authors identified a direct relationship between time spent outdoors and reduced risk of chronic disease.[28] For the sake of your health, put down your phone and go play outside. Gardening, fishing, bird-watching, hiking, camping, visiting a dog park, or playing with your kids all bolster your health, extinguish stress, and add value to your life.

NUTRITION

One of the most common questions my patients ask is, "What is the best way to eat?" And I don't have a single, straight answer. That's because nutrition is nuanced. Of course, food plays an important role in fueling our bodies, but the reach of nutrition in life doesn't just begin and end with grams, percentages, and calories. Food also brings us social, spiritual, emotional, and cultural value. We have likes and dislikes, and not everyone can access all types of foods all the time. There are also circumstances when eating certain foods may be totally fine or even beneficial for some people but dangerous for others, such as in the case of food allergies. Additionally, therapeutic dietary modifications may help in managing certain conditions such as the Crohn's Disease Exclusion Diet,[29] the Autoimmune Protocol,[30] or using a ketogenic diet to manage seizure frequency in epilepsy.[31] These examples are dietary extremes, so they are not appropriate for all people, all the time. Likewise, depending on the circumstances, they may not even be appropriate for a person who has Crohn's disease, autoimmunity, or epilepsy, especially if that person has a history of disordered eating. In such cases, therapeutic dietary modification, even when evidence based, may actually harm a person's health by triggering a relapse into dangerous food-related behaviors. One of the most important pillars of medicine is to first do no harm, so it's essential to recognize that dietary changes do not offer an appropriate means for managing a health condition if they create psychological distress. In clinical practice, I screen every patient for disordered eating and do not recommend dietary change, even if it may help manage a hormonal concern, because the potential risk to that person's health outweighs the potential benefit of the dietary intervention. If you think you might have an eating disorder, please make an appointment with your doctor, a therapist, and a dietitian to get the help you need.

SIGNS AND SYMPTOMS OF EATING DISORDERS

Unfortunately, stereotyping runs rampant in our culture, and preconceived notions about what it "looks like" to have an eating disorder is no exception. In many cases, providers overlook the possibility of eating disorders in their patients if they aren't extremely thin; however, people with eating disorders come in all shapes and sizes. The degree of suffering has nothing to do with the way a person looks and everything to do with behavior, relationship to food, and mental distress. I look for the following red flags when screening my patients for eating disorders:

- Do you frequently diet or attempt to lose weight (with or without success)?
- Do you ever feel like you overeat, binge eat, or lose control around certain foods?
- Do you intentionally skip meals, or deny yourself food when you feel hungry?
- Do you exercise, restrict food, use laxatives, or induce vomiting to "make up for" food that you ate? Do you try to "earn" your food through exercise?
- Do you meticulously count calories, grams, or macronutrients, or check labels on your food for reasons other than diagnosed allergies?
- Are you concerned that food may harm you?
- Do you constantly think about food, exercise, or the size and shape of your body?
- Do you ever feel guilty for the food that you ate, or for exercising less/differently than you prefer?
- Do you feel like you can accept the size and shape of your body?

If you answered yes to any of the above questions, I would encourage you to seriously and honestly consider the role of food and exercise in your life. If thinking about food or the size and shape of your body, making food-related decisions, or exercising causes you feelings of distress, you may be suffering from an eating disorder. While having an eating disorder or engaging in disordered patterns with regards to food or exercise is nothing to be ashamed of, it's not normal, you don't need to continue suffering, and there is help available to you. Please make an appointment with a therapist, your primary care doctor, and a certified eating disorder registered dietitian.

Eating disorders and allergies aside, some basic nutrition principles apply to all women in terms of laying a healthy foundation for hormonal health. These include sufficient calories, macronutrient balance, and micronutrient diversity.

Calories

The idea of a standard, two-thousand-calorie diet didn't become ubiquitous until the 1990s as a consequence of the Nutrition Labeling and Education Act, the goal of which was to substantiate nutrition claims to be consistent with FDA regulations. So, a vague survey was sent out to estimate and quantify most people's diets with the goal of standardizing nutrition data and labeling.[32] This information was never intended to suggest that most people do, or should, follow a two-thousand-calorie diet, but that's exactly how the labeling practices evolved. In reality though, many women need to consume many more than two thousand calories per day in order to meet their basic energy requirements, obtain sufficient vitamins and minerals from food sources, and support fertility while maintaining an active and engaging lifestyle. As such, energy needs among women to maintain basic processes of the body vary by as many as two thousand calories, and that doesn't even factor in athletics and intense exercise.[33]

We really don't have a reliable way to predict how many calories an individual woman needs to maintain period health and fertility, and I really discourage calorie-counting for this reason. It's not an evidence-based way to structure an eating plan and often runs the risk of triggering food-related anxiety and obsession. Instead, I advocate for eating regular, balanced, palatable meals and snacks throughout the day according to hunger and fullness cues (addressing any disordered eating concerns if you struggle to do so) and including a variety of fresh foods. Then, let the calorie cards fall as they may.

Macronutrients

We use the term macronutrients to describe chemical components of food that the human body needs in relatively large quantities. For the most part, these nutrients provide sources of calories and structurally serve as building blocks for tissue growth and repair. They also participate in the many metabolic processes in the body. Macronutrients include dietary protein, fat, and carbohydrates, and I also include fiber on the list. All women need all of them every day. This means that the popular low-fat diet of the 1980s and 1990s and the low-carbohydrate diets of the 2000s are not optimal for women and their hormones. While these dietary strategies may aid in weight loss, that weight loss usually doesn't last,[34] and has no inherent benefit to a woman's overall health and fertility. Rather, these dietary extremes usually end up harming women rather than helping them.

I recommend consuming carbohydrates in relation to the other main macronutrients in a ratio of about 1:1 at a minimum. This means that for every gram of carbohydrate you would also have at least one gram of protein, fat, fiber, or a combination of those. This comes from research demonstrating the fertility benefits of low glycemic load,[35] and the glycemic-lowering effect of combining carbohydrate foods with other macronutrients, especially protein.[36] However, just as I don't advocate for calorie counting, I don't recommend counting grams of protein, carbs, fat, or anything else. Instead as a reference, I include the following rough estimates to give you an idea of a minimum, or how you might approach proportions on your plate. Aim to fill about one-quarter of your plate with high-quality animal protein at each meal, with no need to choose especially lean cuts. Organic, free range, or grass-fed beef, chicken, pork, turkey, venison, bison, fish, and eggs are all excellent sources of protein and, when sourced well, include substantial levels of essential fatty acids too. I also recommend including nuts and seeds and moderate amounts of organic, grass-fed, or A2 dairy. Include carbohydrates as another quarter of your plate and fill the remaining half of your plate with vegetables and fruit, seasoned generously with healthy oils.

A2 DAIRY

The main proteins found in milk include casein and whey, but casein further subdivides into A1 and A2 β-casein. Compared to A1 β-casein, A2 β-casein is more similar to the proteins found in human breast milk and we can therefore digest it more easily because we possess the enzymes required to break it down. Because of this, A2 β-casein is not associated with inflammation, gastrointestinal problems, and metabolic syndrome in the same way as A1 β-casein. You can find A2 milk by looking at the labels of milk at your local grocery store, or working with a dairy farmer who raises A2 cows.

Blood Sugar Balance

We'll explore the details of how each of these macronutrients benefits our health in a few pages, but I also want to highlight the importance of following an eating plan with balanced ratios of macronutrients. Combining carbohydrate foods with protein, fat, and fiber helps keep blood sugar steady throughout the day, supporting your hormonal health. Every year, researchers release new findings regarding the importance for fertility of keeping a blood sugar–balanced diet. This means including rich sources of healthy fats and protein, as well as sufficient carbohydrates consumed in such a way to minimize the glycemic load.[37]

Whenever you eat foods containing carbohydrates, these nutrients absorb into your bloodstream and cause your blood sugar to increase. While some carbohydrates do this more slowly than others, they all have this effect. In response, your pancreas releases insulin, which helps those carbohydrates enter cells so that they can convert to cellular energy. Because the glucose moves *from* the bloodstream and *into* cells, your blood sugar level decreases when insulin enters the bloodstream. Keeping blood sugar under control involves a delicate balance between absorption of dietary carbohydrates and the activity of insulin. However, the more frequently your blood sugar spikes, the more insulin you make, and these cumulative effects of high insulin lead to insulin resistance and inflammation.

With insulin resistance, your body requires an increased level of insulin in order to accomplish the task of moving glucose from the bloodstream and into cells. This is where the term insulin resistance comes from: cells resist the effects of insulin and consequently insulin levels must rise to bring about the same physiological effect. While blood sugar levels may overall remain normal in the case of insulin resistance (though they may also be high, which translates to type 2 diabetes) the insulin level always elevates. High insulin increases the growth of the body's fat cells,[38] and also negatively impacts ovarian production of hormones, increasing testosterone levels[39] as seen in PCOS, and decreasing progesterone levels.[40] High insulin also increases inflammation in the body, which is bad news for period health and fertility, and increases the risk of developing metabolic syndrome, type 2 diabetes, and cardiovascular disease.[41]

Part of the reason insulin resistance translates to chronic disease, apart from the effects of insulin alone, is that high blood sugar often accompanies it. Persistently high blood sugar creates inflammation beyond what insulin provokes, and high sugar levels directly create toxicity to cells. This does not mean that sugar itself is toxic but, rather, that excessive sugar levels in the bloodstream at one time damages cells. Following dietary proportions of roughly 1:1 for carbohydrates to protein, fat, and fiber effectively lowers the glycemic load of a meal, preventing glucose spikes.[42] This means that when carbohydrates combine with protein, fiber, and fat in a meal, they absorb into the bloodstream more slowly, and we subsequently require less insulin to keep blood sugar levels in check. This serves to both protect against blood sugar levels from becoming damagingly high due to rapid absorption of carbohydrates and subsequently prevents the need for increasing levels of insulin.

Eating to support blood sugar also offers benefits beyond preventing high glucose and high insulin. We also need to keep our blood sugar from dropping too low because that creates problems, too. We use the term "reactive hypoglycemia" to refer to a phenomenon in which a person's blood sugar drops too quickly after a meal,[43] leading to symptoms like jitteriness, shakiness, irritability, worsened anxiety, fatigue, and nausea, to name a few. While this is the opposite of insulin resistance, as people suffering from reactive hypoglycemia have a heightened response to insulin, it still increases risk for metabolic syndrome and other chronic diseases. That's because it ultimately sends your blood sugar on a roller coaster. When blood sugar drops, it stimulates your appetite, particularly for sweet foods, in order to keep glucose levels from getting too low. (If blood sugar drops low enough, you will pass out.) If you aren't able to eat or choose not to, your body tries to compensate by activating the stress response and releasing cortisol into the bloodstream. This hormone converts glycogen—a storage form of carbohydrate for emergency purposes, stored in the liver and muscles—into glucose and dumps it back into the bloodstream so that our bodies can skate by on "sugar fumes" until we eat a meal or snack. While this often gets the job done in terms of preventing loss of consciousness, all the other negative effects of increased cortisol remain. It ultimately worsens the blood sugar problem too, as cortisol causes blood sugar to spike *without actually eating any sugar*. You should also note that caffeine, particularly when consumed on an empty stomach apart from food, also has this effect. For this reason, I recommend eating breakfast before consuming any caffeine, or better yet—switch to decaf.

Paradoxically, blood sugar can spike when following a low-carbohydrate diet too, or with irregular eating patterns such as skipping meals or with prolonged periods of fasting as seen with "intermittent fasting" and "time-restricted eating." Research demonstrates that combining protein with meals helps reduce glucose spikes at any given meal as well as in subsequent meals except in cases where a person skips a full meal.[44] So, it's not just a matter of eating enough macronutrients in sufficient proportions but also eating frequently and sufficiently throughout the day. I recommend eating a meal or snack every two and a half to three hours.

Following a 1:1 ratio of macronutrients and eating regular meals and snacks keeps insulin production under control, which is good news whether you are insulin resistant, hypoglycemic, or just an otherwise healthy woman looking to protect her hormone health and prevent chronic disease. While there's no need to count too meticulously, as the general previously outlined meal plating method sufficiently covers the minimums required for healthy hormones, whenever you eat carbohydrate foods you should ask yourself, *Where is my protein, fiber, and fat?* If you have those three ingredients, your snack will have staying power, and your blood sugar will remain balanced for hours afterward.

Protein

Protein is an essential building block for maintaining healthy cells and fertility. Every system of the body, including the hormonal system, requires protein as building blocks. Protein also digests relatively slowly, so it helps you to feel both filled and satisfied by your meals with steady, sustained energy. Proteins are made up of amino acids, of which there are twenty, and we need to consume nine of those from our diets—so called "essential amino acids"—in order to maintain our structure and function. Animal proteins are considered "complete proteins" because they contain all nine essential amino acids. Plant proteins, though still excellent sources of amino acids, are not complete proteins and therefore need to be combined with other foods throughout the day in order to meet protein requirements. This is partly why animal foods are a better source of protein than plant foods.

Some controversy exists regarding the recommended amount of daily protein intake. Why? Because there's a difference between eating enough protein to prevent deficiency of amino acids and eating enough protein to benefit the body, optimize physiology, and stave off chronic diseases, such as those caused by hormonal imbalances. Protein deficiency at its worst manifests as a severe disorder called kwashiorkor, which is characterized by swelling and the shutdown of the bodily systems, ultimately leading to death. This is very different from an imbalanced diet that is protein sufficient but lacks optimal protein. To cover these bare minimum protein needs, the recommended daily allowance (RDA) for protein is set at about 0.36 grams per pound of body weight. (For a 150-pound woman, this would equate to approximately 55 grams.)[45] This does not by any means indicate that you need to limit protein intake to this amount, or that this level should be seen as optimal, because it's not. Flip back to our discussion of blood sugar balance for a refresher on the importance of protein for the safe and healthy consumption of carbohydrates. Some organizations incorrectly interpret this bare-minimum requirement as a maximum and suggest that plant-based and otherwise low-protein diets are optimal for human health when in reality they pose barriers to hormonal health.

WHY ANIMAL PROTEIN?

In general, I do not recommend a vegetarian or vegan diet. While you may have important cultural or religious reasons for avoiding certain animal foods and it is absolutely a personal choice whether to include them in your diet, nutritional patterns that restrict animal protein are not optimal for hormonal health. These dietary paradigms make it very challenging to obtain all the macronutrients in their optimal proportions from food without having to rely on supplements. Because meat and eggs are made up almost entirely of fat and protein, it's easy to combine them into blood sugar–balanced meals and snacks. Protein in plant foods, on the other hand, rarely exists apart from carbohydrates. Take beans, for example. Often recognized as one of the best sources of whole food vegetarian protein, a half-cup serving contains 8 grams of protein but 20 grams of carbohydrate. This means that in order to achieve the 1:1 ratio of protein to carbohydrates, you'd need an additional 12 grams of protein. Sources of pure protein of this nature are extremely limited in plant-based foods, making it difficult to build blood-sugar-balanced meals without relying disproportionately on supplements.

On the contrary, animal foods are rich in protein and fat, making them an excellent companion for carbohydrate-dense plant foods to build well-rounded meals. Animal foods also richly source otherwise hard-to-come-by nutrients like the fat-soluble vitamins A, K, and E, zinc, iron, omega-3 fatty acids, and B vitamins. In particular, vitamin B12 and the omega-3s eicosapentaenoic acid (EPA) and docosahexaenoic acid (DHA) only naturally occur in animal foods. This means that vegetarians cannot sources them in their diets without supplementation. In the case of EPA and DHA, these supplements almost always come from animal sources anyway, though B12 can be synthesized in a lab. However, considering that optimal fertility depends on following an optimal human diet, logic points to the idea that humans were designed to consume animal foods in order to thrive as a species.

Additionally, despite the many controversies, strong bodies of research demonstrate the superiority of animal-based proteins in human health. For example, animal protein outcompetes plant-based proteins in maintaining lean muscle tissue and strength in young adults[46] and it has been shown to improve hormonal fertility markers in young women.[47] Diets that specifically include poultry and fish have been linked to improved fertility outcomes as well.[48] Of course, too much protein may also cause problems so it's important to balance protein intake along with carbohydrates and fats as sources of energy. Protein intake shouldn't exceed 3.5 grams per pound of body weight,[49] though most people don't consume nearly this much. Instead, utilize the meal-plating outline described above to divide your plate, and if you go back for seconds, do so accordingly.

Carbohydrates

Carbohydrates are complicated. They are a good and necessary component of your diet, but as with anything, too much of a good thing can lead to problems. With carbohydrates, it's all about how you eat them. In our previous discussion of blood sugar balance, you may be tempted to conclude that you should avoid carbohydrates. But this is not the case! As much as we need to mind the glycemic index of food, at the same time we need to make sure we have a sufficient intake of carbohydrates. Like low-calorie diets, low-carbohydrate diets lead to anovulatory cycles and amenorrhea (missed periods). Without sufficient carbohydrate intake, not just total per day but regularly throughout the day, the body fails to produce essential thyroid and sex hormones, causing metabolic rate and fertility to suffer in favor of increased cortisol levels.[50]

Ultimately, we need carbohydrates because they offer the most basic natural energy source for our cells. Though complex carbohydrates like starches and whole grains differ from simple sugars, they all ultimately provide glucose to our cells for energy. The brain alone runs entirely on glucose and consumes upward of 20 percent of the body's energy.[51] Just as caloric and carbohydrate deficits impair cognitive executive function, caloric and carbohydrate-restricted diets suppress ovarian function via the HPATG axis.[52] Low-carbohydrate diets are also less likely to satisfy you, and may actually increase hunger levels or potentially trigger disordered eating behavior such as binge eating.

Beyond the energy they provide, carbohydrate-containing whole foods also contain valuable nutrients that are essential for fertility and vitality, like essential fatty acids, fiber, and micronutrients. Different from refined carbohydrates found in manufactured food products in grocery stores, which often lack micronutrients unless added through the production process, whole foods like squash, potatoes, yams, and fruit are rich in both macronutrient carbohydrates as well as essential vitamins and minerals. Sweet potatoes and carrots offer beta-carotene, an antioxidant and precursor to vitamin A, and bananas are one of the most ubiquitous food sources of potassium. This doesn't mean that we should make packaged food products completely off-limits by any means, though. Just as you can consume both Oreos and strawberries in a 1:1 blood sugar–balanced way with some thought and intentionality, no food is forbidden for a healthy diet. Doing so would make the experience of eating chaotic and distressing. Nourishment from food involves not just the building blocks of nutrition but also the emotional, spiritual, and social elements of food. Sometimes that means going out for ice cream with your kids, ordering dessert on date night, or enjoying popcorn while watching your favorite movies in your coziest pajamas. That's real life, and there's room for it in the conversation about hormonal health. The habits cultivated by behaviors you engage in most days, most of the time matter the most.

Fats

Like carbohydrates, dietary fat has endured its own misappropriated bad reputation over the past several decades. However, unlike the low-fat craze of the 1990s, we now know and appreciate the vital role that dietary fat plays in stabilizing blood sugar, improving satiety, and supporting hormones. Dietary fat also serves as the building block for making hormones in the first place. More specifically, hormones derive from cholesterol, which is a type of fatty material that is either consumed or manufactured by a person's liver when provided with the right material ingredients. So, when a woman follows a fat-restricted diet, it likewise limits her body's ability to produce the necessary levels of estrogen, progesterone, and other essential hormones. This impacts fertility, of course, as well as the experience of menstruation, period health, and overall well-being. Deficiency of essential dietary fatty acids has strong implications for hormones. But not all fats are created equal.

You might already be familiar with the two main categories of dietary fats: saturated, which form solids at room temperature, and unsaturated, which form liquids. The term "saturated" refers to the chemical structure of these oils and whether or not the chemical bonds that link the individual molecules together are straight or bent. If they are straight, the molecules can "stack up" and form a solid. Think about this like neatly arranging blocks in a box. If you line them up nice and straight, they all fit. They also essentially form one, big, solid block because the tight packing restricts their movement in the container. This is not the case if you just haphazardly dump them in, however. In a messier arrangement with corners and edges all over the place (akin to the kinks in the molecular structure of unsaturated oils), you could stir the blocks around in the box, or pour the particulate pieces out, rather as you would a liquid.

Not all unsaturated fats are exactly the same, however, and that's where the block-box analogy falls short. Individual unsaturated fatty acids differ from each other according to where in their molecular structure the bend—or bends—can be found. So, we've named omega-3 fatty acids as such because the "kink" or double-bond is located third from the end of the molecule, whereas omega-6 fatty acids have their final kink sixth from the end. Again, despite the ill-gotten reputation of dietary fat, particularly the saturated variety, our bodies need all of them. Unsaturated fatty acids are particularly important in cell membranes, which we want to be relatively soft and more like a liquid at room temperature, and saturated fats are essential for our brains, which we would prefer not to be a mushy, liquid puddle. Likewise, we need both omega-3 and omega-6 fatty acids to keep our bodies healthy, we just need to exercise mindfulness regarding that balance.

In Western, industrialized countries, the diet tends to disproportionately favor omega-6 fatty acids, which are found in plant-based seed oils derived from soy, corn, canola, and cottonseed. While these omega-6 fatty acids naturally exist in the diverse plant and animal foods that would make up a whole food diet, other oils, including omega-3s and saturated fats, naturally accompany them when eaten as part of a whole food. In manufactured foods, like cereal products (think crackers, chips, cookies or actual cereal that you would buy at a grocery store) or items from restaurants that use these oils for frying and cooking, the omega-6 oils exist in disproportionately high levels. This doesn't even take into account the incorporation of these oils into store-bought salad dressings, cooking oils, or butter replacements. Eating a diet high in these manufactured foods subsequently shifts the fatty acid profile of our own bodies, thereby forcing our immune system to adapt to using different building blocks than it would prefer to use for maintaining and repairing our cells. This results in heightened levels of inflammation, accounting for the reason we sometimes describe these seed oils, rich in omega-6s, as pro-inflammatory. When in balance with the other important types of fats, they cause no problems. But when taken out of their whole food context and used in place of other fats like butter, lard, tallow, olive oil, dietary nuts, and seeds, or fatty fruits and vegetables, particularly in combination with dietary restriction of healthy animal fats and fish, they become inflammatory. The manufacturing process used to produce these seed oils also renders them free of fat-soluble vitamins like A, K, and E, which would otherwise be present in a whole food source of fat. This results in an oil-based food product that offers none of the other benefits found in fat-rich whole foods.

These issues are magnified further when considering that the high omega-6 diet comes at the expense of omega-3 fatty acid foods. Research shows that omega-3 fatty acids play an especially important role in hormonal health. Diets rich in animal-based omega-3s such as eicosapentaenoic acid (EPA), docosapentaenoic acid (DPA), and docosahexaenoic acid (DHA) are associated with decreased risk of anovulatory periods and increased luteal phase progesterone levels.[53] Likewise, an excess of omega-6 fatty acids, particularly in relation to omega-3s, correlates with infertility in women of all ages.[54] We also can't forget the profound influence of omega-3 fatty acids over risk of developing cardiovascular disease and cancer.[55]

We find omega-3 fatty acids in both animal and plant foods, but not all foods have all of them. The three main omega-3s include EPA and DHA, found primarily in fish, and alpha-linolenic acid (ALA), which comes from both plant and animal foods. We need all of them in our diets. While our bodies can convert DHA into EPA and ALA in some capacity, this process lacks efficiency and does not occur at a high enough level to provide for a diet that does not include both plant *and* animal sources of omega-3s. In fact, the plant-based sources of ALA are actually the most difficult for the body to use and studies show that it does not build up in the body's tissues the same way that EPA and DHA do.[56] To maintain healthy levels, nutrition experts at Harvard University recommend consuming at least 12 ounces of low-mercury fatty fish per week.[57] If you don't achieve this level in your diet, you probably need to supplement with fish-based omega-3 fatty acids such as krill oil or wild-caught, cold-water cod liver oil.

So, now for the elephant in the room: what about saturated fats? To answer this question, we need to go back in history more than seventy years. The diet-heart hypothesis originated in the 1950s in which researchers identified an association—albeit weak one—between dietary intake of saturated fat and cardiovascular disease. However, subsequent clinical trials were unable to prove a causative relationship. Rather, large bodies of scientific evidence concluded that dietary intake of saturated fat alone has no effect on cardiovascular risk factors, including cardiovascular disease, stroke, cardiovascular mortality, or total mortality. These findings were suppressed in the media for decades until, in the early 2010s, journalists brought them to light. The damage had already been done, however, with policy and public opinion suffering the inertia of the unsubstantiated allegations against saturated fat.[58] The overshadowed truth is that the optimal human diet requires saturated fat as a component: it helps promote the formation of lean body mass,[59] serves as the precursor for beneficial cholesterol and hormone production, and improves satiety from meals.[60] Oh, and about cholesterol—it's also not the villain we once thought, either, and if you restrict dietary cholesterol, your liver will make up for it by producing its own.

Fiber

We don't technically classify fiber as a macronutrient. That's because fiber really is a form of carbohydrate. However, unlike other carbohydrates, we can't break down fiber to use it for energy. Instead, it passes through our digestive systems largely untouched until the good bacteria living in our gut encounters it and starts to break it down to use for food. In addition to serving as fuel for our good bacteria to keep our microbiome healthy, fiber also bulks up stool to help pass waste products out of our bodies.

Although it all falls under the same umbrella term, *fiber* doesn't just describe one thing. Rather, nearly infinite different types of fibers exist. Think about fiber like a chain-link of carbohydrate molecules. A simple, straight chain would be a regular carbohydrate that humans digest. On a molecular level, fiber exhibits an extensive branching pattern, with additional chains branching off of the original chain at different points. Think of fiber like a large, bulky, treelike structure. These branch points could occur at chain link number 5, number 25, or number 525, and those branches could then also branch at any point, and so on and so forth. Each different pattern of branching constitutes a different type of fiber found in different types of foods. They're all a little different from each other but they're all fiber and they're all important. In fact, the greater the number of different types of fiber you include in your diet, the better.

How much fiber should you get? Well, we don't have a consensus on that either. Most health sources recommend a minimum of about 30 grams of fiber per day, but many people need much more than this. The source of fiber matters too; if you get 30 grams of fiber per day from carrot sticks alone, that's great—but you're missing out not only on the delicious taste and vitamins found in other vegetables, but the different types of fiber too. This is another reason why dietary diversity matters. Researchers from the American Gut Project don't reserve the magic number of 30 just for grams of fiber but also for the number of different plant food servings to consume *per week*. Eating in this way supports microbial diversity of your gut and all the benefits that come along with that—of which there are many, including in the realm of hormonal health.[61]

What counts as a plant? Anything that grows in the ground, really. Fruits, vegetables, nuts, seeds, grains, legumes, and more. Keep in mind, too, that kale is different from spinach even though they're both salad greens, so they both count toward your weekly 30.

QI, BLOOD, AND TRADITIONAL CHINESE MEDICINE

Modern medicine offers so much in terms of its ability to identify health problems and support human well-being. Especially in the realm of hormones, up-to-data scientific data is essential for understanding how medical and lifestyle practices influence fertility and women's health. However, other medical paradigms exist beyond just the Western approach, which falls short in many ways. As an example, it's possible to have perfect lab test results, follow a balanced and supportive lifestyle with optimal nutrition, exercise, sleep, and stress-management practices, and still struggle with period problems or fertility. That's where other medical perspectives become essential. Numerous studies show the profound influence that Traditional Chinese Medicine (TCM) techniques, including acupuncture, have over women's reproductive health, fertility, and hormones. Through TCM-related lifestyle changes or acupuncture alone, we can bring about measurable changes in hormones like estrogen, LH, and FSH without ever swallowing a pill.[62] That's powerful medicine, and it speaks to the importance of increasing accessibility of TCM techniques for wellness.

Note that Eastern and Western medicine are not mutually exclusive, meaning that we can address a patient's hormone concerns—such as heavy periods with clots, for example—through a modern paradigm, diagnosing estrogen excess and high inflammation, but also concomitantly through a TCM model, diagnosing Kidney Yin Deficiency, Liver Qi Stasis, or blood stagnation. If those phrases made you do a double take, you're not alone—the language of TCM can be very confusing if you aren't familiar with it, as most people in the West aren't (barring those who have actually studied it).

Despite the language barriers and the challenge of opening your mind to a completely new idea, I find that the benefits of TCM to period health and fertility are powerful enough to warrant the hard work of learning about these new ideas. So, in this section, I am going to attempt to translate more than 2,200 years of East Asian medical theory into a few practical ideas that you can use to balance your hormones and fix your periods.

Yin and Yang, Balance and Harmony

One of the primary facets of TCM is the importance of balance and harmony. In modern medicine, we talk about hormone balance, but Chinese medicine emphasizes the balance of yin and yang. TCM considers yin and yang the two forces of life, and everything that exists reflects different qualities of yin or yang. Yin and yang describe the two sides to everything: male and female, day and night, hot and cold, water and fire, and so on. It's like the two sides of a coin, two partners in a relationship, and the way that a human exhibits both physical as well as spiritual qualities. For any given pairing, TCM considers a yin quality and the other a yang quality. Neither matters more than the other, but TCM observes that the two need to be in balance or harmony with each other or else disease or disharmony develops. While Western medicine measures pathology as lab values falling outside of a reference range (such as low progesterone, or high estrogen, for example), TCM observes patterns of imbalance or disharmony between the two sides—yin and yang—of life's five elements and the body's five organ pairs.

The Five Elements Theory

The Five Elements theory is another central principle of TCM. This theory proposes that five different elements comprise everything in the universe. These include earth, metal, water, fire, and wood. Likewise, the human body contains five major organ pairs that correspond to each of those five elements. Within these organ pairs, TCM refers to one organ as the "yin" organ and the other as the "yang" organ. These yin and yang organs work together to maintain balance. In addition to the associated organ pair, each element also corresponds to a tissue of the body, a sensory organ, an emotion, a season, an aspect of the environment, sound, taste or flavor, and a time of day. Just as the organ systems of the body interact with each other, the elements and their associated aspects of life all also interact with each other. Each element nourishes or generates another element and

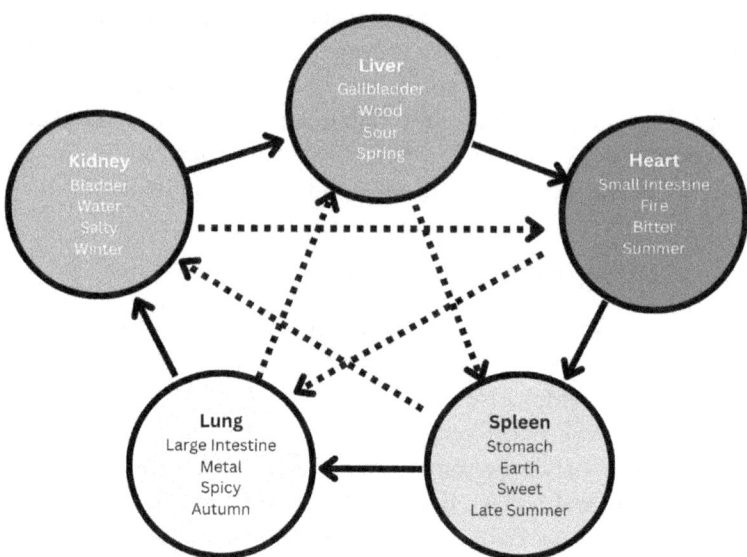

Figure 6.1 Five Elements Theory of Traditional Chinese Medicine

restrains or overcomes another. We classically map out these relationships through a pentagram. See figure 6.1.

These relationships play a crucial role in fertility, hormonal health, and period health because, like the perspective in Western medicine, TCM recognizes that the systems of the body do not exist in isolation from each other. Rather, every system and organ pair at least indirectly influence all the others through the flow of energy among them. In TCM, we call this energy "qi." Without the activity of the various organ systems in TCM supporting the whole body, functions like fertility and reproductive health devolve into disharmony. So, while both medical perspectives recognize the vital interrelationship of bodily systems, the language used to describe those connections differs. Western medicine observes hormones and neuronal connections, whereas TCM describes yin and yang, the five elements, and the flow of qi.

The classification of the organs themselves reflects another key difference between TCM and a Western medical approach. In Western medicine, we understand organs according to their anatomical structure—a physical location within the body. In TCM, the organs describe function. As an example, when we talk about the liver in Western medicine, we are referring to the large, lobe-shaped gland located in the upper right quadrant of the abdomen. In TCM, however, the "liver" refers to the processes of the body responsible for digestion, absorption, emotional regulation, circulating qi and blood, and modulating reproductive function.[63] While some of these overlap with the functions of the Western, anatomical liver (especially digestion and absorption), not all of them do. All of the organs in TCM differ from their Western counterparts in this way. Additionally, the way each organ relates to qi and blood in TCM defines its main overarching function.

QI

From a Western medical perspective, material travels throughout the body in lymph and blood, two fluids with distinct channels for movement. Traditional Chinese Medicine (TCM), however, recognizes a third type of fluid, called qi (pronounced: chee), which represents energy. While the term "energy" doesn't completely embody qi in the field of traditional Chinese medicine, it's about as close as we can get within the limitations of the English language. Qi doesn't refer to energy in terms of vigor, or as a "lack of fatigue," but rather with regards to the force that sustains and drives activity. Think of it more like electricity that powers the body and its processes versus the wherewithal to accomplish a task. In this sense, qi is often also described as "life force energy."

Qi can't be seen or measured through Western scientific means. (Ironically, though, countless Western studies have validated the efficacy of TCM treatments, all of which involve a qi-focused paradigm.) Unlike lymph or blood, qi is not a physical material, so it's not solid, liquid, or gas. However, we consider it a fluid, meaning that it flows throughout the body in distinct patterns or channels called meridians. These meridians correspond to the major organ systems in TCM, spanning along the midline of the body, or to or from an arm or leg. Acupuncture points run along these meridians, which serve as portals for acupuncturists or practitioners of TCM to interact with and influence qi for the purpose of rebalancing it. For example, if a TCM practitioner identifies a deficiency of spleen qi, they would recommend stimulation of acupuncture points related to the spleen's activity. Additional TCM-aligned lifestyle recommendations may include dietary strategies, recommendations regarding body temperature, exercise limitations, a prescription for rest, or avoiding certain types of unfavorable environments.

The full body of Traditional Chinese Medicine theory expands far beyond what one could cover in this book, or any other for that matter—thousands of TCM texts spanning thousands of years have been written throughout history. Rather than attempt to summarize that impossible level of information, the goal of the next few paragraphs is to help you understand how to apply the Five Elements theory and the principles of yin and yang to support your own health, fertility, and hormones.

Principles of Yin/Yang: Applying Logic to Create Balance and Harmony

As we've already discussed, the concept of yin and yang in Traditional Chinese Medicine is all about balance. Some of the pull between yin and yang to maintain harmony in life comes naturally. For example, if you're in a cluttered space, you might become agitated, craving order and tidiness. Or, if you spend a lot of time in a cool room, you may yourself become cold and turn on the heat or wrap a blanket around yourself. Some other facets of yin and yang may not be as intuitive though, perhaps because you aren't keenly aware of them, or because of cultural patterns that contradict them. Here's an example of how that could occur: in American culture, we tend to idolize diets and "clean eating," particularly around the start of a new year. Consistent with New Year's resolutions, many people start new diets that emphasize things like vegetable-rich smoothies and salads full of leafy greens and raw foods. While these are generally healthy ingredients, TCM would say that the New Year is a bad time to consume such foods because in most parts of the country, January temperatures run about the coldest that they're going to get all year. Because of the cold environment, yin–yang theory would suggest that putting cold foods like smoothies and salads into our stomachs furthers the temperature imbalance, creating disharmony, depleting the spleen and qi, stagnating the blood, and impairing blood flow to the digestive and reproductive organs. Instead, a person should consume slow-cooked, animal-protein-rich soups and broths as well as red-colored foods like cherries and red meat. It's the cultural practice of dieting around the New Year holiday that may put a person's lifestyle at odds with the foundational elements of TCM. But there are many other ways this could occur. Regardless of the reason for the disconnect, the following lifestyle practices help lay a foundation to align behavior and habits with the yin–yang theory of TCM. Oh, and in case you were wondering, *yin* is the female aspect of the two pairs, though all people and things have both yin and yang qualities, ideally in perfectly balanced harmony.

- *Temperature and humidity*: cold reflects yin and hot reflects yang; moisture is yin and dryness is yang. During winter months, sleep with a humidifier in your room to combat dryness, and prioritize long, steamy showers. In the summer, make sure to use your dehumidifier, and consider shorter, cooler baths in lieu of steamier showers. If you tend to feel generally cold, reduce excess yin by avoiding prolonged periods spent in cold or damp spaces as well as cold drinks and cold or uncooked food. Instead, support yang by prioritizing warm food and beverages, particularly those that have been roasted or slow cooked. Consider regular use of saunas and spend time warming yourself in front of a fire or with a heated blanket. Prioritize outside time on warm, sunny days, especially those with a low humidity index. On cold/rainy or winter days, try to avoid recreational activities that include water or cold temperatures to balance exposures to cold and dampness that are outside of your control. If you tend to run hot, or find yourself intolerant of warm environments, avoid yang excess by limiting outdoor time in peak heat of the day in favor of evening nature time. As much as possible, stay in appropriately climate-controlled and cool rooms when inside buildings. Support yin by including room-temperature cooked foods and moderate amounts of raw or lightly cooked foods such as steamed vegetables. Avoid foods cooked at very high temperatures, like roasted or grilled meats and vegetables as well as fried food. Even if served cold, the temperature quality (and qi) used for cooking matters.
- *Light and darkness*: black and darkness are yin, and light, white, and brightness are yang. On long winter days, keep the lights in your workspace or home brightly lit until the evening hours, and consider incorporating natural light such as that from the sun during the day or candles/fireplace whenever possible during the evening and early morning hours. I recommend limiting screen use in general, but the summer months with long days and more comprehensive light exposure make this practice especially beneficial. During the summer, avoid artificial light and allow natural light to illuminate for you whenever possible.
- *Activity*: fast pace and high activity are yang, slowness and inactivity are yin. If you have a fast-paced job with high demands or are busy around your house with day-to-day responsibilities and a tight schedule, you should prioritize restorative activity and a gentle pace of life whenever you have the chance. Consider yoga, brisk walking, and stretching for exercise, and make provision to avoid rushing

throughout your day. Give yourself ample time to slowly wake up in the morning and wind down in the evening. Likewise, if you have a slow-paced job, particularly with inactivity such as a desk job, consider bursts of higher-intensity exercise added regularly throughout the day, such as high-intensity interval training (HIIT) workouts and weights, running, or the 7-Minute Workout. Take walking breaks every couple of hours.

- *Mental and physical*: mental load is yin; physical load is yang. Aim to balance mental and physical demands throughout your day. If you carry a lot of psychological stress, balancing that with regular exercise, or exercising in shorter, more frequent iterations throughout the day may benefit you. If you have a very physical job, or a particular lack of mental stimulation in your day, you may benefit from regularly seeking new skills and hobbies, utilizing logic games or puzzles in your leisure time, and/or looking for creative outlets. At the same time, if you regularly engage in active hobbies and exercise, or regularly find yourself on your feet for work, you may benefit from prioritizing sedentary leisure activities.
- *Sound*: quiet is yin, loudness and sound are yang. Do you have a balance of these two in your life? If you spend much of your day around crowds of talking people, you will benefit from calmer settings for leisure, such as quiet restaurants and more visual rather than auditory stimulation. Likewise, if you tend to spend much of your days in solitude, support yang with background music, or consider more public leisure activities, like visiting museums or attending concerts.
- *Exchange of ideas*: storage and receiving are yin, giving and utilization are yang. Do you balance your own intuition against the ideas or instructions given to you by others? Do you pause and listen as quickly as you speak your mind? Consider where you may benefit from fine-tuning this balance.

The Five Elements Theory in Practice

The Five Elements theory of Traditional Chinese Medicine incorporates the principles of yin, yang, balance, and harmony. However, rather than merely recognizing the importance of duality within each element, the five also interrelate with, sustain, and limit one another. In essence, the five elements need to maintain balance among themselves. In the way that too much heat in comparison to cold would indicate a manifestation of excess yang in relation to yin, too many qualities of a given element in a person's life may indicate excess of that particular element, its associated organs, or related harm to the associated tissues and functions of the body. As nearly every bodily function affects fertility, menstruation, and period health, imbalances among the five elements lead to abnormalities with the menstrual cycle. In a few chapters, we will discuss a cycle syncing method rooted in TCM, which allows you to align your lifestyle and menstrual cycle according to the Five Elements theory.

Remember that a person is not yin or yang, or earth, wind, or fire. Neither is any given health problem, like PCOS or estrogen dominance. Rather, all people reflect all elements in TCM and have both yin and yang qualities. Imbalances among these elements and their relationships lead to disharmony and disease, including the types of period and fertility problems that led you to pick up this book. So, while a Western diagnosis such as endometriosis doesn't necessarily have a TCM protocol for treatment, certain patterns of disharmony often accompany these problems, and such will be the focus of the TCM-influenced cycle syncing we'll discuss in a few chapters.

TOXINS AND ENVIRONMENTAL EXPOSURES

Up until now, our discussion of the foundational elements to support hormonal health has focused on strategies of inclusion—things you can add to your life to benefit hormones—rather than things to stay away from. I've written it this way intentionally, as psychology shows how trying to avoid something paradoxically creates desire for it. (You know, the example of how "Don't think about a pink elephant" makes you visualize exactly that.) This is particularly true in nutrition, where forbidding certain foods makes them seem particularly appetizing, sparking cravings and mental turmoil—even anguish—associated with avoiding them. In clinical practice, I find that it's much easier for my patients to make changes when we focus on the things we add to our lives rather than what we strip away. However, there is one exception: toxins.

No pill, no nutrition plan, no exercise regime, or sleep schedule, and no lifestyle pattern informed by Traditional Chinese Medicine can undo the harm caused by acute or chronic exposure to pesticides, plastics, parabens, and other hormone-disrupting chemicals that saturate our industrialized, modern world. Unfortunately, these chemical exposures aren't limited to the devastating albeit relatively uncommon disasters that make the news, such as lead contamination of water in Flint, Michigan, or the East Palestine train derailment in Ohio. They also show up in small, seemingly insignificant ways in our daily lives, the amalgamation of which creates an enormous toxic burden that disrupts cycles, contributes to inflammation, and otherwise throws off hormonal balance. These toxins include surfactant chemicals, which make soap and shampoo sudsy, and which disrupt hormonal regulation in the body.[64] We also see problems with fragrances, such as those added to perfumes and hair and beauty products, which increase both estrogen and inflammation levels as well as breast cancer risk in substantial, measurable ways.[65] We also can't forget the plastic compound bisphenol A (or BPA), which leaches into food and water from plastic packaging, increasing cancer risks and perpetuating estrogen dominance[66] or the estrogen effects of chemical contaminants in drinking water, including those caused by birth control pill runoff.[67] The list of health effects, both hormonal and otherwise, would frighten anyone, and my intention in outlining them here is not to create undue fear. Rather, it is to highlight the fact that we cannot take for granted that our groceries, water, personal care items, household cleaning products, food packaging, and more are free of contaminants that could harm our hormones and contribute to problems with periods and fertility. Because they aren't free of them. Instead of creating a laundry list of how, exactly, these chemicals create harm, look for simple swaps you can make in your home to protect yourself from the accumulation of chemicals that may hurt your hormones and health in general. Here are a few you can get started with:

Food

PESTICIDES

Pesticide content in food has been under scrutiny for decades, and with good reason. Exposure to glyphosate, 2,4-dichlorophenoxyacetic acid (2,4-D), atrazine, DEET, and other agricultural chemicals disrupts reproductive hormones in both men and women, affecting production, release and storage of hormones, their flow throughout the body, clearance of old and broken-down hormones through the liver and gut, and the way that hormones interact with cells when they reach them. They also negatively affect thyroid function and the activity of the central nervous system.[68] To reduce exposure to pesticides, choose organic whenever possible. Of course, the challenge with this is that organic plant and animal foods are typically more expensive than their conventional counterparts—but you can shop around. Even discount stores like Costco and ALDI have extensive organic selections, many of which are less expensive than conventional produce items at traditional retailers. If you aren't interested in making the full switch to organic, prioritize items that tend to have the highest levels of pesticides. The Environmental Working Group, an independent agency that evaluates environmental contaminants on human health, publishes a list they've dubbed "The Dirty Dozen," which in 2023 included the following foods as having the highest levels of pesticide contamination: (1) strawberries; (2) spinach; (3) kale, collard and mustard greens; (4) peaches; (5) pears; (6) nectarines; (7) apples; (8) grapes; (9) bell and hot peppers; (10) cherries; (11) blueberries; and (12) green beans.

PLASTIC PACKAGING

During production, manufacturers add chemicals to plastic packaging materials to improve flexibility, durability, and barrier properties. When these plastic materials are used in food packaging, the added chemicals such as BPA and phthalates migrate into the food, absorb through the digestive tract when consumed, and interfere with hormonal systems. They have been reported in research to produce "adverse reproductive, neurological, developmental, and immune effects."[69] The solution is to avoid plastic food packaging whenever it's realistically possible to do so. In general, I recommend focusing your attention on the packaging you use most often, which for most people is the food storage containers used when cooking at home. Plastic Tupperware, storage bags, and wrappings all run the risk of leaching endocrine-disrupting plasticizers into food. Repurpose your plastic storage containers for nonfood functions such as organizing drawers or storing knickknacks, and switch to glass or stainless-steel storage ware. Use silicone zipper bags or parchment paper in lieu of disposable plastic baggies and also take care to avoid plastic (and foil) wrapping for food. Many companies sell universal silicone discs designed to cover bowls and cups that don't have matching lids and make a great substitute for press 'n' seal or cling wrap.

COOKWARE

While you can't buy plastic pots, pans, or baking dishes (for good reason), many of the coatings and materials used to make cookware pose similar risks to plastic. Polytetrafluoroethylene (PTFE) and perfluorooctanoic acid

(PFOA), the chemicals used in Teflon and other nonstick pans, flake off and dissolve slowly over time into the foods that are cooked in them. Once ingested, they accumulate in the body and cause endocrine (hormone) toxicity and reproductive harm.[70] Switch out your nonstick pans for cast iron, ceramic coated cast iron, stainless steel, and glass bakeware. For baking, consider laying down unbleached parchment paper rather than aluminum foil if you need a nonstick barrier underneath your baked goods.

Water

FILTRATION

Birth control chemicals and pesticide runoff aren't the only concerns when it comes to drinking water safety. Heavy metals such as lead and arsenic, bleach, plastic derivatives, copper from piping, and other industrial contaminants accumulate in meaningful levels in water sourced from both city municipalities and private wells. The simple solution? Use a filter. Stainless steel filtration systems with charcoal filters and reverse osmosis are both great options for keeping contaminant levels to a minimum. You also could consider using a faucet attachment. These slow down the water flow but are a good solution if a larger system isn't an option.

ARE YOU GETTING ENOUGH CLEAN WATER?

You should aim for about half your body weight in ounces per day. As an example, a 150-pound woman should consume around 75 ounces of filtered water per day. Caffeine and alcohol both count against this ounce-per-ounce, and you should include an extra 16 ounces for every hour of exercise you perform.

Personal Care Products

Plastic packaging isn't the only source of endocrine-disrupting chemicals that you need to be aware of when it comes to protecting your hormonal health. Products such as shampoos, soaps, lotions, toothpaste, and other personal care items also source endocrine disruptors, particularly those that exacerbate estrogen-progesterone imbalances. You may have already seen labeling on your own products or items at the store that contain phrases such as "made without phthalates" or "paraben free." The obscure names of these chemicals are alarming enough to warrant avoiding them, but these advertisements come with good reason. All of these are endocrine disruptors, which means they interfere with hormonal balance and affect sexual development. They also cross the placenta and affect developing babies. Phthalates specifically inhibit egg maturation in ovarian follicles, decreasing egg quality. They also correlate with premature ovarian failure, inducing menopause prior to age forty, and negatively impact both puberty and pregnancy.[71] Meanwhile, parabens are xenoestrogens, meaning they look like estrogen and interfere with the activity of estrogen in the body, and they absorb through the skin at a high rate.[72] Once in the body, they interfere with production and release of estrogen and are known to cause irregular periods and decreased odds of successful pregnancy.[73] However, phthalates and parabens aren't the only chemicals of concern with personal care products. Sodium lauryl sulfate, benzyl alcohol, fragrance chemicals, and countless others also pose risk. There are thousands upon thousands of potentially problematic chemical additives in everything from hand soap to perfumes to deodorant, and it's virtually impossible to know whether a given product is likely to cause a hormone imbalance just by glancing at the label. Instead, I recommend using an external resource to screen the products for you based on their ingredients such as the Yuka app or the Environmental Working Group's (EWG's) *Skin Deep* website. The EWG website alone profiles nearly 100,000 products, scoring them on a scale of 0 to 10 (with 0 being the "cleanest" and 10 being the "worst") as well as the individual chemicals in those products, as listed on the label. As an example, a hair conditioner from a major grocery retailer rated 3:10 is stated on the EWG website to have earned that score based on a combination of its additives including: behentrimonium chloride, a potentially immunotoxic conditioning agent rated 7:10; sodium benzoate, a preservative, rated 3:10; a surfactant called polysorbate-60 which has a high risk of contamination with ethylene oxide, rated 3:10; as well as a handful of other ingredients rated 1 and 2. As stated on their website, "Cosmetics and personal care products are not required to be tested for safety before being allowed on the market. The *Skin Deep* scoring system was designed to help the public understand whether a product is safe to use or whether it contains ingredients of concern."[74] In addition to outlining the safety profile of major brands, Yuka and EWG's *Skin Deep* database also offer recommendations for clean products at all price points for everything from makeup, sunblock, and toothpaste to shampoo for all hair types.

Cleaning Products

Cleaning products, like personal care products, often also contain endocrine-disrupting detergents, preservatives, and other ingredients that harm hormones. Beyond the direct hormonal relationships, though, these chemicals often (and by design) contain additives that negatively impact the microbiome, too. We've already discussed the immense importance of a diverse and robust microbiome and accidentally killing off those good bacteria because you spray down your countertops with bleach is the last thing you'd want to do. Like lotions and hand soaps, the chemicals in cleaning products absorb through our skin, enter our blood streams, and interact with hormone receptors and microbes that way. However, we also are likely to ingest them, especially when they are used to clean dishes, countertops, and other surfaces that we may touch before consuming or preparing food. The Environmental Working Group operates a second website called the *Guide to Healthy Cleaning*, which is dedicated completely to profiling household cleaners, laundry detergents, dishwashing soaps, and even furniture cleaners. The letter grades range from A through F, with the EWG-certified seal awarded to the cleanest of cleaning products. While this site is particularly useful for dishwashing liquid, laundry soap, and some of the more specialized products such as hardwood floor cleaners, I recommend the simple combination of baking soda and vinegar for the majority of your household cleaning. Not only are these products safe enough to actually consume but they outperform many of the cleaners on the market, natural or otherwise. The added bonus is that they're extremely inexpensive. Instead of specific sink-cleansers or counter sprays, make a simple paste with baking soda and water, and use it along with a scrub brush to scour soap scum, bathroom mildew, and buildup in sinks, on countertops, and around bathroom utilities. After wiping or rinsing off the excess, spray the surface with a one-to-one ratio of vinegar and water (in a regular spray bottle). The acid will neutralize the baking soda to prevent white residue and kill any lingering microbes. If the vinegar smell bothers you, wipe down the surface a third time with a wet rag, or you can simply let it air dry. You can also use the vinegar-water mixture to wipe down windows and stainless-steel appliances instead of ammonia-based cleaners, to sterilize humidifiers and essential oil diffusers, and as a replacement for bleach in the clean cycle of your laundry machine. If you were really in a gardening pinch, vinegar also kills weeds. So, you can spray it around your pavers and mulch to keep dandelions and ivy from encroaching on your bushes. Just be mindful that it is a nonselective strategy, so it will damage your tomato plants and petunias in addition to weeds. Because of this, it's best used for walkways and other paved surfaces where no plants are typically invited.

Environmental Exposures

GROCERY RECEIPTS

A lesser-known source of endocrine disruptors, thermal receipt paper used to print grocery and retail receipts, contains BPA levels up to 1,000 times higher than the plastic lining of canned goods.[75] This chemical can absorb through your skin when handling receipts, or transfer to food if you don't wash your hands first. In today's digital age, most receipts are available through email or text in lieu of print, so opt for that whenever you can. If you do handle a receipt, wash your hands as soon as possible, or keep a pack of baby wipes in your purse or car to wipe off your skin after handling.

CLOTHING

Many clothing textiles are doused with flame retardants and pest repellants during warehouse storage. Unfortunately, with the exception of the state of California, clothing manufacturers are not required to disclose if these chemicals have been applied. In most cases, they probably have. While there are some brands of clothing that advertise being free of flame retardants, the best thing you can and should do is simply wash your clothing after purchase, before your first wear. Use the warmest water the textile can tolerate without damage and a hefty dose of soap.

FURNITURE AND FOOTWEAR

Cloth furniture often is subject to treatment with pest repellants and flame retardants the same way that clothing is, but unlike a T-shirt, you can't throw your couch in the wash. Instead, you can wipe it down with a damp rag prior to use. However, the additional concern of both furniture and footwear is the foam. Many furniture products contain labels that indicate "off-gassing," which is the process of chemical gas products releasing into the air that diffuse from the cushioning on chairs, couches, and shoes after manufacturing. Typically, you can detect the smell of these gases, and the labels warn against inhaling them. Usually, these products come with tags that say something along the lines of, "Be sure to allow this product to air out in a well-ventilated room for 48–72 hours." A good guideline if you can't find the tag (or threw it away) is to keep the product sequestered in a room with closed doors but open windows until the smell is completely gone, plus another twenty-four hours.

DO-IT-YOURSELF (DIY) PROJECTS

Many projects around the house or for craft purposes involve paints, solvents, lacquer, varnish, and other chemical products that are simply unavoidable if the task is to be completed. Rather than give up your favorite woodworking hobby or throw in the towel on your oil painting class, be mindful to ensure that your workspace is well-ventilated with windows and fans. Try not to breathe the fumes directly and, if applicable, wear a well-fitted mask. Read the warning labels on the products themselves regarding ventilation and time of exposure, and don't ignore them (no matter how tempting it may be). While it's important for everyone to heed label warnings for hormonal health and otherwise, it's especially important for pregnant women, as many of these chemicals (such as paints and varnishes) contain explicit prohibitions for use during pregnancy.

While we can control many things with regards to our exposure to hormone disruptors, we can't control everything. If we live in a densely populated area, we can't do anything about the diesel and car exhaust from nearby highways. Likewise, it's not our fault if someone down the street puts sealcoating on their asphalt driveway and the fumes drift through the entire neighborhood on a sunny spring day. The pesticide spray at nearby farmland, the mosquito lawn treatment at our neighbors' house, or the asbestos insulation hiding in the attic—we generally can't change these factors without moving to a private island off the coast of California. But even then, we are still subject to forces beyond ourselves. The moral of the story is this: pay attention to the areas that you can reasonably control, but don't stress about the rest. Pollution puts our bodies at risk just as it does other creatures and growing things that dwell on the earth, but it's still possible to live a hormonally balanced and otherwise healthy life despite it. Do what you can, and let the rest go. Enjoy takeout from your favorite restaurant, even if the hot food arrives in Styrofoam containers, because you know that 98 percent of the time, you use safe cookware and food storage in your own home. Enjoy your favorite fashions despite the chemical additives because you know your own laundry soap is paraben free, and you'll wash the garment before wearing it. Filter your water, but don't fret if the waiter serves you tap water while out with friends. Do what you can to create a healthy foundation for your sleep, nutrition, exercise, and other habits, but don't forget to enjoy your life too.

7

REALLY GETTING TO KNOW YOURSELF

Once you have a healthy foundation in place, you'll have a better understanding of how sleep, stress, nutrition, exercise, and other lifestyle habits affect your hormones, your period, and your fertility. You might even find that from adjustments made based on the previous chapter alone, your cramps improve, your cycle regulates, and you feel worlds better. But then again, you still might not. Of course, not every ailment can be solved by simply living a healthy life. Sometimes, *stuff just happens*, and that's where medicine comes into play—and I'm not talking about popping the pill. Rather, I'm talking about making a diagnosis, figuring out the root cause of the issue, and then making a plan to treat that underlying problem so it's fixed once and for all. That's where the final section of this book will come into play. But first, we need to get a little more cycle-specific with our lifestyle habits.

Here's a question for you: Do you know when you ovulate? Remember from our discussion about hormones, we outlined how ovulation is the main event of the menstrual cycle. Ovulation allows you to make progesterone, which is one of the most important hormones in the body, affecting everything from your brain to your skin, to breast health and the comfort of your periods. Without ovulation, you can't make progesterone. Without progesterone, nothing else in your body works the way it should; and if you're on the pill, you can't make progesterone. Whether or not you have periods and when is pretty obvious. But do you know for sure that you're ovulating, and when?

One of the ways you can find out if you're ovulating is by making an appointment with your doctor, who will run some tests. First, she will perform an ultrasound to evaluate your ovaries and look for developing follicles. This is the first clue, demonstrating that your brain communicates effectively with your ovaries. Then, around the twenty-first day of your cycle when hormone levels theoretically reach their highest (if you ovulate right in the middle of a twenty-eight-day cycle), she will run a blood test to measure your progesterone level and make sure it's above 4.44 nanograms per milliliter (ng/mL). A level this high indicates a strong likelihood of corpus luteum activity, the main way that we produce progesterone, only possible if a follicle has matured and released an egg. If your doctor wanted to figure out exactly when you ovulate, as is often important in in vitro fertilization (IVF) egg retrieval cycles, she will perform these tests every day for several days, sometimes for weeks.

Having blood tests and ultrasounds performed every day or couple of days is extremely invasive, expensive, and stressful, so most doctors don't do that unless absolutely necessary. In fact, most doctors don't even perform day-twenty-one progesterone tests for regular period problems because most of them simply prescribe the pill for irregular cycles, midcycle spotting, or other problems associated with ovulatory dysfunction. But if you want to avoid the pill *and* fix your period problems, it's really important that you figure out if you're ovulating and when. This allows you to make lifestyle changes specific to the phase of your cycle that you're in or to use herbal and supplement strategies based on certain phases of your cycle without guessing, so that you can treat your period problems naturally. It also helps you understand why you may have more energy and motivation on certain days compared to others, and you'll be able to plan ahead rather than constantly playing catch-up with your health. Knowing when you ovulate also empowers you to make decisions about contraception and sexuality to help you avoid pregnancy without disrupting your ever-so-important hormones. On the flip side, knowing when you ovulate also helps you conceive more quickly and easily, if this is your goal. Knowing how your body works empowers you in so many ways, and we will discuss all of them and more in this chapter.

PREDICTING AND CONFIRMING OVULATION

Several methods exist for tracking ovulation without any need for formal testing in a doctor's office. You can use all of the tracking methods outlined below from the comfort of your home, with a little bit of inexpensive equipment, or even none at all. Basal body temperature, cervical fluid, and resting heart rate all fluctuate predictably throughout the menstrual cycle based on changes in estrogen and progesterone, and we can likewise use these simple measurements to identify whether and/or when ovulation has occurred. Urine test strips for measuring levels of luteinizing hormone give you valuable information for predicting ovulation. Some of these measures are more accurate than others and are consequently more appropriate for helping to promote or avoid pregnancy. But all of them are available to use easily from home. Let's discuss each one so that you can decide which among them is most appropriate for you, depending on your goals.

Basal Body Temperature

The term "basal body temperature" refers to your body temperature when you are completely at rest. Physical activity and moving around, of course, produces body heat, but your body also produces heat from basic metabolic processes partly as a by-product but also partly to keep you warm enough. (Humans are warm-blooded creatures, after all!) Because resting body temperature fluctuates so much throughout the waking hours based on different types of activities, we consider body temperature taken at rest—or as close to sleeping as possible—as a truer reflection of metabolic activity.

One of the many roles played by progesterone is to increase metabolic rate via the hypothalamic-pituitary-adrenal-thyroid-gonadal (HPATG) axis. Progesterone produced following ovulation signals the brain to increase thyroid activity, changing how the body uses energy, ultimately leading to greater body heat production. This includes during rest. In fact, the thermogenic increase follows a predictable change of around 0.3 degrees between the follicular and luteal phases of the cycle. (This increase in metabolic rate also explains why you may feel hungrier during your luteal phase: your body actually uses more energy to make body heat!) By tracking body temperature daily throughout the menstrual cycle and identifying the temperature shift, you can not only confirm ovulation but also the precise day on which it occurs. The subsequent rise and fall of body temperature correlates directly to the rise and fall of progesterone levels throughout your cycle.

If you know when you ovulate, you know a lot of other things about yourself too, such as when you are fertile. If you use an app to track your periods, it probably gives you an estimate of fertile days—meaning, the days you can potentially conceive if you have unprotected sex. However, unless it's an app for tracking ovulation in addition to periods, the fertile days provided on the app are just estimations. These estimations come from the assumption that your luteal phase is fourteen days long and predict that ovulation will occur on the day corresponding to your average cycle length minus fourteen. For example, if you really do have a twenty-eight-day cycle, the app predicts ovulation on day fourteen. But if you average thirty days, it will predict ovulation to occur on day sixteen. If you average thirty-five days, it will predict ovulation on day twenty-one. The fertile days given correspond to the five days that sperm can survive in the female reproductive tract (waiting in anticipation of an egg), plus two additional days corresponding to the day of ovulation and the day after—adding up to a seven-day-total window.

While these app estimations are good for giving a general idea, they can't and shouldn't be used to assume real-life information about your cycle. Apart from the days that you record your period, the app knows nothing about your menstrual cycle or whether or not you ovulate in the first place. Second, the apps operate on averages. Take, for example, a situation where a woman has a forty-day average cycle, but half the time her cycle is fifty days long and the other half of the time it is thirty days long. With an average of forty, the app will predict that she ovulates on day twenty-six. (40 – 14 = 26). If she truly has a fourteen-day luteal phase, the reality is that some months she will ovulate on day sixteen, and, in other months, on day thirty-six. If she were to time intercourse based on this estimate—whether to promote or avoid pregnancy—she would do herself a great disservice. The limited assumptions don't stop here, though. The apps are also *estimating* that every woman has a fourteen-day luteal phase when, in reality, they don't. It's true that in many cases the luteal phase lasts fourteen days, but it is shorter than that in many cases too. A short luteal phase is a problem for fertility and signifies a hormone imbalance. We even have a term to describe a luteal phase of less than ten days, "luteal phase deficiency." If you are concerned that you have luteal phase deficiency, please refer to the treatment section (chapter 11 of this book).

In the case of a short luteal phase, the average-cycle-minus-fourteen rule definitely doesn't apply. Rather than on day fourteen, a luteal phase of twelve days corresponds with ovulation on day sixteen in a twenty-eight-day cycle. You can see how this spells trouble for fertility and family planning, but it is also important to know about changes in luteal phase length and timing of ovulation due to the implications it has for progesterone production and other areas of your health. For example, if you experience a short luteal phase in combination with premenstrual spotting, breast tenderness, and scanty flow, you are likely experiencing progesterone deficiency and need help.

Because charting basal body temperature allows you to confirm the day of ovulation, you can compare charts from sequential cycles to figure out if you tend to ovulate on the same day of the month. If you do, you can then apply the 5 + 2 rule for predicting fertile days based on *your own* chart information rather than an app's estimate and know your likelihood of conception on any day of your cycle with certainty. Plus, you can identify the length and timing of your follicular phase in addition to your luteal phase, thereby empowering yourself with the knowledge of where you are and what's going on with your hormones at any given time. If you're on your period, you know hormones are at their bare minimum. After your period ends but before ovulation, you know that estrogen has taken the spotlight. If you know it's ovulation day, you know that estrogen has just dramatically dropped off after reaching its peak. In the first week or so after ovulation, progesterone and estrogen begin to rise, and as your temperature declines in the days leading up to your next expected period, you know that your hormone levels are dropping off too. If the temperature doesn't decrease on time as predicted, it may be a very early sign of pregnancy and an early clue that you should take a test in a few days, because even pregnancy tests aren't as accurate as basal body temperature is! Once you get an idea of different changes in your brain and body during these different times of the month, you can really know what is and isn't normal for you. That's why I recommend that women chart their temperature even if they aren't trying to conceive, if they aren't sexually active at all, or if they don't have any concerns about their periods. There really is no comparison for the detailed and accurate information it provides and how that knowledge then empowers you to know and care for yourself.

Charting your basal body temperature is pretty straightforward—often surprisingly so, given how powerful of a tool it is. You don't need to start on the first day of your cycle (which corresponds with the first day of your period), though I do recommend this starting point if you've never charted before because it makes it easier to read and evaluate your data. Once you decide which day you're going to start, set your thermometer on your nightstand and in the morning, as soon as you wake up, take your temperature and record it on your chart. Because the goal is to evaluate temperature as close to rest (sleeping) as possible, try to take it as soon as you realize you're awake, without rolling over in bed, sitting up, drinking water, using the bathroom, or engaging in any other type of activity. This will help prevent an artificially elevated reading from activity-related body heat production. Please also note that an average basal body temperature less than 97.8 degrees Fahrenheit when measured orally strongly suggests hypothyroidism. If you notice this, please make an appointment with your health care provider and ask for a complete thyroid panel.[1]

BASAL BODY TEMPERATURE THERMOMETER

Because basal body temperature is so specific of a measurement, you need to use an extra-sensitive thermometer that goes to two places past the decimal. So, rather than measuring 98.6 degrees Fahrenheit, it would measure 98.65 degrees, for example. This additional decimal of specificity makes the readings more accurate and trustworthy. Although they aren't the norm, basal body temperature thermometers aren't very expensive, only about $15, and can be purchased online through most major health retailers. The thermometer also needs to be an oral thermometer rather than forehead or ear, though some women choose to take their temperature vaginally.

If you're going through the effort to take your temperature every day, you'll want to take a few steps to make sure it's accurate. In addition to using a specifically basal body temperature thermometer that reads to two decimal places, consider the following when you record your chart:

- *Time of day*: Ideally, you will take your temperature around the same time every day, weekend or otherwise. This will help your readings to be the most accurate, because body temperature naturally rises a bit the later you sleep in. Once you get the hang of it and are more familiar with your own chart's patterns, you might be able to get away with sleeping in an extra hour or so on weekends without it affecting your overall chart patterns. But when you're first starting out, I recommend strictly following the time-of-day rule. If you really don't want to get up with your 5:30 a.m. work alarm on weekends, it's totally okay to go back to bed after taking your reading! You'll simply have a more accurate chart if you have a predictable time of day for taking your temperature, even if you're half asleep while you do it.
- *Duration of sleep*: you'll want to make sure to take your temperature recordings after a period of at least four hours of uninterrupted sleep, because this is the amount of time that allows body temperature to drop the lowest. If you have a restless night or wake up to use the

bathroom, don't worry—your chart won't be completely ruined. This is just a way to make sure that, most of the time, your readings are as accurate as possible. The Fertility Friend app allows you to indicate if a given reading is potentially inaccurate, such as the inconsistencies that result from irregular sleep patterns, consuming alcohol, illness accompanied by fever, and more. There will always be outliers, but the most important thing on a chart is the overarching pattern, established by accurate readings on most days.

- *Alcohol and other drug use*: substance use affects body temperature. Alcohol, specifically, is a nervous system depressant, so it slows down bodily processes and reduces body temperature. For this reason, on mornings after you've had a drink, your body temperature may be lower. You can indicate this on the Fertility Friend app, and I would also recommend doing so if you record your data manually.
- *Mouth breathing*: if you are congested or otherwise tend to breathe through your mouth, your readings may not be accurate. The air flowing through your mouth will cool things off, and your readings will be artificially lower. If you often wake up with a dry mouth or notice mouth breathing, you should consider taking your temperature vaginally for accurate data.
- *Stress*: besides affecting sleep quality and increasing restlessness or insomnia, stress also increases body temperature. That's not to mention its tendency to throw off ovulation and fertility, too. Make a mental note for yourself that your chart might be a little off that month if you're enduring a particularly heightened period of stress.
- *Illness*: it probably goes without saying that a fever is going to increase your temperature readings. Make a note on your chart if you are ill in a given month.

Interpreting Your Chart

With charting basal body temperature, there are two main phases of your cycle that you're looking for: before the temperature shift and after the temperature shift. In an ovulatory cycle where data was measured accurately (according to the above considerations), body temperature readings will predictably increase at least 0.3 degrees but as many as 0.5 degrees or more during the luteal phase (after ovulation) above what they were in the follicular phase (before ovulation). The day before the first increased temperature reading corresponds to the day of ovulation. (Note: rarely, the temperature increase is only about 0.2 degrees, which is not ideal and may also be a sign of low progesterone.)

You will notice that your chart doesn't follow a perfectly smooth line, however. Temperature naturally fluctuates a little bit, plus or minus a few decimal points from day to day. Because of this, the chart data will look a little jagged, especially in the follicular phase. When the temperature shift following ovulation takes place, *all* of the subsequent readings will be *at least* 0.3 degrees above the highest follicular phase readings. If, for example, the highest temperatures in your follicular phase are 97.9 degrees, all of the luteal phase readings will be at least 98.2 degrees or above. That is, until the temperature starts to drop again as your period approaches. For many women, temperature readings slowly fall as the first day of the next cycle draws near. This corresponds to a decline in progesterone occurring at the end of the luteal phase. However, some women's temperatures don't drop off until a day or two after their periods come, and that's normal too.

Another reason I like the Fertility Friend app is because its software analyzes chart data and gives an estimation of when ovulation was likely to have occurred with red crosshairs appearing on the chart, corresponding to ovulation day, after a period of three elevated readings are recorded. This can be helpful if you are new to charting and are not yet used to deciphering the data patterns. It also makes chart reading easier in general. If you choose to record your data manually on graph paper or with a different app, you may find it beneficial to combine your basal body temperature data with other markers of ovulation such as cervical fluid changes or luteinizing hormone (LH) strips, which we will detail in a bit. We refer to the practice of combining techniques like this as a "symptothermal method" (symptoms + thermal/temperature data) and is considered by the *Merck Manuals*—a leading medical resource—to be the most accurate means for tracking fertility.[2]

Once you have recorded about three months of data, you will know if you tend to ovulate around the same time each month and how long each phase of your cycle typically lasts. For example, if you always notice the temperature shift occurring on day seventeen of your thirty-day cycle, you will know that your follicular phase is sixteen days long (including ovulation on day sixteen) followed by a fourteen-day luteal phase (beginning on the first day of the elevated temperature). Then, your fertile days, meaning the days you would be most likely to become pregnant, would include the day of ovulation, the five days preceding, and the one day after. If you were actively trying to conceive, you'd want to have sex about every other day throughout that range. Likewise, you would want to be sure to avoid

Really Getting to Know Yourself 117

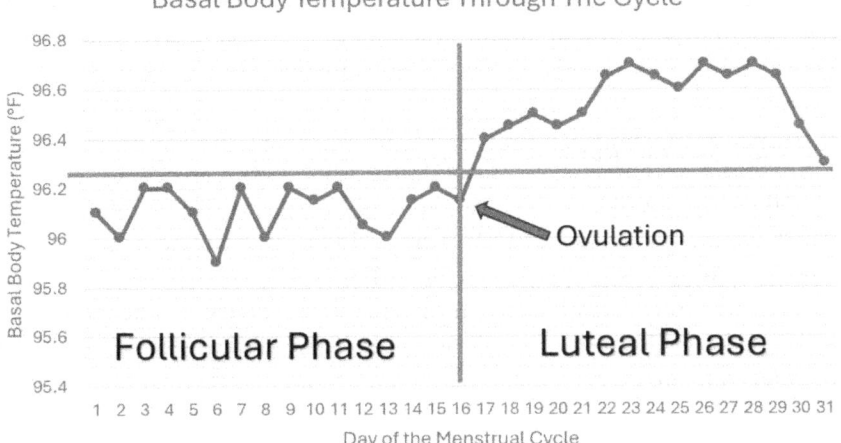

Figure 7.1 Fluctuation in Basal Body Temperature Throughout the Menstrual Cycle

unprotected sex throughout that seven-day period if preventing pregnancy is your goal, though I recommend using a barrier method of contraception as well. Continue to do so until you have confirmed ovulation through three consecutive elevated luteal-phase readings to be especially careful and account for any unexpected changes to the day of ovulation. Take a look at the sample BBT chart (figure 7.1) to practice identifying the temperature shift and day of ovulation.

LIMITATIONS OF BBT

Although basal body temperature (BBT) charting, when performed correctly, offers extremely accurate data regarding the timing of ovulation after it occurs, it can't perfectly predict it. This is because the temperature shift only takes place *after* the corpus luteum develops and produces progesterone. While for most women, ovulation typically occurs around the same time in every cycle, this can normally vary by a day in either direction, and can be affected by things like illness, travel, and the other factors that influence the HPATG axis. It's also important to recognize that if you have irregular cycles, varying in length from each other, ovulation is also likely to occur at a different time in each given cycle. With conditions like polycystic ovarian syndrome (PCOS), in particular, menstrual cycles are notoriously long and unpredictable, so predicting ovulation far in advance really isn't possible. However, regardless of chronic health conditions such as this, charting BBT still offers the same benefit of knowing if and when ovulation has occurred in any given cycle. As I hope is clear by now, this information offers countless benefits beyond merely predicting fertile days.

Resting Heart Rate

Because progesterone production following ovulation influences all metabolic activity via the HPATG axis and not just body heat production, we consequently see variation in the other vital signs as well. (The vital signs include body temperature, heart rate, blood pressure, and respiration rate.) These vital signs can also serve as an indirect, qualitative measure of progesterone production and ovulation, but not all of them are as practical as basal body temperature. Respiration rate is nearly impossible to measure accurately on your own because it's something you can cognitively control; as soon as you direct attention to how frequently you take a breath, you end up overriding the natural underlying bodily signals at least a little bit, even if you don't mean to. For this reason, respiratory rate is not considered an accurate or valid reflection of metabolic and hormonal activity, and pulse-oximetry is usually used instead.

Unlike respiration rate, we cannot control our blood pressure with our minds. (Wouldn't that be nice?) And while it does vary throughout the menstrual cycle, it does not mirror the changes in progesterone seen with other vital signs.[3] Even if it did, most people don't have blood pressure cuffs at home, and it would be extremely difficult to finagle the cuff onto your arm while maintaining a near-sleeping level of restfulness anyway. So, that option is out. Heart rate, on the other hand, does change throughout the cycle in the way that body temperature does—increasing after ovulation and dropping around the start of menses due to changes in progesterone and the HPATG axis. However, using heart rate to observe ovulation differs from BBT in two key ways: accuracy and ease.

Heart rate fluctuates rapidly throughout the day, and even moment by moment. Heart rate actually changes more quickly than body temperature, so it is more likely to give a falsely elevated reading compared to BBT. It also fluctuates more dramatically in response to stress, illness, or other environmental and lifestyle factors. Even hydration level can influence heart rate, so it's much more sensitive to variation from lifestyle habits than BBT and is therefore not as reliable. We also don't have any large-scale studies validating it as a tool for specifically confirming ovulation, so there isn't an agreed-upon definition of how much heart rate needs to change after ovulation in order to confirm that an egg was released.

That being said, resting heart rate (RHR) *does* change predictably throughout the menstrual cycle[4] and, hence, can be used as a qualitative measure of ovulation. In other words, if you measure your resting heart rate throughout your cycle, it can give you a pretty good idea of whether and when you ovulate, albeit not *exactly* when. Even though it's less accurate and less precise with the information it provides, the advantage of measuring resting heart rate compared to basal body temperature is that it's easier to do, and you might already be doing it. Most fitness watches and other smartwatches these days include a resting heart rate monitor function, which tracks your heart rate throughout the day and night if you wear it while sleeping, and records the data in the associated app. This is how the watches estimate duration and quality of sleep, for example, based on nocturnal movements and heart rate variability over the course of sleep. Wearing these watches at night also allows for vital sign measurements to be taken while you actually are asleep, which is ideal when tracking basal activity such as heart rate. (If you don't wear a smartwatch, you can track your resting heart rate similarly to BBT, except by using a pulse-oximeter on your pointer finger rather than an oral thermometer.)

In comparison to BBT, RHR begins increasing sooner in the cycle, before ovulation occurs, in response to the spike of estrogen that helps pull the trigger for ovulation. Then, once the egg is released, progesterone propagates the rise of RHR until about a week before your period, when it pretty quickly moves back to the follicular phase levels. If you conceive during a given cycle, however, RHR (like BBT) will remain elevated, and can serve as an early pregnancy clue. It also may help you time intercourse if you are trying to conceive, as the period in which RHR starts to increase usually coincides with the onset of fertile days. As you can see in figure 7.2, the distinctive shift and wavelike pattern indicates a transition in heart rate, triggered by ovulation and progesterone.

Because RHR is not as accurate or precise as BBT, I don't recommend using it alone as a method of contraception. However, if you're not up to the task of charting BBT but still want to keep general tabs on when in your cycle you're ovulating (such as if you choose to follow a cycle syncing method described later in this book, or you just like to monitor your reproductive health) this is a great low-maintenance option. If you have a fitness watch that syncs with your phone, you probably don't need to do anything at all to record your data. If you're already using a fitness watch, evaluate the graphed form of your RHR data and if it looks like a sine wave over the past several months, you're probably ovulating. Make a note of

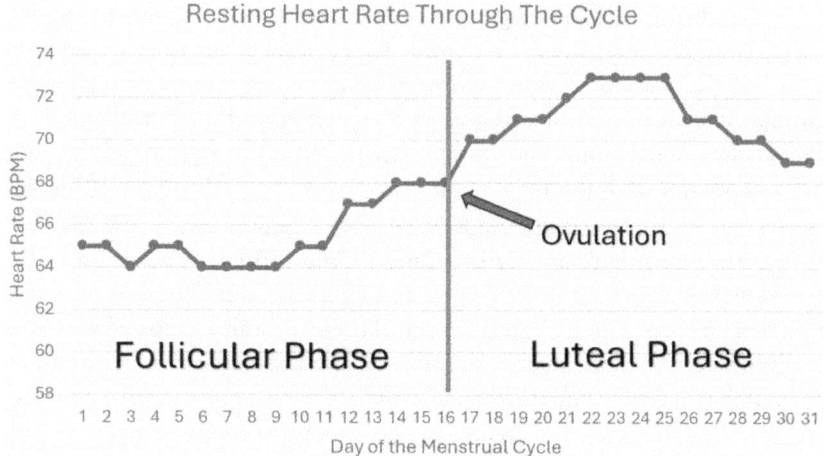

Figure 7.2 Fluctuation in Resting Heart Rate Through the Menstrual Cycle

how your heart rate fluctuates based on where you are in your cycle and use that information to stay one step ahead!

Cervical Fluid

If numerical data like RHR and BBT don't fit your lifestyle, but you still want to monitor your cycle, tracking cervical fluid might be the non-tech solution you need. A few chapters back, we outlined the fact that hormonal changes throughout the cycle translate to changes in the consistency and chemical composition of cervical fluid—the discharge naturally released throughout the month that serves in part to clean and protect the vagina. It also plays a secondary role of aiding sperm motility or preventing anything from entering through the cervix, depending on the time of the month. Due to the fluctuations in hormones, mainly estrogen, throughout the menstrual cycle, cervical fluid changes in very obvious ways. You can monitor the quality of cervical fluid over the course of the month to gather clues about when you may be ovulating, and consequently help you gauge the relative lengths of the follicular and luteal phases of your cycle.

The most notable type of fluid released from the vagina is menstrual blood, but as that clears away, you will notice a clear, white or pale-yellow discharge on toilet paper when you wipe or left over in your underwear. The amount and consistency of this cervical fluid responds mostly to fluctuations in estrogen levels. If you recall from our conversation about physiology, estrogen dominates the follicular phase, though the peak rise and fall of estrogen occurs in a relatively short space of time immediately preceding ovulation. This is when cervical fluid changes are most obvious and also when they are most important for fertility. Here's how cervical fluid fluctuates in response to hormonal changes throughout the menstrual cycle:

- *Menstrual phase*: During this phase, estrogen and progesterone both reach their minimum, and cervical fluid is indistinguishable from menstrual blood
- *Follicular phase*: Following the cessation of menstrual bleeding, cervical fluid is sticky and dry. You may not notice it at all. As estrogen very slowly increases, the water content and amount of cervical fluid produced likewise slowly increases. Typically, the mucus is whitish or pale yellow but may reach a thinner consistency (like the texture of milk) by around day nine or ten of your cycle.
- *Late follicular phase*: Estrogen rises dramatically toward the end of the follicular phase, and cervical fluid becomes thin, watery and clear, though sometimes it maintains a pale whitish/watery color. It may also take on a stretchy texture. This type of cervical fluid is referred to as "watery" and is semi-fertile. Typically, this cervical fluid is seen within the five-day fertile window leading up to ovulation. If you are avoiding pregnancy, don't have unprotected sex during this time.
- *Ovulatory/Fertile phase*: A few days before ovulation, when estrogen has peaked, cervical fluid becomes abundant, clear, and stretchy, similar to the texture of raw egg white. (For this reason, fertile cervical fluid is often referred to as "egg white cervical mucus, or EWCM.") Although late follicular/watery cervical mucus may be stretchy too, the hallmark characteristic of fertile EWCM is the ability to stretch up to two inches without breaking apart when you stretch it between your fingers. The watery and gelatinous quality of this type of cervical fluid both aids sperm motility and provides sperm with extra sugars and nutrients to aid survival through the reproductive tract. When you see this type of cervical fluid, you are likely to ovulate within twenty-four to forty-eight hours.
- *Luteal phase*: Immediately following ovulation, estrogen levels plummet again, and the egg dissolves within thirty-six hours if it hasn't been fertilized by a ready, waiting, and able sperm. Since there is no longer a need to allow sperm (or anything else) into the uterus, cervical fluid changes quickly and dramatically from the stretchy, clear EWCM and instead becomes thick, sticky and white, resembling Elmer's glue. This is referred to as "creamy" cervical fluid and is an

inhospitable environment for both sperm and unfriendly microbes. When you see this type of cervical fluid, ovulation has passed, you are no longer fertile, and your next period is less than two weeks away.

Cervical fluid offers the benefit of real-time information about your fertility. While BBT and RHR offer fertility predictions based on the previous months' data, cervical fluid changes reflect what's going on with your cycle *right now*. You can certainly use these patterns to make predictions for future months, but when that month comes along, your cervical fluid will still either confirm or refute that prediction. Tracking cervical fluid changes as a fertility awareness method has been endorsed by the Catholic Church as a method for contraception because of how accurate it is. The Creighton Model Method is one such system for tracking fertility to promote or prevent pregnancy based on cervical fluid changes and has been shown in the research to be 98.8 percent effective as a form of contraception.[5] The Creighton Model System also offers an app where you can track data if you decide to monitor your cervical fluid changes over time, though paper and pencil of course work too. To check your cervical fluid, examine your toilet paper after using the bathroom in the morning, or gently insert a clean, dry index finger into your vagina and inspect the characteristics of the cervical fluid that way. Family planning aside, tracking cervical fluid, like BBT or RHR, offers you invaluable information about your body, its hormones, and your fertility as a vital sign.

SOME ADDITIONAL NOTES ABOUT CERVICAL FLUID

- If you notice vaginal discharge that is dark yellow, green, gray, blood-tinged, or thick and white, like cottage cheese, you may have an infection. Please refer to chapter 5 to review what is and isn't normal and make an appointment with your health care provider as needed.
- If you don't notice any vaginal discharge at all, you may be suffering from a hormonal imbalance, particularly one characterized by low estrogen levels. Please refer to the treatment section to address this.
- Scanty or diminished cervical fluid is common during breastfeeding, hypothyroidism, and other hormone imbalances. It may also decrease in response to dehydration or use of antihistamines such as Claritin, Xyzal, Benadryl, and Zyrtec. If you are well hydrated, not using the above medications, not breastfeeding, and are already taking steps to

improve hormone balance and still would like support to increase your cervical fluid production, consider the following supplements:

- Evening primrose oil (EPO): Oral supplementation with EPO increases blood flow to the cervix, softening it and increasing mucus production.[6] This helps prepare the cervix for dilation during childbirth but also relieves symptoms of vaginal dryness during menopause.[7] Because EPO increases the effects of estrogen,[8] it is thought to increase cervical mucus, especially fertile cervical mucus, through this mechanism. I recommend that my patients take 500 milligrams (mg) of EPO three times daily with food, during the follicular phase only.
- L-arginine: Supplementing with 1,000 mg daily improves blood flow to the cervix and subsequent mucus production.[9]
- Vitamin B6: Some studies have shown improvements in cervical fluid through supplementation with 500 mg of extended-release vitamin B6, however toxicity risks emerge when supplementation exceeds 100 mg daily. I recommend that my patients consider combining 100 mg daily of vitamin B6 with L-arginine and/or evening primrose oil to improve production and quality of cervical mucus.[10]

Cervical Position

Although much more difficult to maintain reliability and objectivity, other qualities of the cervix also change throughout the month in cycle-specific ways. As a reminder, your cervix is the thick, muscular opening to your uterus, which protrudes into the vagina. In response to estrogen levels, the position of the cervix, its texture, and the diameter of the opening fluctuate. Therefore, evaluating the position, texture, and diameter of the opening of your own cervix gives you information about where you are in your cycle and what's going on with your hormones. Keep in mind that unlike BBT or RHR, this is qualitative data and cannot specifically confirm that ovulation has occurred or when. However, it does give you a pretty good indication of what's probably going on.

In order to use cervical texture and position to track your cycle, you need to get comfortable with performing an internal exam. To do so, insert one or two clean (freshly washed, with nails trimmed) fingers into your vagina while your pelvic floor muscles are relaxed, such as when sitting on the toilet or in a squatting position. You know you've found your cervix when you encounter a smooth, firm protrusion of tissue at the top of your vaginal canal with an indentation or opening in the middle. Practice evaluating the size of the opening, but don't insert your finger (or anything else) into it. Continue finding your cervix and gently evaluating its texture a few times per day for several days to get an idea of what it feels like and how it might change based on your sitting position. Then, once you've found a comfortable position and time of day when you can regularly check your cervix, start tracking your data so you can learn about your cycle.

Here's how your cervix changes throughout the month, and what that information tells you about your menstrual phase:

- *Menstrual phase*: During menstruation, your cervix moves lower in the vagina and opens up to let blood out. You will notice that you don't need to insert your fingers in as far to find it, and the opening will be wider. The texture of your cervix will be firmer, like the texture of your nose.
- *Follicular phase*: During the follicular phase, the cervix starts to slowly move higher up in the vagina, so you'll have to insert your fingers further to find it. After your period, the entrance will close, but the texture will slowly become softer.
- *Ovulatory phase*: During ovulation, the cervix is at the highest point throughout the cycle. The texture will be soft, like the texture of your lips when they're relaxed, and it will remain open.
- *Luteal phase*: Following ovulation, the texture of your cervix will slowly start to firm up again and will slowly move down through the vagina as your period approaches. It will remain closed for the first week, but if you are not pregnant, it will slowly start to open again as menstruation begins.
- *Pregnancy*: If you conceive in a given menstrual cycle, the texture of your cervix will become soft due to increased blood flow, but it will remain tightly closed. It also will move back up to the top of the vagina, rather than moving downward as it does during menstruation. If your period is late and your cervix is high, soft, and closed, it could be an indication that you are pregnant and you should take a test.

Luteinizing Hormone Test Strips

Most commonly used to aid conception efforts, you can also predict ovulation fairly accurately by using at-home test strips for luteinizing hormone. Recall from chapter 9 that luteinizing hormone surges mid-cycle, triggering the release of an egg from a ripened follicle. After luteinizing hormone has traveled through the bloodstream to communicate with the ovaries, our kidneys filter it out of our blood and excrete it in the urine, where it can be collected and measured. You can purchase urinary test strips for luteinizing hormone over the counter or online very inexpensively. Using them is just as simple: collect a morning sample of urine in a small cup, because urine will be most concentrated in the morning. Then, dip the test strip in your urine and wait a few minutes (usually five, or according to the test strip's instructions).

These test strips function pretty similarly to a pregnancy test, with a test line and a control line to make sure the test is valid. However, there's one key difference: LH strips will always have two lines because you always are making at least a small level of LH. So, on a non-ovulatory day, you'll see two lines on the test strip. The control line will be very dark, and the test line will be relatively pale in comparison. As LH surges before ovulation, however, the test line on the LH strip will become as dark as, or darker than, the control line. This is considered a "positive." If you take many tests over the course of the day when you have identified a positive, you may get many positive results. However, the most important test is the one in which you first see the positive, because it's this cue that lets you know your brain has already told your ovaries to pull the trigger on ovulation. Therefore, it's after the *first* positive result that you should start counting down to ovulation—about eight to thirty-six hours.[11]

If you've never used LH strips before, and if you aren't aware of when in your cycle you ovulate (because you aren't tracking BBT, cervical position, or other markers), I recommend practicing with the LH test strips by using one every time you urinate starting at the end of your period. If you have a regular cycle of normal length, you'll be using these strips for a little over a week before you see a positive test line. Once you get that positive result, ovulation will likely occur in a day or so. You should know that LH strips don't confirm ovulation, as it's merely measuring the pituitary signal—not providing real-time information about the activity of your ovaries. Every so often, the brain signals to the ovaries to release an egg but they don't. This would result in one of two things: an anovulatory cycle or a second LH surge, later in the month, which finally gets the job done. In the latter case, it's the second LH surge that matters. Situations such as these are relatively uncommon but are more likely to occur for you if you have PCOS or insulin resistance, as these conditions often result in resistance of the ovary to signaling from LH. This means that the brain sends the signal, but the ovaries don't respond very well.

WHICH METHOD IS BEST FOR YOU?

Tracking your cycle through BBT, RHR, cervical mucus, cervical position, and LH strips are all easy, inexpensive, and empowering methods for understanding what's happening in your body throughout the month. They help you know what's happening hormonally without the need for invasive testing like blood work or ultrasounds, and that information goes a long way in helping you lay a healthy foundation or identifying problems when they arise with your period health. However, there's no need to use

Table 7.1 Summary of Methods for Cycle Tracking

	BBT	RHR	CM	CP	LH
Overview	Take your temperature every morning with a BBT thermometer; record the data on graph paper or an app.	Record your resting heart rate upon waking, or allow a fitness watch to do it for you	Observe cervical mucus on your fingers or toilet paper after using the bathroom	Palpate your cervix daily throughout the month using one or two clean fingers	Urinate on LH test strips (available over the counter) several times daily for several days, around ovulation
Benefits	Extremely accurate, and predicts ovulation in regular cycles	The most passive method	Real-time information both for predicting and confirming ovulation	May predict ovulation	The most reliable and objective way to predict ovulation at home
Limitations	Cannot predict ovulation in irregular cycles, sensitive to factors in the environment, equipment is required	Does not confirm ovulation and cannot predict it accurately; equipment is required	Cannot confirm data specific to the day of ovulation; may be more easily influenced by other biological changes	Data is qualitative, and subject to user error; should not be used as a method of contraception	Cannot confirm ovulation has occurred; cannot be used as a contraceptive method
Best For	Women who want to track their cycles numerically with accuracy and precision, whether for family planning, to inform cycle syncing, or to evaluate their health	Women who want to know they are likely ovulating, but don't plan to use it to inform the timing of intercourse	Women who prefer not to purchase equipment, who are in tune with their bodies, or who are Catholic, as this family planning method is endorsed by the Catholic Church	Women who want real-time data about ovulation, impending menstruation or early pregnancy, for women who are very comfortable evaluating their bodies in this way	Timing intercourse when trying to conceive, but can also be used to predict when ovulation typically occurs in a given cycle

all of them all the time. So, which method is best for you? The answer to that question depends on your goals. Review table 7.1 to decide which method works best for you in the context of your own life.

Once you've chosen a method that appeals to you, get started! After you've gathered data for a few months, you'll be able to apply the information in a practical way to understand the length and timing of your follicular phase, ovulation, luteal phase, and menses, and know which phase of your cycle you are in on any day of the month. If you know where you are in your cycle, you'll also know what's going on in your body at a hormonal level—or not going on, if you experience abnormal symptoms. What's more, you will be able to customize your lifestyle habits even further to support hormonal balance specific to each phase of your cycle. We call this *cycle syncing* and the next chapter is all about what it is, how it can help your period, and how you can implement it in your own life.

8

HARNESS YOUR HORMONES

By now, we've covered more information about the hormones behind your menstrual cycle and how they work than most college anatomy and physiology courses. So, you're basically an expert in female reproductive health. Or rather, you're equipped with the tools and information you need to become an expert in *your own* reproductive health, because that's really the goal: understanding your body and how it works and knowing how to know if your hormones need help. So, now's the time to stop trying to ignore or cover up the coming and going of your period and instead start making your cycle work for you. Whether your periods are perfectly normal (à la chapter 5), or you have some serious concerns about your hormonal health, this chapter will outline practical steps that you can take to synchronize your life with your menstrual cycle for the sake of hormonal balance. I'm not talking about putting your life on hold when your period comes but rather using tangible strategies for self-awareness every day of the month. It's called the *cycle syncing* method and in addition to its ancient roots in Traditional Chinese Medicine (TCM), it has modern scientific support, and meaningful application for your own life, today.

In order to sync with your body, you need to know where you are in your cycle. That's where the previous chapter comes into play. Start tracking not only your periods but ovulation as well. Then, you'll know not just whether you're "on your period" or otherwise, but you'll also have awareness of when you're in each of the five phases of the menstrual cycle: menstrual, follicular, ovulatory, luteal, or premenstrual. Based on the anatomy and physiology we already covered, you know what's *supposed* to be happening in each of those phases and from the cycle tracking methods we just discussed, you'll know *if it actually is* happening for you. In this chapter, you'll learn how to make lifestyle changes to support the expected hormonal fluctuations that take place in each of those phases so that you can feel your best at all times of the month. In many cases, these foundational habits are enough to stabilize a wayward hormonal flow, fixing everything from cramps and spotting, fatigue and premenstrual mood changes, to bloating and cravings. Cycle syncing will also help you understand why you might feel super energized at certain times of the month, less interested in intimacy or social events at others, or perhaps even hungrier, sleepier, or more introverted. Aligning your life with your cycle will help you to embrace these fluctuations as fundamental experiences of being a woman rather than problems to be fixed. Then, you can focus your time and attention on the real problems, whether they relate to your period or otherwise.

Unfortunately, the conversations about periods in our culture don't pay homage to the true power that the menstrual cycle provides us as women. We often think of them as too messy, or too inconvenient. We discredit our experiences, saying we're "just being hormonal" and write off the significant health implications that come from living life out of attunement with our bodies and their needs. But the dynamic, three-dimensional hormonal experiences your body was designed with is your, and every woman's, right. Don't let anyone convince you that embracing your physiology, exactly the way it was made, isn't worth doing every single day of the month (even if it might seem challenging or inconvenient in someone else's eyes). At the end of the day, honoring your hormones is one of the very best things you can do for your health.

THE FIVE-PHASE CYCLE

The Western medical perspective only recognizes two distinct phases of the menstrual cycle with marked transitions at ovulation and onset of your period to divide the cycle into roughly four weeklong phases. We outlined these four "windows" in our discussion of physiology in chapter 4 but expanded on them when we introduced the perspective of Traditional Chinese Medicine and its accompanying theories of yin, yang, and the Five Elements. Reflecting the wood, fire, earth, metal, and water of the Five Elements theory, the yin follicular phase and yang luteal phase give way to five separate stages that closely mimic the four phases observed in Western medicine, except separating the ovulation time into its own distinct phase:

- *The menstrual phase* lasts the duration of menses and corresponds to the element of water
- *The follicular phase* corresponds to the period of time following menstruation but before ovulation. Although in Western medicine, the follicular phase technically encompasses menstruation, we differentiate the two for the sake of cycle syncing. This stage of the cycle—the part of the follicular phase that takes place after your period ends—corresponds to wood in TCM.
- *The ovulatory phase* includes the day before, the day of, and the day after ovulation, corresponding to fire in the Five Elements theory.
- *The luteal phase* follows ovulation. While the luteal phase technically encompasses the entire time period after ovulation and before menstruation begins, in the cycle-syncing method, we will use it to refer to the first half of your luteal phase, when progesterone levels are increasing. This corresponds to the TCM element of earth.
- *The premenstrual phase* is the second half of the luteal phase, when progesterone levels are decreasing and your period approaches. This phase corresponds to the metal element.

Based on a combination of TCM theory and the known influence of lifestyle habits over hormone levels as evidenced by modern scientific research, cycle-syncing strategies align your lifestyle habits with your hormones. By making TCM-informed adjustments to nutrition, exercise, stress-management strategies, and your social calendar according to the phase of your cycle that you're in at any given time, you can support the production and detoxification of the hormones designed to dominate during that phase. This honors what your body is already trying to do, takes the pressure off of you to perform at the same level, in the same way, every single day, and creates space for the very real influence of your hormonal fluctuations over not only your own well-being but also the way you work, relate to others, and more. Let's get started.

The Follicular Phase:

WOOD, SPRING, LIVER; YIN DOMINATES OVER YANG

- *Days*: Six through thirteen in a twenty-eight-day cycle, or if you chart your cycle, the day after your period ends until the day before ovulation usually occurs.

- *Hormonal review*: The follicular phase is all about getting ready for ovulation. At the start of this phase of your cycle, hormonal levels are at the minimum level they will reach throughout the whole cycle. Pituitary hormones follicle-stimulating hormone (FSH) and luteinizing hormone (LH) begin to rise in these days following your period, sharply spiking right before moving on to ovulation. Estrogen follows suit, transitioning from a very low level to a dramatic height as the follicular phase ends. Therefore, the goal of this phase is to support the production of estrogen, LH, and FSH, and minimize inflammation and stress which inhibit hypothalamic-pituitary-gonadal (HPG) axis signaling and estrogen production. It's also a good idea to focus your attention on your gut and microbiome, which are responsible for detoxifying old hormones so that they do not build up in your bloodstream and cause disruptions. If you are prone to irregular cycles, the follicular phase length sets the stage for the timing of events in the remainder of the cycle.
- *TCM review*: During the follicular phase, ovarian follicles ripen, the uterine lining begins to build, and your liver functions to shunt blood to the uterus and ovaries to support this. If this blood flow becomes stagnant, the TCM perspective suggests that symptoms such as pain, cramping, bloating, indigestion, breast tenderness, and headaches may appear. Imbalances in wood energy will also likely lead to irregular cycles, as the wood organ—liver—is responsible for regulating the menstrual cycle. Supporting the follicular phase from the TCM perspective therefore involves supporting blood flow and detoxification and avoiding factors that inhibit either the wood element or the rise of yin, both of which dominate during this phase.
- *Energy and sleep*: Estrogen is an extremely energizing hormone, as it upregulates thyroid and adrenal activity, which both play a role in metabolism.[1] During the follicular phase, estrogen most certainly is on the rise. Take advantage of this high-energy, high-metabolic phase by tackling your to-do list, especially long-awaited projects, or those that require more of a physical effort. It also is a great time to try new things, like a new exercise class or hobby that you've been interested in. You may find that you don't need as much sleep to feel rested and rejuvenated in the morning. However, because the wood element corresponds to the 11 p.m. to 3 a.m. period, you would be better off waking earlier rather than staying up especially late, as this is when your liver's detox efforts will be most active. Because of the increased motivation and resolve you see during this phase, it's also a

great time to kick bad habits that drain your energy, or work on letting go of vice, such as overuse of screens, coffee addiction, smoking, drinking, or mental rumination.
- *Emotional health*: This increased energy also translates to increased sociability. Even if you naturally tend to be more introverted, you will likely feel the greatest interpersonal draw during this time. Consider making an effort to schedule your social engagements and obligations during this phase of your cycle, as you will likely find them to be more energizing and engaging than at other times of the month. Note that because anger is tied to the wood element and liver function in TCM, you may be more prone to that emotion during this time, particularly if wood energy becomes stagnant or "stuck." When you are in social settings, take care to set boundaries so that you are less likely to be pushed toward irritability and anger when you encounter an offense. To support your emotional health during this time, set intentions, make plans, and take time to ensure that you are living life according to your goals. Use this peak in physical and emotional energy to refine your mental focus, creativity, and confidence.
- *Nutrition*: Because so many hormones rise up during this phase, and because activity and energy levels tend to run high, it's especially important to make sure you eat enough. This is not the time to cut calories or skip meals, as both of those create an additional stress response, suppressing LH, FSH, and healthy estrogen production. Supporting gut health with prebiotic fiber and fermented probiotics also helps the gastrointestinal system and microbiome with their detoxification efforts. You also should avoid alcohol or excessively greasy foods during this time, as these tax the liver and may impair its function from a TCM perspective. Because the follicular phase is a time of rising yin, emphasize foods like cooked vegetables, stews, and bone broths. For foods that support the wood element and liver, think "green" and "spring," especially fermented (sour) foods like kombucha, kimchi, sauerkraut, and small servings of salad greens with citrus-or vinegar-based dressings. You will also want to include larger servings of gently cooked greens and sprouts, like steamed broccoli with a squeeze of lemon, or a massaged kale salad served at room temperature. If you are prone to anemia and use iron supplements, replenishing your blood supply with iron-rich foods or a supplement may be important during this crucial time, following menstrual blood loss while the liver is especially active. (Note:

please do not take an iron supplement if you have not tested and identified an iron deficiency, as unnecessary supplementation can be dangerous.)

- *Exercise*: High energy equals a high need for healthy energy outlets, such as exercise! If you are thinking of starting a new workout routine, this is the week to do it. If you're already in a habit of moving regularly, you will benefit the most from higher-intensity workouts during this phase, such as running and other cardio or high-intensity interval training (HIIT) workouts, though you may find the resistance of weight training to be frustrating. If so, avoid that type of exercise during this time. You'll get a two-for-one deal with exercise and social activity if you work out with a friend, whether that be attending a group fitness class, pairing up as gym buddies, or just walking and talking together.
- *Sexuality*: If you are trying to conceive, this is the time to focus on intimacy with your partner. The week leading up to ovulation is when you are the most fertile, which will be confirmed by increased cervical fluid and a slow ramp up of your resting heart rate. You will likely also notice that your libido increases during this time due to the rise of estrogen, which makes sense biologically considering that this is the time that sex would most likely lead to procreation. If you aren't looking to expand your family, make sure you use some form of contraception during this week. But that doesn't mean your increased libido is all for naught! Yes, libido involves sexuality but also your drive, passion, interest, and excitement—all of which can also be channeled elsewhere in healthy ways. So, be sure to take advantage of your full feminine power during this phase of your cycle.
- *In summary*: Springtime brims with anticipation and potential—for fertility, for big goals and plans, for new growth, and abundant energy. Put the inertia to good use as the train picks up speed.

The Ovulatory Phase:

FIRE, SUMMER, HEART; YIN

- *Days*: Fourteen to sixteen in a twenty-eight-day cycle, or if you chart your cycle, the day before, day of, and day after ovulation; a positive LH strip and the appearance of egg white cervical mucus (EWCM) marks the start of this three-day phase.

- *Hormonal review:* During ovulation, the dominant ovarian follicle ruptures, releasing an egg that will travel to the fallopian tube where it either becomes fertilized or dissolves. Immediately prior to the start of the ovulatory phase, estrogen and then LH peaked to their highest levels. The subsequent days then involve the sharpest decline in both estrogen and LH, back to low baseline levels. Following the release of the egg, the remnants of the ovarian follicle convert into the corpus luteum, a gland that will soon begin releasing progesterone.
- *TCM review:* Just as in the Western perspective, ovulation marks an important time of transition in TCM. However, rather than referring to the transition from an estrogen-dominant phase to a progesterone-dominant one, TCM describes the movement from a predominantly yin phase into yang dominance. In TCM, the fire element and the associated season of summer transition to peak energy and movement. Plants and trees achieve their full, vibrant green, and the sun shines brilliantly between the branches. Hormones surrounding ovulation also maximize during this time, mirroring the fullness of the fire element. The fire organ is the heart, which functions to circulate blood throughout the body to ensure an adequate supply of nutrients to all of our cells. It also "houses the spirit." (Think of this like the relationship between heart, soul, and feelings in the Western paradigm.) The heart organ also connects directly to the uterus via a special meridian called the *Bao Mai*, which is how TCM explains the relationship between mental and emotional stress and the menstrual cycle, particularly through suppression of ovulation. Imbalances in the fire element typically manifest as mid-cycle anxiety, hot flashes and sweating, mental restlessness, palpitations, and insomnia. Supporting the fire element involves cultivating appropriate outlets for fire while at the same time taking care not to extinguish or suppress it too much.
- *Energy and sleep:* This is when energy reaches its absolute peak, given the height of estrogen at the start of the ovulatory phase. This will be the most extroverted few days of your cycle, and you may find you are most productive between 11 a.m. and 3 p.m.—the time frame that corresponds to the fire element. Expect to be most efficient and do your best work during this time. It will also benefit your sleep to spend time outdoors in the sun during this time of day, especially during the summer months.

- *Emotional health:* The emotions of the fire element are joy, along with the accompanying laughter and verbal energy. This is a great time to unwind with upbeat friends, engaging in playfulness and fun, or enjoying a comedic book, podcast, or TV show. You will likely appreciate the humor in things more easily, so it may be a good time to reflect on recent disappointments to transform your perspective into something more positive. Support your heart energy and fire by counting your blessings and expressing gratitude verbally to those you love. Because this is a verbal season, you might consider taking initiatives to lead and direct during this time, or by being the one to reach out to friends and family to plan a spontaneous get-together.
- *Nutrition:* Coming away from the height of estrogen, ovulation is a time to detox and cleanse. Cruciferous vegetables naturally contain chemicals like diindolylmethane (DIM) and indole-3-carbinol (I3C), which are powerful detoxing chemicals. Enjoy broccoli, cauliflower, brussels sprouts, and kale, blanched or lightly steamed so as to not extinguish fire or tax the small intestine through rawness. Lighter foods will also balance summer heat, and you will feel your best by choosing fish, seeds, quinoa, and other lighter carbohydrate foods like fruit.
- *Exercise:* To maximize the benefit of your full energy, consider resistance or weight training at this time. You'll make the most efficient progress and "gains" from heavy lifting around ovulation. You may find you have the best performance during workouts, thanks to the internally robust hormonal environment.
- *Sexuality:* With summer fire, think "burning passion." Ovulation epitomizes fertility, and your libido will likely mirror that. This phase exemplifies the peak of sexual energy, and is the time when fertilization occurs, given the opportunity.
- *In summary:* The energy of fire and summer represents fulfillment and achievement. The egg bursts forth from its follicle, passion peaks, joy bubbles over into laughter. Run, jump, and let your happiness be known.

The Luteal Phase:

EARTH, LATE SUMMER, SPLEEN; YANG BEGINS TO RISE

- *Days:* Seventeen through twenty-one in a twenty-eight-day cycle, or if you chart your cycle, the day after the temperature rise until the midway point between ovulation and your next period

- *Hormonal review*: After ovulation, the corpus luteum begins producing progesterone at increasing levels for about a week (in typical cycles). Estrogen also increases somewhat during this time, as the uterine lining matures in preparation for possible pregnancy. Rising progesterone signals through the hypothalamic-pituitary-adrenal-thyroid-gonadal (HPATG) axis to increase thyroid activity, rev your metabolism, and increase body temperature.
- *TCM review*: As yang energy rises, so do warmth and dryness. This mirrors Western physiology, as basal body temperature (BBT) rises during this period and cervical secretions dry up. Corresponding to the earth element, the spleen and its associated activities dominate during this phase. The spleen relates to the menstrual cycle by keeping blood flowing in its proper channels—not allowing bleeding to occur before its time. (This is akin to the balancing nature of progesterone in maturing the uterine lining and controlling its thickness.) Furthermore, another role of the spleen is to distribute nutrients from food to the other organs. Failure of the spleen to complete this task may result in a depleted or deficient uterine lining and subsequent fertility problems. Think of the earth element like creating a fertile, rich soil to sustain a potential pregnancy. The purpose of this phase of the cycle is all about nourishing new life. Supporting the earth element therefore involves quality nutrition, avoiding anything that depletes resources, and allowing energy to flow freely throughout the body.
- *Energy and sleep*: Energy levels after ovulation remain fairly steady for about a week. When estrogen and progesterone are in balance, the metabolism hums along at a steady pace, helping you feel up and able to meet the demands of life while still staying cool, calm, and collected. You may not be brimming over with extra energy, but you'll have enough to work well and rest well too.
- *Emotional health*: "Levelheaded" is the word for this phase of the menstrual cycle. Typically, the week after ovulation is associated with feeling calm and regulated, though the luteal phase overall tends to reflect more introverted and intuitive characteristics. You may find yourself equally inclined to spend time with others as you are to recharge by yourself, so prioritize a bit of both this week but in moderate doses.
- *Nutrition*: Because of the relationship between the spleen and stomach in TCM, rest is essential. Make the intention to keep mealtimes peaceful. Don't mix eating with work or responsibility. Put your

phone down and stay present with your meal. Eat slowly and thoroughly chew your food to support your digestion. Avoid any food or beverages that are particularly cold, as these deplete spleen energy and draw away late summer warmth. Yellow and sweetness belong to the earth element, so enjoy mineral-rich foods like roasted squash, carrots, sweet potato, and other root vegetables that have sweet flavors but also complex carbohydrates like fiber. Emphasize light proteins such as legumes and fish. Consider avoiding sour foods during this time, as they relate to the wood element, which limits earth.

- *Exercise*: The key with exercise during this phase is to keep it steady. Stay consistent with your favorite exercise routine and prioritize a predictable schedule, whether that be daily walks, alternating rest and active days at the gym, or something else. With the activity of the spleen and stomach reigning during this phase, the body is hard at work transforming food into qi and transporting it throughout the body. Regular exercise during this phase, whatever that may look like for you, will keep qi moving to nourish all systems of the body.
- *Sexuality*: Libido will likely diminish over the course of this week. Communicate with your partner about how you're feeling to maintain a sense of connectedness and consider intimacy in all of its many forms.
- *In summary*: Late summer is all about winding down and wrapping up the hustle and bustle of ovulation activity. Stay the course and enjoy the "afterglow" but don't put pressure on yourself to maintain the same level of performance as the previous week.

The Premenstrual Phase:

METAL, AUTUMN, LUNG; YANG DOMINATES OVER YIN

- *Days*: Twenty-two to twenty-eight in a twenty-eight-day cycle, or if you chart your cycle, the midway point of your luteal phase until your next period
- *Hormonal review*: Progesterone peaks halfway through the luteal phase and begins to drop as menstruation approaches. Estrogen also enters another decline, though this time less dramatic than what occurred prior to ovulation. If conception and implantation were to take place, it would be during this time. In the absence of pregnancy, the corpus luteum gland itself degrades during this phase and the blood vessels lining the uterus similarly break down. Body temperature and

metabolic activity remain elevated above follicular phase levels, but they enter a decline, which may cause noticeable changes in energy levels and mood.
- *TCM review*: Autumn is the time of harvest, organization, and storing up while metal represents structures and establishing systems. This element also corresponds to the immune system, elimination (detox), respiration, and distribution of bodily fluids. This includes menstrual blood and other bodily fluids involved with preparation for the cellular breakdown and shedding that will occur during menstruation. The body (and the mind) are "tidying up" loose ends from a TCM perspective during this phase, which creates a foundation for clearing away and detoxing old physiological material. Out of balance, the metal element and its associated premenstrual hormones may trigger grief, constipation, weakness, or intestinal inflammation, symptoms commonly labeled as PMS in the Western tradition.
- *Energy and sleep*: Energy begins to slow down leading up to your period, with a gradually increasing need for sleep and rest. Now is the time to start winding down your schedule—both socially and with work—not the time to take on new challenges or push yourself. Tie up loose ends in your home responsibilities and take some extra time to wind down in the evenings with dim lights, perhaps even candlelight.
- *Emotional health*: Everything winds down in this week of the cycle, including mood and social activity. Because the luteal phase is associated with turning inward, this may sometimes manifest as pensiveness or worry if taken to the extreme. Support healthy mental processing through journaling, or talking one-on-one with a trustworthy, close friend or partner. You may find yourself more drawn to deep, reflective conversations with a close friend rather than small talk or group gatherings. Consider a meditation practice or deepening your prayer life during this time. Take initiative to prevent feeling drained by paring down your social calendar and turning your home into a haven. This is also a good time to reflect on your work and personal life boundaries and make a plan to protect your emotional health.
- *Nutrition*: Foods to support the metal element include mineral-rich navy beans, almonds, and cooked sulfur-rich vegetables for detoxing hormones, such as radish, onion, and mustard greens as well as celery, cucumber, and broccoli. These pungent foods support yang as it declines during this phase, which is helpful for sustaining a

pregnancy-friendly environment. Consider avoiding bitter foods, as these relate to the fire element which limits metal.
- *Exercise*: The most important perspective during this week is to listen to your body. You may feel the need to reduce the intensity of workouts or cut them shorter, with activities like brisk walking, calisthenics, and yoga taking precedence over more intense varieties. Consider taking walks immediately following meals to support digestion and movement of qi.
- *Sexuality*: Many women notice a significant decline in libido during this week, which mirrors the decline in fertile days. Often the pelvic area will become slightly tender and swollen, so communicate with your partner about what is comfortable to you. If you notice a troubled mind, you can build a foundation for intimacy with your partner by sharing your emotions and feelings to draw you two closer together.
- *In summary*: The metal element relates to grief, letting go, and getting things in order. In autumn, we let go of things that no longer serve us and focus our energy on planning for the cold days ahead. Tie up loose ends, process what you need to and prepare yourself for a smooth transition to menstruation.

The Menstrual Phase:

WATER, WINTER, KIDNEYS; YANG

- *Days*: One to five in a twenty-eight-day cycle, or the number of days of your period
- *Hormonal review*: This is the best-known time of the cycle, in which the endometrial lining of the uterus sloughs off and washes away. Estrogen and progesterone both fall to their minimum during this time of the cycle, and a woman is at her least fertile. Technically menstruation kicks off the start of the next follicular phase, with early signaling from the brain stimulating the next round of follicles. Blood loss during this time depletes nutrients such as iron, B vitamins, and minerals.
- *TCM review*: The water element represents winter, a time for rest and reflection. Instead of energetic activity for the whole body, qi invigorates the uterus to release and start anew. The emphasis this week is on conservation and restoration with an inward focus. Overactivity or pushing yourself depletes water and creates imbalances

that manifests as chaotic social interactions, loss of confidence, and becoming withdrawn or detached. During the menstrual phase, the uterus clears away old tissue and prepares to start afresh. Both emotionally and physically, this time can be used to heal, renew, and prepare for a new cycle of activity in the coming spring. Yang dominates during this phase but slowly begins to decline as yin will soon take over. This initiation of the transition from yang to yin directs energy inward and downward toward the uterus where most of the activity occurs during the menstrual phase.

- *Energy and sleep*: Like winter hibernation, our bodies have a greater need for rest during the menstrual phase. You may find yourself needing a longer stretch of sleep than during other phases of the cycle, so honor that by winding down and getting into bed earlier. You may also find yourself feeling tired from the loss of blood and nutrients through menstruation, with less stamina and energy. Prioritize rest and restorative activities this week.
- *Emotional health*: The emotion associated with winter and water in TCM is fear, which can quickly become a source of chaos and depletion if this element is not supported. If you are prone to anxiety and stress, it is essential that you make provision for self-care and attunement with what your body tells you this week. Deep breathing exercises support the water element, so make a habit of practicing them regularly. Take time to honestly check in with yourself. Let go of what no longer serves you and focus your energy on what will sustain you long term.
- *Nutrition*: Hydration during the menstrual phase is key. Avoid alcohol and caffeine, as these are dehydrating, and be sure to include natural sources of salt and minerals to maintain blood volume and energy levels. Salty soups and stews are a great option for both fluids and nourishment. They are also easier to digest, which gives the body a bit of a break amid the activity taking place in the uterus and internal organs. Because of the iron lost through menstruation, include grass-fed red meat, eggs, and iron-rich plant foods like spinach, kale, bok choy, lentils, and beans. It's also a good idea to focus on anti-inflammatory foods such as those rich in omega-3 fatty acids (like fish, walnuts, and chia seeds) and to balance the coolness of winter with warm, slow-cooked meals. Consider limiting sweet foods, as they relate to the earth element, which limits water.
- *Exercise*: You should take a break during this phase, whatever that looks like for you. Compared to the rest of the month, exercise

during the menstrual phase should be the lightest that it ever is. Consider slow walks in nature, restorative yoga, and deep stretching.
- *Sexuality*: Libido reaches its minimum during this phase of the cycle.
- *In summary*: Winter is about minimization, letting go, and giving in to the flow. It's a time of conservation and rest, so honor that. Lean into the wisdom of a slowed down season before the time comes to open up to a new cycle of activity.

Cycle syncing looks different for each of us because our individual lives are so different. From the above information, pick and choose what works for you. If you hate green leafy vegetables like spinach and kale, that's not a problem! You don't have to eat them just because you're in your follicular phase. There are several other ways to support your body nutritionally during this time, as well as the balance of yin and yang, your liver, and the dynamic hormonal environment throughout the month. They are all listed here, however, to empower you in whichever modalities you choose to use. Additionally, it's important to know that cycle syncing doesn't solve all period problems. For many women, diagnosable conditions persist with fertility and menstrual health even after implementing a cycle-syncing plan. That's what the last section of this book is about: knowing all your options for treatment so that you can make the best, most informed decision for you in the context of your own life and values, once you've set a healthy foundation in place.

9

BIRTH CONTROL

Know Your Options

One of the overarching themes of this book is empowerment: making sure that you are the one in charge of making decisions about how to manage your health. In this chapter, we'll be discussing all the possible options for contraception, including the risks and benefits of each respective type. Think of this like an elevated version of what you did (or didn't) get in sexual education. In this chapter, the word "contraception" refers to methods for preventing pregnancy, but physicians often prescribe them for the purpose of medically managing menstruation. Please keep in mind that in most cases, the way you choose to manage your period problems is not a moral issue. You're not any better or worse for choosing to use a birth control pill to control heavy periods than you would be if you chose to use some of the more conservative lifestyle methods that we will discuss in the treatment section. The only problem would be if you didn't know other options existed. So, this chapter offers an overview of both hormonal and hormone-free methods of pregnancy prevention and notes about other ways that certain methods might be prescribed by physicians. Read them all and make the decision that best suits your life and values. As you do so, here are a few reminders:

- It's your body, and therefore your choice how you manage your health and fertility. This means it's not your doctor's, not the internet's, or anybody else's. Don't let someone coerce you into doing something you don't feel comfortable with.
- In hormonal contraceptives, there is only one type of estrogen used (ethinylestradiol), and there are very real health risks that come with it. The most serious of these risks include blood clot formation,

which can be fatal, as well as increased risk of endometrial and invasive breast cancer. Contraindications (meaning it should not be prescribed) for ethinylestradiol use include: estrogen receptor sensitive cancers; coronary artery disease; history of blood clots; migraine headaches; seizure disorders; history of dementia or neurocognitive disorders; high blood pressure; uterine leiomyomas; endometriosis; urinary incontinence; high cholesterol; gallbladder disease; liver disease; tobacco use; and pregnancy.[1]

- Ovulation is important for your health. It is the only way to produce progesterone, and you cannot get real progesterone from any form of hormonal contraceptive. (This is a common misconception, even in physician offices!) You do not need to alter your anatomy and physiology in order to plan your family or manage your menstrual health. You have many options!

CONTRACEPTIVE METHODS

Sterilization

Sterilization techniques are surgical procedures intended to render a couple infertile, or unable to reproduce. They can be performed on both men and women, though it's not necessary for both members of a couple to undergo a sterilization procedure in order to prevent pregnancy in the long term. The sterilization techniques discussed in this chapter include vasectomy and tubal ligation/removal.

VASECTOMY

Overview: Male procedure, prevents pregnancy for women in monogamous relationships

Details: A surgical procedure in which a small piece of tissue, called the vas deferens, is removed from a male's scrotum. This prevents sperm from traveling from his testes (where they are produced) into the semen during ejaculation. This is usually an outpatient procedure performed with local anesthetic (you don't need to be "put under") with a minimal incision and quick recovery.

Note: There is a waiting period of about six months following the procedure in which a barrier method should also be used, as residual sperm may make their way into semen and render a male still fertile during this time. Often, physicians performing the procedure offer follow-up semen testing to ensure that sterilization has been completed. In certain cases, a man may elect to have his vas deferens reconnected to restore fertility, though this is not always effective.

TUBAL LIGATION/REMOVAL

Overview: The fallopian tubes are surgically blocked to prevent an egg from entering and becoming fertilized

Details: Tubal ligation is a surgical procedure performed under anesthesia in which small incisions are made in a woman's abdomen, allowing the surgeon to cauterize, clip, cut, or remove a portion of the fallopian tubes on both sides. In some cases, the entire fallopian tube is removed. Because the fallopian tube is where fertilization occurs, if an egg cannot travel there then it cannot be fertilized.

Note: Many women elect to combine a tubal ligation or removal procedure with a planned C-section if they don't intend to birth additional children. In certain cases—depending on the type of surgical procedure performed—a tubal ligation can be reversed, though a return to fertility in this circumstance is not guaranteed.

Benefits:

- It is more than 99 percent effective.[2]
- It is completely hands-free.
- This procedure does not affect hormones.

Drawbacks:

- Tubal ligation/removal is surgical, so there's a risk of infection or complication (such as pain or scar tissue formation) though this risk is very low.
- It's not always covered by insurance, and because it's a surgery, the out-of-pocket cost can be prohibitive.
- It is intended to be permanent, which may be a problem if you ever change your mind.

146   Chapter 9

Most appropriate for:

- couples who are sure they do not want future pregnancies, or for whom additional pregnancies may be dangerous.

Intrauterine Device (IUD)

An intrauterine device (IUD) is a small, T-shaped device placed in the uterus as a form of contraception. This is accomplished by preventing ovulation, impairing sperm motility, making the uterine lining inhospitable to the implantation of a fertilized egg, or a combination of these. IUD placement is an in-office procedure, and it can be removed at any time. They are the longest-lasting reversible form of contraception.

HORMONAL

Types: Skyla, Kyleena, Mirena, LILETTA

Overview: Hormonal IUDs release a synthetic form of progesterone—called levonorgestrel (LNG)—into the uterus that acts locally to thin the uterine lining, making it less likely that a fertilized egg would implant. The synthetic progesterone also thickens cervical fluid, slowing down sperm motility and making it more difficult for them to reach the egg. Depending on the type of IUD used and the dosage of LNG contained in the IUD, a woman using an IUD may or may not continue to ovulate with the device in place. Because these IUDs thin the uterine lining, many women notice lighter periods or sometimes do not have periods at all.

Details:

- The Skyla IUD lasts for up to three years and releases 14 micrograms (mcg) per day of LNG when inserted. This is the lowest dosage available of the hormonal IUDs on the market so there's the greatest likelihood of a woman continuing to ovulate. About 6 percent of women using the Skyla IUD stop having periods while this IUD is in place.[3]
- The Kyleena IUD lasts for up to five years and releases 17.5 milligrams (mg) of LNG when inserted. About 12 percent of women stop having periods while this IUD is in place.[4]

- The Mirena IUD lasts for up to eight years and releases 20 mcg per day of LNG when inserted. About 20 percent of users stop having periods while this IUD is in place.[5]
- Because of the high dose of LNG, women are less likely to ovulate when using the IUD. Within the first year, only 45 percent of women have ovulatory cycles, though this increases to 75 percent by year four.[6]
- The Liletta IUD lasts for up to eight years and releases 20 mcg per day of LNG when inserted.[7] By the sixth year of use, 78.5 percent of users have ovulatory cycles.[8]

Note: In rare cases the body may expel the IUD on its own. If this occurs, future IUDs would not be considered a reliable method of contraception.

Benefits:

- Many women still ovulate while using hormonal IUDs, which allows the body to produce its own hormones.
- This form of contraception lasts for several years and is hands-off, so it doesn't require active use to be effective.
- All IUDs are estrogen free, so they do not present the risks associated with estrogen-containing contraceptives.
- Compared to other hormonal contraceptives, the exposure to LNG with IUDs is much lower.

Drawbacks:

- Irregular bleeding or spotting is very common with hormonal IUDs.
- Amenorrhea (absent periods) is also a possibility, which eliminates your ability to use your period as a means for tracking your overall health.
- In rare cases, IUDs may cause pelvic inflammatory disease or ovarian cysts, which may be painful, cause scarring, and affect eventual return to fertility.
- Because many users ovulate while using an IUD, fertilization is possible. Because one of the effects of LNG in IUDs is thinning the uterine lining to prevent implantation of an otherwise fertilized egg, some women may have reservations about using this form of contraception for moral reasons.

- If pregnancy occurs while an IUD is in place, it causes serious risks to the safety and development of the baby.
- Because the IUD is a physical object within the uterus, some women experienced worsened menstrual cramping because of it.

Most appropriate for:

- couples who would like to prevent pregnancy for several years at a time and are not at risk of sexually transmitted infection;
- women with heavy periods who would like to use a hands-free pharmacological option for reducing menstrual flow; and
- women with endometriosis because the progestin may help with symptoms like pain, and they reduce bleeding that may be severe with endometriosis.

NONHORMONAL

Types: Paragard

Overview: The nonhormonal IUD option is the copper IUD.

Details: Instead of releasing hormones into the uterus, the copper IUD slowly leaches copper metal into the uterus, which is toxic to both sperm and fertilized eggs. It also changes the cellular structure of the uterine lining, preventing implantation of a fertilized egg. The copper IUD can last for up to ten years.

Note: In rare cases the body may expel the IUD on its own. If this occurs, future IUDs would not be considered a reliable method of contraception. Because of the risk of copper toxicity from using Paragard, users should ask their health care provider to test their copper levels regularly. Sometimes Paragard is prescribed as a form of "emergency contraception," and can prevent implantation of a fertilized egg that would otherwise progress to pregnancy when inserted within five days of unprotected sex.

Benefits:

- Copper IUDs are hormone-free, so users still ovulate normally and do not face the health risks associated with hormonal contraceptives.

- It can be used while breastfeeding.
- It does not interact with other medications.
- You still ovulate while using copper IUDs, which allows your body to continue producing its own hormones.
- This form of contraception lasts for several years and is hands-off, so it doesn't require active use to be effective.

Drawbacks:

- Copper IUDs bring a meaningful risk of copper toxicity that leads to neurological problems, kidney and liver failure, gastrointestinal symptoms, and anemia.
- Because the IUD is a physical object within the uterus, it may cause painful menstrual cramps for some women.
- Mid-cycle spotting is very common with the copper IUD and causes periods to become about 50 percent heavier for most users.[9]
- Copper IUD insertion can cause a hole to form in the uterus, called uterine perforation. This occurs in about one out of every five hundred users.[10]
- Because the copper IUD prevents implantation of a fertilized egg, this may be a moral concern for some women.

Most appropriate for:

- women who do not plan to become pregnant for several years, who do not already have a problem with heavy menstrual bleeding or cramping and are not at risk of sexually transmitted infection.

Implant

The implant is a form of contraception inserted into the body that renders a woman temporarily infertile due to the drugs it releases.

Types: Nexplanon

Overview: A small rod inserted under the skin that slowly releases a form of synthetic progesterone called etonogestrel to prevent ovulation. The release rate ranges between 35 and 70 mcg/day, which is higher than any of the IUDs available.[11]

Details: The implant is very small, so after it's inserted as an in-office procedure, you won't see or feel it. The high dose of progestin tricks your brain into thinking you've already ovulated, so it won't send signals to ripen and release another egg. It also thickens cervical mucus, making it more difficult for sperm to travel. The implant lasts for up to five years and is considered about 99.9 percent effective.[12]

Note: The way the implant works is by preventing ovulation.

Benefits:

- hands-free contraception.

Drawbacks:

- Irregular bleeding and spotting are very common for the first year, though it may continue for as long as the implant is in place. This can be stressful and negatively impact quality of life.
- The implant prevents ovulation, which means you cannot produce your own hormones.
- Removing the implant involves a minor surgical procedure, cutting the skin to then take it out.
- Other common side effects include mood swings, weight gain, headaches, acne, and depression. Frequently, these effects are significant enough to prompt women to have the implant removed.[13]

Most appropriate for:

- women looking for hands-free contraception who are unable to tolerate or are not interested in using an IUD.

Injection (The Shot)

The birth control shot involves injection of medication to suppress ovulation.

Types: Depo-Provera

Overview: Injection of a synthetic progestogen called medroxyprogesterone that suppresses ovulation for about three months. It's considered about 96 percent effective with typical use.[14]

Details: The shot involves a 150 mg dose of artificial progesterone injected into a muscle. This is more than ten times the dose used in the lowest-hormone IUDs, so the effect of a single injection lasts for a long time.

Note: The way the shot works is by preventing ovulation. It is not recommended to be used for longer than two years.[15] The Depo-Provera shot was banned for use in the United States between 1978 and 1992 due to concerns about cancer risks.[16]

Benefits:

- hands-free contraception

Drawbacks:

- The shot can't be undone once you receive the injection. So, if you have uncomfortable side effects, you're stuck with them until they wear off.
- Irregular bleeding is a common side effect, along with increased appetite.
- Return to fertility after using the shot is delayed, with a median time frame of ten months but up to thirty-one months.[17]
- The Depo-Provera shot causes loss of bone mineral density and increases risk for osteoporotic fracture later in life. This is a black box warning on the drug insert.[18]

Most appropriate for:

- I do not recommend the injection; there are safer contraceptive options available.
- Sometimes the injection is recommended as a management technique for painful period cramps, however other hormonal and non-hormonal strategies also offer this benefit.

The Birth Control Pill (Oral Contraceptives)

Oral contraceptives are prescription pills containing artificial hormones, taken daily to prevent ovulation. Following each pack of hormone pills, users then take placebo pills for a few days, which allows for uterine bleeding to occur, simulating a period. There are two main categories of pill: combined pills containing synthetic forms of both estrogen and progesterone, and progestin-only pills. Of the combined pills, the majority are monophasic, which means they contain the same amount of hormone every day of the cycle. Others, called multiphasic pills, vary the amount of hormone throughout the cycle to more closely mimic a natural cycle with the goal of reducing side effects. Additionally, some types of pills reduce the frequency of bleeding to once every three months, but most produce bleeding at twenty-eight-day intervals. This is the most common type of prescription contraceptive used in the United States.[19] In general, birth control pills are understood to be about 91 percent effective with typical use.[20] The pill must be taken daily at the same time to be effective.

There are more than one hundred different types of birth control pills, which differ from each other in terms of the amount of hormone as well as the type of artificial progesterone that they contain. As noted above, ethinylestradiol is associated with risks, including increased chances of developing breast cancer, blood clots, cardiovascular disease, and many of the other health conditions described in earlier chapters of this book. Estrogen-containing pills are classified according to dosage. In today's market, these include high-dose pills that contain 50 mcg or more of ethinylestradiol, moderate-dose pills in the range of 30 to 35 mcg, and low-dose pills between 15 and 20 mcg. A relatively newer pill sold under the brand name Lo Loestrin Fe is considered a "very low dose" or "ultra-low dose" pill, containing only 10 mcg of estrogen. In general, the higher the dose of estrogen, the higher the risks to your health. While the progesterone analogue in birth control pills (and other hormonal contraceptives) is the component primarily responsible for preventing ovulation, it's also what's responsible for quality-of-life side effects like weight gain, mood changes, acne, and irregular bleeding. To combat this, pill manufacturers include an estrogen analogue (i.e., ethinylestradiol) to make the product more tolerable.[21] Choosing a pill with a lower level of estrogen makes it safer, but it has a greater likelihood of uncomfortable side effects.

The different types of progestins in birth control pills are classified according to generation, which refers to the timing of when the chemicals were developed and released into the market. All progestogens bind to progesterone receptors, which is how they bring about their progesterone-related effects, but they also interact with other hormone receptors, like androgens and stress hormone receptors, because they are not actually the same as the real progesterone your body makes.[22] Binding to progesterone receptors in the body is how they prevent ovulation and act as contraceptives, but binding to other receptors is how they produce side effects. Here is an overview of each type of progestin and some key areas of interest:[23]

- First-generation progestins fall into two categories. The first category (called estranes) includes norethindrone, norethindrone acetate, ethynodiol diacetate, and norethynodrel. They are derived from testosterone and have a tendency to interact with testosterone receptors in the body. Because of this, they bring about the effects that testosterone would, such as acne, weight gain, and facial hair growth. For this reason, pills containing these progestins are not a good choice for women who already deal with androgenic symptoms related to high testosterone, such as in the case of polycystic ovarian syndrome (PCOS). The estranes also have the benefit of reducing some of the clotting risks associated with the estrogen component of combined pills, but they convert into estrogen-like compounds as they are metabolized, so this increases some of the other estrogenic risks, like breast cancer.[24] The second derivation (called pregnanes) come from a hormone called 17-OH progesterone and include medroxyprogesterone acetate, which is used primarily in the Depo-Provera shot. It is not typically used in oral contraceptives but may be found in oral tablets prescribed for other reasons. Overall, first-generation progestins are the least potent, so they are most likely to cause irregular bleeding and spotting.
- Second-generation progestins (gonanes) are also derived from testosterone but hit the market at a later time. These progestins include levonorgestrel and norgestrel. These are slightly more potent than the first generation, so they actually have a higher degree of androgenicity than the first generation estranes. However, they offer a lower risk of breakthrough bleeding.[25] Therefore, pills containing these progestins are not a good choice for women who already deal with androgenic symptoms, such as in the case of PCOS. However, they also have the most protective effect against estrogen-related clotting risks when used in combined pills. So, compared to the first generation, they're more likely to cause quality-of-life side effects but less likely to cause life-threatening ones.[26]
- Third-generation progestins (also called gonanes) are similar to the second-generation gonanes in that they are also derived from testosterone, but they have been chemically modified to have fewer testosterone-like effects. They're also more potent than the first generation so the spotting risk is lower. While this makes them more tolerable, they do increase the risk of forming blood clots compared to older generations.[27] These are the opposite of the second generation: though still derived from testosterone, they are less likely to cause quality-of-life side effects, but more likely to be associated

with life-threatening ones. Third-generation progestins include desogestrel, etonogestrel, norgestimate, and gestodene.
- The fourth-generation progestin on the market is drospirenone, which is anti-androgenic. It is very chemically similar to the drug spironolactone, which is a diuretic also commonly prescribed in the treatment of acne. This makes it a great option for women with androgenic acne, or other androgen-related symptoms such as those seen in PCOS. The downside is that, like third-generation progestins, drospirenone fails to counteract the clotting risks from estrogen in combined pills. However, it also increases blood clotting risks on its own, so it has the greatest risk of blood clots of all four generations.[28]

MONOPHASIC COMBINED PILLS

Overview: These pills contain both artificial estrogen and artificial progesterone, with the same dose daily for about three weeks, followed by several days of placebo pills in which bleeding occurs.

Details: Monophasic combined pills include ethinylestradiol (estrogen) in combination with a progestin from any of the four generations. Depending on the pill, levels of the synthetic estrogen and progesterone vary, and the number of days of placebo pills may also vary. In any given pill, however, the level of hormone is the same each day (barring placebo days, of course). There are also some extended cycle options, which prevent bleeding for three months at a time.

Note: Monophasic pills have been around the longest, so we know more about their relative risks. For this reason, they're most commonly recommended by health care providers.[29]

Benefits:

- They may help improve symptoms in women who have premenstrual mood disorders, particularly those characterized by anxiety.[30]
- They are less likely to cause breakthrough bleeding to develop over time.[31]

Drawbacks:

- Because the hormones are the same each day, users may experience muted emotions or depressive symptoms.

Most appropriate for:

- new users of the pill, because their symptoms will likely be the same each day of the month, making it easier to track side effects and how the pill makes them feel; and
- monophasic combined pills are the most commonly prescribed form of pill and are often prescribed by physicians to manage irregular, painful, and heavy cycles, as well as those associated with premenstrual mood changes.

Multiphasic Combined Pills

Overview: Hormone levels in the pills vary throughout the month to more closely mimic a natural cycle.

Details: Multiphasic pills can exist as biphasic or triphasic. Biphasic pills involve two phases with increasing doses of estrogen and progestin. Triphasic pills maintain the same level of estrogen each day with increasing levels of progestin throughout the month. Both types are followed by a placebo pack when bleeding occurs.[32]

Note: Quadriphasic pills exist but they are not commonly prescribed.

Benefits:

- They may be more likely than monophasic pills to reduce premenstrual symptoms of breast pain and swelling.[33]
- They have a lower overall monthly dose of hormone, so they theoretically have fewer health risks.[34]

Drawbacks:

- Multiphasic pills are alleged to be associated with higher accidental pregnancy rates with multiphasic pills compared to monophasic.[35]

Most appropriate for:

- women who want to limit their exposure to artificial estrogen but are not motivated to avoid it completely.

Progestin-Only Pills

Overview: Also known as "the mini pill," these contraceptives contain only progestin, no estrogen. The majority of them do not have a placebo week, but most users still have monthly bleeding.

Details: These pills primarily function as contraceptives by thickening cervical mucus to prevent sperm motility. About 40 percent of users still ovulate when using this type of pill, so they theoretically come with a higher chance of pregnancy.[36] However, with typical use they are shown to have about the same effectiveness as combined pills. Because it does not contain estrogen, the mini pill comes with a greater risk of side effects like weight gain, acne, and mood changes. Irregular and breakthrough bleeding are very common with these contraceptives, though some women do not experience any bleeding at all, including the monthly bleeds typically seen with combined pills.

Note: Users are more likely to experience contraceptive failure from not taking the pill at the same time when using the mini pill compared to combined pills.[37]

Benefits:

- Women who cannot use estrogen-containing contraceptives (such as smokers or women over thirty-five) are eligible to use the mini pill.
- The potential to still ovulate allows you to make your own hormones, which is a good thing.
- In 2023, the Food and Drug Administration (FDA) approved a second-generation progestin-only pill containing norgestrel for over-the-counter use. Opill is therefore available without a prescription.

Drawbacks:

- Side effects are common and severe, which often prompts users to stop using them.

Most appropriate for:

- women who want to use a birth control pill but don't want to or cannot use pills containing estrogen, or who are unable to get a prescription from a physician.

The Patch

Overview: The patch is a topical form of contraceptive in which hormones absorb through the skin to prevent ovulation. The patch functions similarly to oral contraceptive pills, except instead of taking them orally, they are applied to the skin through a piece of sticky material, like a Band-Aid. You apply a new patch each week and on the fourth week, you don't use one, which is when bleeding occurs.

Details: There are three patches available: Xulane, Zafemy, and Twirla, which has a slightly lower dose of estrogen than the other two. All of them contain the third-generation progestogen—norelgestromin—in combination with ethinyl estradiol (35 mcg for Xulane and Zafemy, 30 mcg for Twirla). Because the absorption of these hormones through the skin can be affected by body fat levels, the patch is only recommended for women who are younger than thirty-five years old, who do not use cigarettes or tobacco products, and who have a body mass index (BMI) less than 30 kilograms per meters squared (kg/m^2) and who weigh less than 198 pounds.[38] Women who use the patch and fall outside of these parameters have a higher risk of unintended pregnancy and a significantly elevated risk of developing a blood clot.

Note: Although you can apply the patch in many potential locations on your body, it is very important not to apply it to breast tissue.

Benefits:

- The patch has less user error than the pill, because you apply a new one weekly rather than daily.
- You can stop using the patch at any time.

Drawbacks:

- The patch increases risks of developing metabolic syndrome, including blood sugar control problems and elevated blood lipids.[39]
- The patch is more likely to cause symptoms like painful periods and breast pain compared to combined oral contraceptives.[40]
- Unlike the pill, there is a potential risk of a local skin reaction.

Most appropriate for:

- women who prefer to use hormonal contraception that is less hands-on than birth control pills but more easily removed than an IUD.

The Ring

Overview: The ring is a hormonal form of contraception, inserted vaginally.

Details: There are two types of ring contraceptives. They both consist of a thin plastic ring that is inserted into the vagina. It sits near the cervix and slowly releases hormone into the local tissues as well as into the bloodstream to prevent ovulation and thicken cervical mucus. Users insert a new ring at the start of each month and remove it after three weeks to allow bleeding to occur. The hormones released by the NuvaRing include 15 mcg per day of ethinylestradiol in combination with a third-generation progestin, etonogestrel. Annovera releases 13 mcg per day of ethinyl estradiol in combination with a fourth-generation progestin, segesterone acetate.

Note: In some cases, health care providers recommend replacing the ring every three weeks instead of allowing for a withdrawal bleed in order to altogether prevent bleeding in women who have very uncomfortable menstrual symptoms.

Benefits:

- The ring has less potential for user error than the pill.
- It has a lower dose of hormone than the patch and unlike the patch, cannot be seen outside the body.
- You can remove the ring yourself, at any time.

Drawbacks:

- Irregular bleeding and spotting are common side effects that are sometimes uncomfortable enough to cause women to stop using the ring.

Most appropriate for:

- women interested in lower-dose, hands-free contraception.

Condoms

Condoms are a barrier method of contraception which physically prevent sperm from entering the vagina during sex. They are nonhormonal and do not affect the fertility of either men or women using them. There are two categories of condoms, called "female" and "male" condoms. In addition to preventing pregnancy, condoms are one of the only forms of contraception that prevent sexually transmitted infections (STIs).

MALE OR "EXTERNAL" CONDOMS

Overview: Male condoms are thin pouches applied externally to the penis to prevent skin and sperm from contacting vaginal tissue.

Details: Male condoms—also simply known as "condoms"—are classically made out of latex, but they also can be made from lambskin, polyurethane, or polyisoprene, which are all good options for people who have latex allergies or who don't prefer the texture of latex. When used correctly, meaning that they are applied prior to sexual intercourse, every time, they are about 98 percent effective. Condom failure results from breaking, which can happen if the condom is stored incorrectly, combined with an incompatible lubricant, expired, or does not properly fit the user. Condoms can be easily combined with other forms of contraception, such as a fertility awareness method, to offer additional protection against pregnancy.

Note: Condoms should generally only be used with water-based lubricants, as oil-based lubricants can cause the condom material to weaken, increasing risk of breakage. The one exception is lambskin condoms, which can safely be used with oil-based lubricants.

Benefits:

- Condoms are effective, nonhormonal, prevent STIs, and have no side effects apart from the possibility of local skin irritation in individuals with latex allergy.
- They are inexpensive and don't require a prescription from a physician.

Drawbacks:

- Both partners need to be in agreement about condoms and how and when they are used.
- Some couples don't prefer the texture of condoms, but there are many material options to choose from. If you don't like one, try another!

Most appropriate for:

- women who would like to use a nonhormonal form of contraception at any time in the month.

FEMALE OR "INTERNAL" CONDOMS

Overview: Female condoms are applied internally to a female rather than externally to a male.

Details: Much less common than male condoms, female condoms are thin polyurethane bags that are inserted into the vagina to prevent skin and sperm from coming into contact with the vaginal tissue during intercourse. They are less effective than male condoms, preventing pregnancy about 95 percent of the time.[41]

Note: Female condoms should not be used at the same time as male condoms. Only one is needed! Female condoms are also commonly used with spermicide, but spermicide significantly increases the risk of contracting a urinary tract infection following sexual intercourse.[42]

Benefits:

- Some people prefer the sensation of female condoms over male condoms.

Drawbacks:

- They are more likely than male condoms to cause some irritation to either partner's genitalia because they are not tight-fitting.

- They are more expensive than male condoms when purchased over the counter.

Most appropriate for:

- women who would like to use a nonhormonal form of contraception at any time in the month, who would like to be the one "in charge" of condom usage.

Diaphragm and Cervical Cap

Overview: The diaphragm and cervical cap are small silicone cups inserted into the vagina to cover the cervix during intercourse and prevent sperm from entering.

Details: The diaphragm and cap create a seal around the cervix and act as a barrier for the entry of sperm. However, sperm may "leak" past this barrier, or survive in and around the reproductive tract, so they're not as effective as other barrier methods of contraception like condoms. The diaphragm is estimated to be around 83 to 84 percent effective when used in combination with spermicide (a cream added inside the cup to kill sperm) and the cervical cap is estimated to be between 71 to 86 percent effective and also needs to be used with spermicide to be effective.[43] A standard-size diaphragm is available over the counter (Caya), but health care providers can prescribe "fitted" diaphragms (Milex). Cervical caps (under the brand name FemCap) are custom fitted by health care providers and available with a prescription.

Note: Spermicide significantly increases the risk of contracting a urinary tract infection.

Benefits:

- The diaphragm and cervical cap do not affect hormones.
- The female partner is in control of insertion and application, and they do not change sensations during sexual intercourse.

Drawbacks:

- Some women may find them uncomfortable.

- They are less effective than other forms of contraception, and without spermicide are even more so.

Most appropriate for:

- women interested in a barrier method of contraception who are not interested in using condoms, though they're not the best option in terms of contraceptive effectiveness.

Sponge

Overview: The sponge consists of a piece of plastic foam inserted into the vagina to block entry of sperm and release spermicide.

Details: Women using the sponge insert it up to twenty-four hours before sexual intercourse. The foam sponge physically blocks sperm from entering the cervix, similar to the diaphragm, but also slowly releases spermicide into the vagina. The sponge is estimated to be between 73 percent and 91 percent effective, though that decreases for women who have previously delivered babies vaginally.[44] The chemical found in the sponge is called nonoxynol-9, which also increases the risk of STIs.[45]

Note: Spermicide significantly increases the risk of contracting a urinary tract infection.

Benefits:

- The sponge is a nonhormonal form of contraception.
- It does not require a prescription.
- The sponge can remain effective while in place for up to twenty-four hours.

Drawbacks:

- It has a high risk for contraceptive failure. If you are serious about preventing pregnancy, this would not be a good option.
- Because it contains nonoxynol-9, the sponge increases risk of urinary tract and sexually transmitted infections. Many women also experience vaginal irritation from this chemical.

Most appropriate for:

- There are other, more effective, less expensive, and safer forms of contraception available.

Emergency Contraception

Overview: Emergency contraception is used after unprotected sex to prevent pregnancy.

Details: Emergency contraception is a method of contraception available to prevent pregnancy if unprotected sexual intercourse has already occurred. The copper IUD can sometimes be prescribed as emergency contraception because it prevents implantation of a fertilized egg that may otherwise progress to pregnancy. (This may be a moral concern for some women.) There are also two pill forms of emergency contraception. The first type contains a high dose of levonorgestrel (and some brands also contain estrogen) intended to prevent release of an egg. These are the same chemicals available in other forms of hormonal contraceptives. (Brand names include Plan B, Take Action, My Way, Preventeza, After Pill, EContra, and more.) Because sperm can survive up to five days in the female reproductive tract, preventing ovulation for a period of time may prevent pregnancy if the egg has not yet been released. This form of emergency contraceptive pill does not work if a woman has already ovulated. The other form of emergency contraceptive pill available is a chemical called ulipristal (brand name: Ella) which blocks progesterone receptors, preventing ovulation and thinning the endometrial lining to prevent implantation. This form of emergency contraception does not work if the egg has already been released but because it thins the endometrial lining, it could complicate a pregnancy if it were to occur.

Note: Emergency contraceptives are not intended to be used as a regular form of contraception. Sometimes ulipristal is prescribed as a treatment for uterine fibroids because of its effects on the endometrium.

Benefits:

- Plan B One Step is available without a prescription.
- This form of contraception can be used if the sexual encounter was not anticipated.

Drawbacks:

- The emergency contraceptive pills do not work if ovulation has already occurred.

Most appropriate for:

- a last-minute attempt to prevent ovulation and subsequent pregnancy.

Withdrawal

Overview: The withdrawal method involves sexual intercourse without male ejaculation during penetration.

Details: Pregnancy is not typically possible without penetration and ejaculation occurring at the same time. The withdrawal method involves a male withdrawing prior to ejaculation so that sperm is not released inside the vaginal canal. This method can refer to otherwise unprotected intercourse until just before ejaculation, or to unprotected penetration that is followed up with a barrier method (such as condoms) prior to ejaculation occurring. The withdrawal method is understood to be about 78 percent effective,[46] but these statistics are difficult to interpret because the chances of pregnancy are not the same for every female on every day of the month. The effectiveness of the withdrawal method depends entirely on the male partner's ability to interpret and control his body during intercourse. While many men are able to discern the timing to prevent ejaculation during penetration, accidents happen. Additionally, some fluid may be released prior to ejaculation without a man's knowledge. If sperm is contained in this fluid, there is a chance of pregnancy.

Note: Communication is essential if this method is to be used as a form of contraception.

Benefits:

- This method does not change the sensations of intercourse, and no equipment is required.

Drawbacks:

- The female partner has no control over the employment of this method. Executing the withdrawal method depends entirely on the male.
- The effectiveness of this method depends on the individuals in the couple.

Most appropriate for:

- couples who don't mind interrupting the moment of intimacy, and who don't mind getting pregnant if it were to occur; and
- women who are okay with not being the ones in control of the contraceptive method.

Lactational Amenorrhea

Overview: Lactational amenorrhea as a method of contraception involves forgoing other forms of protection against pregnancy while a woman is breastfeeding.

Details: Following childbirth, a hormone called prolactin surges, which both stimulates the breasts to produce milk and inhibits the HPATG axis, preventing ovulation. When women breastfeed exclusively, meaning they do not supplement feeds with other forms of nutrition such as infant formula, prolactin secretion effectively inhibits ovulation, thereby rendering a woman infertile. The research shows that prolactin release from exclusive breastfeeding inhibits ovulation and prevents pregnancy about 98 percent of the time.[47] While many women do not have periods at all for the entire time they are breastfeeding, return of menstruation may occur within that first six months postpartum. If it does, however, they are overwhelmingly anovulatory cycles, so pregnancy would not be possible anyway. There is not currently good data about the effectiveness of the lactational amenorrhea method of contraception beyond six months postpartum. Some women experience the return of fertile periods and even become pregnant while they are still breastfeeding whereas others may not resume menstruating for several months after weaning.

Note: Because breastfeeding inhibits ovulation, it also leads to lower estrogen levels. Many women experience vaginal dryness when breastfeeding, which may require additional lubrication to make sex comfortable.

Benefits:

- This is completely hands-free contraception without any required equipment.

Drawbacks:

- It is only reliable for about six months
- Exclusive breastfeeding is required; it is not effective if the baby's nutrition is supplemented with formula or solids.

Most appropriate for:

- postpartum women (less than six months) who are exclusively breastfeeding.

Fertility Awareness Methods (FAM)

Overview: Selective abstinence from unprotected intercourse at fertile times of a woman's cycle as determined by tracking basal body temperature and/or changes in cervical fluid.

Details: Fertility awareness methods involve tracking your cycle to identify when you are fertile and abstaining from unprotected sex during those times. As a review from our discussion in chapter 7, sperm can survive in the female reproductive tract for up to five days following intercourse, so pregnancy is possible if ovulation occurs within that time frame. The egg itself survives for up to two days, so this creates a seven-day window in which pregnancy from unprotected sex could occur in any given cycle. As a method of contraception, couples would either agree to abstain from intercourse during this weeklong window or use an additional method such as condoms to prevent pregnancy. This method is estimated to be more than 99 percent effective at preventing pregnancy.[48] See chapter 7 to review how to track basal body temperature and cervical fluid changes to identify the timing of ovulation in any given cycle.

Note: This method can also be used in the opposite way: to time intercourse to favor pregnancy. Instead of abstaining during the seven-day window, have sex about every other day during that time to maximize chances of conception.

Benefits:

- Highly effective, hormone-free contraception that is inexpensive and doesn't interrupt the heat of the moment.
- Empowers the female partner.
- Can easily be combined with a barrier method to be available at all times of the month.

Drawbacks:

- Requires diligent cycle tracking.
- Requires communication and commitment from both partners.
- Women who have irregular cycles and/or inconsistent ovulation such as in PCOS, while breastfeeding (after six months) or in perimenopause would not be able to reliably use this method for contraception.

Most appropriate for:

- women who have regular cycles and good communication with their partners.

10

FERTILITY AND FAMILY PLANNING

In the previous chapter, we reviewed all the contraceptive methods in detail. Numerous great options exist depending on your goals and values, but none of them is appropriate if you actually want to conceive! In addition to failing to address contraceptive methods comprehensively, sexual education in adolescence and early adulthood often does not adequately prepare couples for success when they move from trying to inhibit pregnancy to trying to promote it. That's what this chapter is designed to fix. In it, we will outline the current statistics on fertility—what they mean for your chances of becoming pregnant as well as what they *don't*—and dive into the details of how you can set yourself up for success in family planning: getting pregnant quickly and staying pregnant, hopefully without the need for additional medical intervention. We will also cover topics like transitioning away from hormonal contraceptives (if you currently use them) and identifying early signs of pregnancy (before a pregnancy test). Think about this chapter as the handbook for trying to conceive. Read it all, then refer back to it later if you need to fine-tune your strategy.

FAMILY PLANNING: THE STATISTICAL STORY

In any given month, unprotected sex results in pregnancy an estimated 30 percent of the time, and 75 percent of couples conceive within six months. Ninety percent of couples successfully achieve pregnancy by the one-year mark, and 95 percent have conceived by two years. There's a relationship between fertility rates and age, with women younger than thirty having the greatest chance of conception in a given cycle. There's a pretty sharp decrease after thirty, with chances of spontaneous conception for women between the ages of thirty-five to thirty-nine running about half of those for women aged nineteen to twenty-six. The main reason for this is a decrease in egg quality. Male fertility also declines with age, so the health of fathers-to-be matters too.[1] Keep in mind that these are the cumulative statistics, which do not take into account things like overall health status, diagnosed medical conditions, or whether or not a woman is ovulating in any given month at all. It also does not factor in things like the timing of intercourse in relation to ovulation, which is really important considering that the fertile window only spans about seven days in any given cycle. Knowing what's going on with your own fertility, such as through the techniques discussed in chapter 7, allows you to maximize your chances of conception in each given cycle. If you really want to figure out what's going on with your own body, your own menstrual cycle, and your own ovulation, you need to start there.

Infertility is defined as "the failure to achieve pregnancy after twelve months of regular unprotected sexual intercourse."[2] Because of age-related fertility decline, some providers make this diagnosis for women over age thirty-five who have been unsuccessfully trying to conceive for half that time—just six months. While "infertility" sounds scary when used to describe your own health, keep in mind that couples conceive after trying for longer than twelve months all the time. We will explore the details of how to maximize chances of conception for a given cycle later in this chapter but keep in mind that if you've been trying for six months, or twelve months, and have yet to see double lines on a pregnancy test, there's no need to panic—even if a health care provider has used the word "infertile" in an appointment with you. You're only "infertile" until you're not anymore; you're only "not pregnant" until you are.

If you have been unsuccessfully trying to conceive for several months, troubleshoot your cycle! Make sure you're ovulating! You can find this out through the techniques we described in chapter 7. If you're not, first make sure you have your foundation in place from chapters 6 and 8, as sometimes that is enough to normalize your cycle. If you still need support, flip ahead to the next chapter, where we dive into treatment. But keep in mind that many nonhormonal reasons also contribute to conception challenges. While ovulatory disorders account for 25 percent of diagnosed infertility cases, 15 percent result from endometriosis (a structural problem as much as a chemical one—see the next chapter for details), 12 percent from pelvic adhesions (a form of scar tissue formation in the pelvic cavity, reversible through surgery), 11 percent from tubal blockages (tubes can be unblocked), 11 percent from other tubal or uterine abnormalities, and 7 percent from a condition called hyperprolactinemia (we'll discuss more about this one later in this chapter).[3] If you find out that you have any of these conditions, it's not a sentence for lifelong barrenness; it's just information about the best next step to support you in your fertility journey.

RETURN TO FERTILITY

The statistics we just discussed would easily overwhelm anyone. Reading them, it's easy to feel like you're doomed before you even start trying to grow your family. But think about it this way: conceiving at all is a miracle. There are so many steps involved and impossibilities to overcome that it's a wonder any of us even made our way to being born in the first place. That being said, the overwhelming majority of couples do conceive eventually! Try to stay patient, trust the process, and do the next right thing. But first things first: if you're thinking of growing your family in the next few years, the time to come off birth control and start preparing your body for a healthy pregnancy is now. Even if your cycle returns quickly after coming off the pill or having your intrauterine device (IUD) removed, there's a lot you can—and should—do to help your body heal from the stress of hormonal steroid drugs, and to ensure you're set up for success when the time comes to actually start trying.

Because many women don't know the details about their fertility before starting to use hormonal contraceptives, they expect to fall pregnant quickly after discontinuing them and wind up surprised or confused when it doesn't happen that easily. But research shows that for women with normal cycles prior to using hormonal contraceptives, it takes time to return to normal fertility. This means you need about eight months to start ovulating again after discontinuing the shot, four months after using the patch, an average of three months after using the ring or birth control pills, and roughly two months after having a hormonal IUD removed.[4] But that's only for women who were having regular, ovulatory cycles without underlying hormonal disorders. For all the women who use contraceptives to manage period problems in addition to pregnancy prevention, there's actually a significant likelihood of fertile cycles taking longer to return—or of them not returning at all until underlying hormonal problems have been sorted out.

COMING OFF THE PILL: WHAT TO EXPECT

If you had uncomfortable symptoms that were suppressed by taking the birth control pill (or using other hormonal contraceptives), expect them to come back when you discontinue. This makes sense; if you had a hormone imbalance to begin with, the pill merely shuts off your body's hormones completely. It didn't "fix" them. So, you'll still experience the same imbalances you did prior to starting the pill in the first place. Likewise, if you experienced negative side effects from taking the birth control pill, such as the weight gain, acne, hirsutism or low libido often caused by the progestins in birth control, they won't necessarily go away right away after you come off the pill, either. The drugs in hormonal contraceptives take time to clear out of your system, and then your body needs time to figure out how to function again after the fact. It's an unfortunate catch-22, where the symptoms suppressed by the pill often come back quickly but the symptoms caused by the pill frequently don't resolve in a timely fashion. We often refer to this as "post birth-control syndrome" or "post-pill syndrome" and this period can involve symptoms like headaches, irritability or weepiness, heavy bleeding, cramping and inflammation, acne, sugar cravings, irregular periods, fatigue, and low libido. While your body clears away the hormone-suppressing drugs and meanwhile resumes its own production of hormones, it makes sense for symptoms to emerge. These symptoms can last for up to a year, but you can limit them by taking steps to balance your body. This is a perfect time to double down on the techniques discussed in chapter 7 to support the natural and expected hormonal fluctuations in the female body. Even still, you can expect some irregular cycles for the first few months, often with a heavier or lighter flow than you experienced while on the pill. You might also experience rapid changes in energy levels and mood, especially if you were taking a monophasic pill, as your body returns to cyclic hormonal *fluctuations.*

If you had an underlying hormonal health issue prior to starting the pill, this post-pill time frame will look a little bit different for you than it would for a woman who didn't have any period problems prior to using birth control. This might cause even more confusion if you had a hormone imbalance but didn't realize it or ever have it diagnosed before you started contraceptive use. In many ways, what you don't know (or didn't know) causes new problems. If you didn't know of any hormonal imbalances prior to starting the pill and coming off it brings negative accompanying symptoms for six months or more despite implementing the foundational elements we discussed in chapter 6, it's a good idea to do some troubleshooting of your cycle (see the following chapter) or make an appointment with a health care provider to have some labs run.

OTHER WAYS TO SUPPORT YOUR BODY

After coming off hormonal contraceptives, you can take some additional steps to help your body clear away the drugs in your system and get back to baseline. Consider implementing the following for at least eight months if you used the implant, four months after using the patch, three months after using the ring or birth control pills, and two months after having a hormonal IUD removed:

- *Liver detox*: Your liver clears away old, broken-down estrogen and progesterone molecules. Dandelion root modulates the enzymes involved in clearing away these steroid hormones.[5]
  - *Dosage*: one to two cups of strongly brewed tea each evening.
- *Estrogen binding*: Estrogen-detoxing chemicals called indole-3-carbinol (I3C) and diindolylmethane (DIM) found in cruciferous vegetables (like broccoli, cauliflower, cabbage, and kale) detoxify estrogen through the liver and gastrointestinal tract, reversing estrogen dominance and the increased cancer risks associated with exogenous estrogen exposure.
  - *Dosage*: If you were using an estrogen-containing contraceptive, the recommended supplementation dosage is 200 to 400 milligrams (mg) per day of I3C[6] and 300 mg of DIM.[7] It's difficult to get this high of a dosage from food—you'd need to eat the equivalent of one-third of a head of cabbage every day[8]—so you'll want to use a supplement. However, the fiber in cruciferous vegetables also helps clear away toxins, so it's a generally good idea to include the actual vegetables too.
- *Replenish lost nutrients*: Hormonal contraceptives notoriously deplete important nutrients, including vitamins B1, B2, B3, B12, C, and zinc.[9]
  - *Dosage*: Utilize a high-quality, daily prenatal vitamin to restore depleted nutrients for at least three months before trying to conceive.
- *The estrobolome*: Gastrointestinal bacteria (i.e., probiotics or the microbiome) modulate the balance of estrogen in the bloodstream by detoxifying broken-down hormones and resorbing the beneficial

ones. More than sixty strains of bacteria have been shown to play a role in modulating the estrobolome.
- *Dosage*: Utilize a high-quality, broad-spectrum probiotic supplement containing strains like *Lactobacillus*, *Bifidobacterium*, and *Enterococcus*. You also can supplement your diet with probiotic-rich foods, like naturally fermented vegetables (i.e., sauerkraut and kimchi) and kombucha. Beneficial yeast strains like *Saccharomyces boulardii* help maintain the health and diversity of gut flora and protect the gut lining, so I recommend my patients supplement with 1,000 mg twice daily for at least two months.

PRECONCEPTION SUPPORT

Once you're off your birth control, it's time to start thinking not only about your own body's health but also how you can maximize the health of your future baby. That starts with the egg. We touched on this already, but your body takes about three months to fully produce the egg released in any given ovulatory cycle. Emphasizing a nutrient-dense diet (the more colorful the better), avoiding inflammatory exposures like alcohol, tobacco, marijuana, and plastic will serve you well in the preconception period to maximize both the health of mom and baby. This probably makes sense, but eating eggs is a great way to support your own egg health, as they provide a rich source of zinc,[10] B12,[11] choline,[12] and coenzyme Q10 (coQ10).[13] Research shows that these nutrients not only increase chances of pregnancy but also increase the likelihood of a successful and healthy one. Omega-3s play an extremely important nutritional role, and depending on the way the chicken was raised, eggs may offer a substantial source of these, too. Research shows that pastured eggs, meaning those produced by chickens who are allowed free range in pastures to eat bugs, critters, and other natural nutrition, have three times higher levels of omega-3 fatty acids than corn-fed chickens.[14] To support your egg health and a healthy pregnancy, eat two per day.

In situations of concern regarding oocyte quality, such as with advanced maternal age (mothers over thirty-five years old) or when using assisted reproductive technology, you can also supplement with these nutrients. Based on the research available, I recommend the following strategies to my patients:

- *CoEnzyme Q10 (ubiquinol)*: 600 mg daily with food[15]
    - Ubiquinone and ubiquinol are the two different forms of coQ10 in the body based on whether or not it has been metabolized a certain way. The body absorbs ubiquinol better compared to ubiquinone and subsequently uses it for fertility-supporting metabolic reactions at improved rates. Currently, only one company worldwide manufactures ubiquinol, which makes it relatively more expensive and harder to find. But, if you're going to take a supplement, the extra effort will make it worth your while.[16]
- *Zinc bisglycinate*: 50 mg daily with food
    - Most of the studies involving zinc supplementation have been performed on animals, and we don't currently have data available from clinical trials regarding zinc supplementation specifically for egg quality in humans. That being said, many studies show the clinical utility of zinc supplementation for specific reproductive disorders in women.[17] Therefore, the recommendation for zinc supplementation here comes from the finding that 50 mg of zinc supplementation improves ovulatory outcomes in women with polycystic ovarian syndrome (PCOS), which is a disorder characterized by incomplete oocyte maturation.[18] Among the forms of zinc on the market, zinc bisglycinate has been shown to be the most bioavailable.[19]
- *Vitamin B12 (Methylcobalamin)*: 2,000 micrograms (mcg) daily with food
    - Studies show that not only does methylcobalamin supplementation improve rates of live birth with in vitro fertilization (IVF),[20] but it also improves neurodevelopmental outcomes in the baby.[21]
    - Approximately 25 percent of people in the United States[22] have a mutation in the gene that codes for the methyltetrahydrofolate enzyme (MTHFR), which leads to abnormal processing of B vitamins and detoxification pathways in the body. This can negatively impact both egg quality and pregnancy outcomes. Therefore, as a general rule, I recommend using the methylated forms of both folate (methyltetrahydrofolate) and vitamin B12 (methylcobalamin), as individuals with an MTHFR mutation cannot process most other forms of these vitamins.[23]
    - While the daily recommended daily allowance (RDA) for vitamin B12 is only 2.4 mcg for women, the ability to absorb B12 from supplements depends on many factors that vary on an individual basis. A supplement at that low of a level does not typically

translate to clinically significant levels of vitamin B12 on lab work. Moreover, we understand high doses of vitamin B12 to be safe.[24]
- Some people do not tolerate high doses of methylcobalamin because it produces or worsens symptoms of anxiety. If you experience this side effect from taking methylcobalamin supplements, you should switch to hydroxocobalamin, also a safe option for people who have the MTHFR mutation.
- *Choline (phosphatidylcholine)*: I recommend that my patients intake a minimum of 450 mg of choline per day[25]
  - Sunflower lecithin offers another source of choline via supplementation, and this form can be continued into the postpartum period to reduce risk of complications such as clogged ducts while breastfeeding.
- *Omega-3 fatty acids (docosahexaenoic acid [DHA])*:[26] I recommend that my patients take a minimum of 600 mg DHA daily, in addition to a diet rich in food-based sources of omega-3 fatty acids.[27]

PRENATAL VITAMINS

In addition to the supplements outlined above, I recommend taking a prenatal vitamin for as many as three months prior to trying to conceive to support the egg that matures during that time. While you absolutely still can safely conceive and carry a healthy pregnancy without having taken the prenatal vitamin for this long, doing so will maximize the likelihood that the egg had everything it needed—nutritionally speaking—to mature throughout its developmental period. In other words, taking a high-quality prenatal vitamin before you get pregnant is ideal.

However, shopping for a prenatal vitamin can get overwhelming really quickly. Thousands of brands exist, often with several different varieties available from any one company! At the end of the day, *any* prenatal vitamin you choose will give you *something* beneficial, and very rarely will it harm you, as manufacturers design prenatals with relatively low levels of these nutrients. That being said, consider the following:

- *Folate and vitamin B12*: Because of the high rates of MTHFR mutations in the United States, folic acid supplementation—rather than *methyl*folate—may be problematic. I recommend choosing a prenatal made with methylfolate instead of folic acid, and methylcobalamin instead of cyanocobalamin.

- *Vitamin D*: Like the nutrients listed in the previous section, you absolutely need vitamin D for egg health, fertility, and a healthy pregnancy. However, not everyone metabolizes dietary vitamin D the same, and excess dietary vitamin D does pose very real health risks. Therefore, we don't have a "one-size-fits-all" recommendation for how much vitamin D to take. In most cases, multivitamins (including prenatal multivitamins) will not provide enough vitamin D to keep your blood levels in the optimal range. You will probably need additional supplementation beyond what your prenatal contains. However, prior to starting a new vitamin D supplement, I recommend having your blood levels tested. Most of my patients need to supplement between 4,000 international units (IU) and 10,000 IU daily.
- *Choline*: Relatively few prenatal vitamins have choline in them, and if they do it does not come anywhere close to the recommended 450 mg per day. You will likely also need to supplement this beyond what's in your prenatal if you do not maintain adequate sources in your diet.
- *Vitamin A*: Because vitamin A builds up in the body, too much is dangerous. This is especially true for developing babies, so the Food and Drug Administration (FDA) warns against excess supplementation with a form of vitamin A called retinyl palmitate. Beta carotene, an orange-pigmented chemical that converts into vitamin A in the body, does not run this risk, so most prenatal vitamins contain this formulation to provide vitamin A. However, a small percentage of the population has a genetic mutation preventing conversion of beta carotene to retinol, the active form of vitamin A, in the body. This leads to deficiency if the diet does not include sufficient animal-based sources of vitamin A, which also poses a risk to the mother and the baby. However, if you consume an abundance of animal foods like eggs and fish (which I recommend that you do), you will get plenty of vitamin A from your diet in the most easily used form.
- *Iron*: Blood volume increases rapidly in the early days of pregnancy, and iron is essential for making healthy red blood cells. However, iron toxicity is also a real risk, and you may not need extra iron before you become pregnant. Most prenatal vitamins have 27 mg of iron in them, but you can find iron-free varieties too. You might consider taking an iron-free prenatal until you find out you are pregnant and then add iron in once you have a positive pregnancy test. Like other vitamins, some forms of iron are better tolerated than

others. Ferrous sulfate notoriously causes constipation and nausea, problems which pregnancy is already known to bring about, whereas you might better tolerate the gentler, more easily absorbed counterpart: iron bisglycinate.[28] I typically recommend my patients take an animal-based iron supplement if they need one, which derives from animal blood, called "heme iron."

TRYING TO CONCEIVE

As is probably obvious by now, trying to conceive (TTC) is not as simple as stopping the birth control pill. Getting pregnant requires a genetically viable sperm and a genetically viable egg to meet (meaning that intercourse needs to occur at the right time in a structurally favorable fallopian tube). The fertilized egg needs to then meet a receptive hormonal and physical environment. A series of delicate steps allowing implantation occur, and then the ovaries sustain the correct levels of hormone to support the pregnancy until the placenta forms and takes over in controlling the chemical environment. *Phew.* That being said, most of that *does* happen pretty quickly for most couples. But when you're TTC on a timeline, every cycle counts. So, making sure that you're meeting all those requirements by tracking your fertility actually increases your chances of conception in a given month by nearly double.[29] This delineates yet another example of why it benefits you to know what's going on—or not going on—in your body in any given month.

Ovulation is an essential piece of the fertility puzzle, and hormones definitely influence the timing and quality of a released egg. However, they also influence the uterine lining and whether or not it's able to allow implantation of the early embryo and sustain the pregnancy. Making sure your hormones are in order (via the foundational elements of chapter 6, or by troubleshooting methods described in chapter 7) really translates directly to the relative chance of pregnancy in each given cycle. But you should pay attention to a few other things as well:

- *Timing of intercourse*: We already covered this briefly, but here's a refresher so it's all in one place: sperm survive up to five days in the female reproductive tract, so you could conceive from intercourse that occurred up to five days prior to ovulation. The egg lasts about forty-eight hours, so there's really about a seven-day fertile window of the five days prior to ovulation, the day of, and the day after. It's a good idea to have sex about every other day throughout this window. However, even though sperm *could* survive for five days, most don't live that long and there's a greater chance of a sperm surviving and thriving all the way to fertilization if intercourse occurs closer in time to when the ovary releases the egg. In fact, researchers identified the *most* fertile window as the two days leading up to ovulation plus the day of ovulation itself.[30] The day of the cycle with the single greatest chance of conception actually corresponds to two days prior to ovulation, so if you only have one chance that month, that's the day to choose.[31] Sperm need enough time to travel up through the uterus and into the fallopian tubes, and if they're already there—ready and waiting when the egg releases—fertilization occurs right away. This probably goes without saying, but if you're looking to maximize your chances, you need to know when you ovulate, and you can do so by charting your basal body temperature (BBT). (Refer back to chapter 7 for details.) Incidentally, the most fertile cervical mucus appears about two days prior to ovulation, and luteinizing hormone (LH) strips turn positive about one to two days before the egg releases. So, if you see the noteworthy clear, gelatinous "egg white" cervical mucus or first see a positive on a LH test strip, make time for intimacy *that day.*

- *Cervical mucus:* In addition to cluing you in about your own fertility, cervical mucus actually helps sperm travel through the uterus and survive while they wait for an egg. That stretchy, "egg white" cervical fluid has the perfect pH and water balance for sperm to survive, and even includes some sugar to keep them happy and fed. For this reason, low levels of cervical mucus (such as in women dealing with low estrogen) may decrease chances of pregnancy in any given cycle. Refer back to chapter 7 for some specific ways to improve your own production of cervical mucus. However, you might also consider using PreSeed™ Fertility Lubricant, which has been designed to match the pH and water content of fertile cervical fluid, supporting sperm survival.[32]
- *Lubricant*: You'd never want to use lubricants that contain spermicide while trying to conceive, but many over-the-counter lubricants also slow down sperm motility and even harm them. Lubricants may also damage sperm DNA. You can reduce your need for external lubricants in the first place by ensuring that your body produces enough of its own natural lubrication. If you experience discomfort during sex, consider using PreSeed™ Fertility Lubricant, or even coconut

oil. While the research is mixed regarding how much coconut oil influences sperm motility, because it is oil-based, you don't need nearly as much to provide comfort as you would when using water-based lubricants, like PreSeed. It's also very inexpensive and widely available. If you're going to use coconut oil as a lubricant, choose the organic, extra-virgin, cold-pressed variety.
- *Contraindicated medications*: In addition to the chemicals widely included in over-the-counter lubricants, many over-the-counter medications interfere with fertility. Here are a few:
  - *Antihistamines* (allergy medications) reduce production of cervical mucus.
  - *Non-steroidal anti-inflammatory drugs (NSAIDs)* like aspirin and ibuprofen can affect ovulation, and they also increase bleeding risk and increase risk of miscarriage by 80 percent.[33] NSAIDs also cause birth defects.

THE TWO-WEEK WAIT

Once you've decided that the time is right to grow your family, you go for it! Then, not a whole lot happens. Or at least, that's the way it seems. Inside, a fertilized egg rapidly develops into just the right shape and size to find its cozy home in your uterine lining. But as an excited mama-to-be, you don't get to directly witness any of it. Instead, you have to just sit and wait until enough time has passed for a pregnancy test to read positive. Commonly known as the two-week wait, this often-agonizing time spent waiting until your next period (doesn't) comes can feel like it takes fourteen eons instead of just fourteen days. But here's a secret—if you know exactly when you ovulated and you know how to read your body's signals, you might figure out that you're pregnant even before a home pregnancy test reads positive. Before we dive into the diagnostics—identifying a pregnancy when it has occurred—let's briefly review what, exactly, happens during this time.

As a bit of a refresher, human reproduction is a complicated math equation. Man + woman = baby, but it's not quite 1 + 1 = 1. It's actually 0.5 + 0.5 = 1 . . . or 2, or 3, if multiples are involved. Your eggs are cells, like the other cells in your body, but they only contain half of your genetic material. While the rest of your cells contain a copy of human genetic code each from your biological mother and father, your eggs (and a man's sperm) each only contain one copy of each. When the two join up, the resulting cell has a full set of genes. During the "two-week wait," this fertilized egg rapidly divides to transform from a single cell into a multicellular person, just like the rest of us. By the time thirty hours have passed, the cell has divided into two, within another fifteen hours, those two become four, and by day three, there are typically about sixteen cells.[34] By around day five after fertilization, there are as many as 150 cells and the baby has earned the new name of "blastocyst." Upon reaching the blastocyst stage, implantation of the fertilized egg could theoretically take place. Implantation involves the blastocyst burrowing into the uterine lining and joining up with the mother's blood supply, thereby allowing the pregnancy hormone, human chorionic gonadotrophin (hCG), to build up in the bloodstream. Implantation typically occurs between six to twelve days after ovulation, with an average of nine days.[35] Implantation as early as day five or as late as day thirteen have been documented, though tubal pregnancies may occur more frequently in cases of very early implantation, and late implantation may be more likely to result in early pregnancy loss. Most successful pregnancies involve implantation between eight and ten days after ovulation.[36]

Once implantation occurs, it takes one to two days for hCG levels to rise enough to detect on a blood test, and another one to two days after that to begin to show up on urine pregnancy tests. If implantation occurs on day ten, let's say, and it takes four days for hCG to read on a pregnancy test, you have a full two weeks of waiting to find out if your family has grown. If you're antsy to find out sooner, your body will give you some clues that would indicate pregnancy well in advance of the day of your expected period. The following techniques empower you to know what's going on in your body without needing to rely on a medical test, like lab work or an ultrasound, to tell you that you're pregnant.

- *Cervical position*: Unlike the low, open, and firm premenstrual cervix, a pregnant cervix will rise high up, remain tightly closed to protect the baby, and become soft due to the increased blood flow.
- *Cervical mucus*: Before a period, estrogen and progesterone rapidly fall from their mid-luteal-phase highs. If pregnancy occurs, however, the brain signals to the corpus luteum to continue producing hormones to sustain the pregnancy. This increasing level of estrogen often changes the quality of cervical fluid to become waterier, transforming from the thickened/creamy or dry premenstrual fluid to thin, milky-white, tinged-yellow or even clear cervical mucus. One of the best clues for you, if you track your cervical mucus, is noticing

a type of fluid that differs from what you usually experience in the days leading up to your period.
- *Sustained high temperatures*: If you track your basal body temperature, you will recall that temperatures typically begin to fall in the few days leading up to a period. If, however, your temperature remains elevated for eighteen days after ovulation without dropping, this almost always indicates pregnancy. Note, however, that a urine or blood pregnancy test would likely identify conception sooner than this.
- *Implantation dip*: If you track your basal body temperature, you will recall that just prior to ovulation, temperatures typically dip a little bit before rising dramatically the following day. For some women tracking their cycles, implantation of the fertilized egg creates a similar dip, in which one or two morning readings reveal a temperature several decimal points lower than the previous temperatures before rising back up again to meet or exceed the other luteal phase temperatures. Note that not all pregnant charts include an implantation dip, so if you don't see this characteristic, it doesn't necessarily mean that you aren't pregnant.
- *Triphasic chart*: If you track your basal body temperature, you will recall that a fertile, ovulatory chart has two phases: pre-ovulatory, when temperatures remain low; and post-ovulatory, when temperatures rise up high. Graphing out basal body temperature values makes this differentiation very obvious. Following implantation, some women see a second shift in data where luteal phase temperatures rise a second time and plateau. This divides the BBT chart into three distinct phases, with that third phase of sustained temperatures indicating implantation of the fertilized egg and subsequent production of pregnancy-related hormones that further increase the mother's metabolic rate. Note that not all pregnant charts include a triphasic shift, so if you don't see this characteristic, it doesn't necessarily mean that you aren't pregnant.
- *Implantation bleeding*: When the fertilized egg implants in the uterine lining, it releases a series of inflammatory chemicals that stimulate new blood vessel growth. These new blood vessels allow it to receive the nutrients it needs for continued development. However, this disruption sometimes leads to extra blood and tissue "spilling" out into the lumen of the uterus, showing up as pale pink or light brown spotting. Many women find this discouraging, believing that their period has started—only the full, red blood never arrives! If you

notice spotting several days prior to when you expect your period and you are actively TTC, don't fret! It could just be implantation bleeding, which may clue you in that you're on the right track. Note that implantation bleeding does not occur in every pregnancy, but up to one-third of women do experience this early pregnancy sign.[37]

- *Implantation cramping*: Similarly to implantation bleeding, the prostaglandins released when the fertilized egg burrows in the uterus sometimes cause some irritability of the uterine muscle. This can manifest as symptoms of twinging, cramping, or pelvic tightness that don't typically present in the premenstrual period. Keep in mind, however, that many pelvic sensations occur at the end of the cycle, and a new onset of cramping may sometimes result from other changes in the body like digestion. So, cramping at this time isn't a symptom specific to early pregnancy, but if combined with other symptoms, may reinforce your suspicions.
- *Increased resting heart rate (RHR)*: Similar to the way that body temperature increases subsequent to rising progesterone levels in early pregnancy, resting heart rate readings also tend to increase. This is true not only in the luteal phase, as we discussed previously, but also in the early stages of pregnancy. In fact, resting heart rate often increases by up to twenty beats per minute in pregnancy.[38] If you track your resting heart rate, whether manually or with a fitness watch, noticing a heart rate that continues to trend upward may signal pregnancy.
- *Urine tests*: We've finally arrived at the infamous home pregnancy test! Pregnancy tests are pretty straightforward—collect a urine sample, insert the dipstick, wait the recommended time on the package instructions, then read the result. One line means negative, two lines mean positive, or if you've used the fancy digital kind, a nice, big, sans-serif "yes" means you're pregnant! Pharmacies typically sell several different types of pregnancy tests that differ from each other in terms of the sensitivity of the test strip to urinary hCG and the color of the dye. Blue dye tests notorious run the risk of false positive results, and these deceptive (and often devastating) miscalculations give reason enough to steer clear of this variety of test. Instead, choose a test that uses pink dye, which significantly reduces the risk of false positives. Different tests on the market detect hCG in urine at different minimum thresholds. Most standard tests can detect hCG at a level of 25 milli-international units per milliliter (mIU/mL), though the First Response Early Result (FRER) test advertises a

sensitivity of 6.3 mIU/mL.[39] So, theoretically, the FRER may identify a pregnancy earlier than other mainstream tests if you're looking to find out as soon as possible. Note, however, that hCG levels increase very quickly in early pregnancy, doubling every couple of days. You can purchase very inexpensive pregnancy tests at dollar stores, or for pennies online in bulk packages. FRER tests often run in packages of $20 or more, so waiting an extra day can save you the price you paid for this book and beyond. One of the perks of using the "internet cheapie" tests (as you might hear them referred to on pregnancy forums) is that you won't really waste your money if you want to take two or three, or that many tests *daily* for several days throughout your luteal phase. Many women enjoy the anticipation of awaiting a pregnancy test result, watching several tests in a row turn from negative to positive with increasingly dark test lines. Given that a pregnancy test might show a positive as early as seventeen or eight days past ovulation, you could potentially cut the two-week wait in half if you start testing early. "Internet cheapie" pink dye tests are the way to go if you plan to do this. On the flip side, serial testing like this, especially if performed month after month, can take an emotional toll. If you find yourself feeling disappointed with early tests, your mental health may instead benefit from waiting to take a pregnancy test until the day after you expect your period. Odds are, you won't get a positive until around the day of your expected period anyway: data from the fertility tracking app Fertility Friend revealed that in a sample of nearly 100,000 BBT charts in which users received a negative pregnancy result prior to a positive result in a given pregnant cycle, the average day that a positive was first received was 13.6 days past ovulation (DPO). On average, these charters first received their negative result at around 10.3 DPO, and only 10 percent of so-called early testers with charts resulting in pregnancy showed a positive test as early as 10 DPO.[40] Again, the likelihood of an early positive test depends on when implantation occurs, and many women who become pregnant in any given cycle don't even experience implantation until 10 DPO (which would result in a positive urine test at around 13 or 14 DPO).

If you're dealing with a fertility problem, trying to conceive may feel like a marathon—or a nightmare, depending on the details. While for many couples, optimizing the timing of intercourse shortens the conception timeline on its own, though of course not everyone shares this experience.

If that's not you, and especially if you struggle with other red flag symptoms in your fertility such as period problems, it's essential that you also address the underlying hormonal imbalance. Understanding the problem with your cycle empowers you to fully treat it, which can allow you and your partner to conceive even if other fertility treatments, which simply override the system, have already failed. So if you want to truly troubleshoot your cycle, reset your hormones, and set your body up for lasting success not only for growing your family but for your whole life, read on—the next chapter will give you everything else you need to finally bring your body back into balance.

11

TREATMENT

Making Your Cycle Work for You

Last, but not least, we have arrived at the treatment section. We've spent the whole of this book working up to this point, where you understand your body and know why the conventional "treatment" for period problems (i.e., hormonal birth control) doesn't work. A few things before we get started though. First, it's really important that you have a healthy foundation in place. You'd be amazed by how many symptoms you can solve just by eating regular, balanced meals, moving your body, sleeping enough, managing stress, and syncing your lifestyle with your natural cycle. Following the healthy habits that we outlined in chapters 6 and 8 will benefit anyone, no matter what else might be going on with their health. But then again, diagnosable health conditions in other areas of your body really do impact periods, as we discussed in chapter 2. Remember that conditions like hypothyroidism or autoimmune diseases won't just disappear if you ignore them. If you have concerning symptoms but you're providing well for your body, it's really important that you have some testing done to make sure that you don't need a higher-level intervention, like necessary surgeries or medications. This book isn't intended to take the place of your doctor in making a diagnosis, though by now you know of many testing options that are available to you. Bear in mind, however, that you will find the most benefit in this chapter if you and your doctor have already identified the driving force behind your period problems (something you can't do effectively while you're taking the pill). Once that diagnosis has been established, it's time to start making your cycle work better for you.

In the conventional model, the next step after ruling out more significant health diagnoses is a birth control prescription. That is a valid option, and the decision about whether to use it is yours and yours alone.

However, if you choose that route, then this chapter is not for you. The purpose of our discussion here is to fine-tune your body's own production of hormones and that just won't be possible if you are taking the pill. Likewise, many of the treatments outlined in this chapter may actually interfere with the activity of the pill and render it ineffective as a contraceptive. Please know that if you use the pill but later change your mind and want to troubleshoot and treat your period problems without medication, this chapter will still be here for you.

But if you've already decided that hormonal contraceptives aren't for you and you want a different approach, you're definitely in the right place. Keep in mind that in this chapter, I outline just a few of the most evidence-based, powerful natural treatment strategies that I use in my clinical practice. This is not by any means an exhaustive list, nor is it a *prescriptive* list. When I use these strategies for my patients, I don't have every patient on every single herb or supplement listed. Instead, I evaluate their period problems in light of the greater context of their health and choose the strategies that will best address the big picture. When considering your own period and your own health, you should do the same.

PROGESTERONE CREAM

In this chapter, we will discuss numerous natural treatment strategies for the most common period problems. Often, the driving force between these symptoms involves an imbalance between estrogen and progesterone. While most strategies aim to address the underlying mechanism behind this imbalance, sometimes the fastest and most effective way to fix the problem is by directly supplementing with hormonal progesterone. Keep in mind that in clinical practice, I only recommend using progesterone supplementation after other, more conservative options have been exhausted. Supplementing with USP progesterone—meaning, it is a form of natural hormone, bioidentical to human progesterone—is not the same as using the progestins found in hormonal contraceptives. These are not the same molecules and do not function the same way in the human body. Unlike synthetic progestogens, which increase cancer risks, natural progesterone lowers cancer risks[1] and counters the effects of estrogen in the body. Topical use of USP natural progesterone cream increases blood levels of progesterone similarly to oral administration but with less than half of the required dosage.[2]

To supplement progesterone, utilize a product that contains micronized, USP progesterone, free of phthalates and parabens. To use it, apply 40 milligrams (mg) topically up to twice daily, which for most products equates to a 0.5 teaspoon total per day. Apply the cream to an area of clean, dry skin without an excess of fatty tissue. Some areas of the body ideal for application include the inside of the wrist or ankle where blood vessels are visible, the sides of your neck, or the top of your chest, above your breasts. Do not apply progesterone cream directly to your breasts or over any area with thicker, fatty tissue because it will accumulate in these areas instead of traveling into your bloodstream. I recommend applying the cream right before bed when it is less likely to be washed off or rubbed away by clothing or sweat.

If you are still having regular periods, I recommend phasic application, meaning that you only apply the progesterone cream after ovulation, during the time when your body would ordinarily be producing its own progesterone. If you have not yet reached perimenopause, do not use progesterone unless you are also tracking your cycle to know when ovulation occurs. This is especially important if you have irregular periods. Using progesterone cream prior to ovulation may prevent or delay ovulation from naturally occurring. If you are perimenopausal or postmenopausal, it is okay to apply the progesterone daily. In either case, start with a 40 mg dosage for three months, only increasing to 80 mg as needed.

Using progesterone cream may lengthen your cycles and cause your periods to arrive a bit later. They will also likely become lighter and may last a day or two longer. If you do not use the progesterone cream daily (or daily within the luteal phase) as directed, you may experience mid-cycle spotting. It is rare for progesterone cream to cause other side effects (unlike synthetic progestogens, which often causes other, significant effects on quality of life) but headaches are reported in a small population of users. Note that oral USP progesterone, often dosed at 200 mg or more daily, is more likely to be associated with side effects.

DIAGNOSING THE ROOT CAUSE

We categorize different period problems according to the underlying hormonal environment. This helps us understand the root cause and treat it directly. In the rest of this chapter, we will break down those individual symptoms, like headaches or period pain, outline the major driving factors behind them, and then discuss both conventional and natural treatment options. Keep in mind that in order to see results, you need to pair the right treatment with the right diagnosis. If the problem hasn't been correctly diagnosed, the treatment likely won't work. For more information about lab tests and how to advocate for appropriate testing in a physician's office, see the appendix at the end of this book. Additionally, the strategies outlined in this chapter aren't treatment protocols in the way that birth control pills are; instead, they're more like algorithms. First you lay your foundation (chapters 6 and 8) and then you fine-tune with choosing one or two treatment strategies to see how they work for you. After about three months, which is about how long it takes to create meaningful hormonal change, you can layer in another strategy or altogether make a replacement. Let's get started!

PREMENSTRUAL SYNDROME (PMS)

Rather than being a diagnosable condition in and of itself, PMS describes an amalgamation of symptoms that often occur during the premenstrual phase such as headaches, premenstrual acne, breast tenderness, mood changes, bloating, sleep disturbances, and changes in appetite. While these symptoms may all result from an overarching hormonal pattern like estrogen dominance, they also each involve specific mechanistic details that we need to address. So, rather than "treating PMS" as a whole, we will address the symptoms individually.

Premenstrual Headaches

Premenstrual headaches or migraines relate to the menstrual cycle in some way. They may be caused directly by changes in hormone levels (most commonly estrogen) or triggered by inflammatory cytokines that are naturally released leading up to menstruation. Hormonal headaches can also occur around ovulation, precipitated by the sharp rise and fall of estrogen just before the ovary releases its egg.

PHARMACOLOGICAL TREATMENT

A prescription for the birth control pill is the most common "treatment" for hormonal headaches and migraines because it overrides the change in hormonal levels and creates a predictable, uniform hormonal environment nearly every day of the cycle. The estrogen in the pill particularly benefits women who experience headaches related to the dropping estrogen levels that follow ovulation and again in the premenstrual period. Ironically, however, migraines are considered a relative contraindication for use of estrogen-containing contraceptives, as both increase the risk of stroke. For this reason, I do not recommend using the birth control pill to "treat" premenstrual headaches. Propranolol, amitriptyline, and triptans are other medications commonly prescribed for migraine headaches, though they are not specific to menstrual migraines and like oral contraceptives, many come with the risk of developing dangerous side effects.

MIGRAINES CAUSED BY ESTROGEN WITHDRAWAL

In the days leading up to menstruation, estrogen declines rapidly. It also dramatically drops off just before ovulation. While we don't have a sure-fire way to test whether *changes* in estrogen are causing your migraines, if you experience a worsening of your headaches around ovulation as well as in the week leading up to your period, it's likely that estrogen is playing a role, and you should start here. If you are perimenopausal, changes in estrogen levels are almost guaranteed to contribute to this symptom for you because the perimenopausal period is characterized by rapidly and dramatically fluctuating levels of estrogen.[3] In that case, you might consider starting with the "Perimenopause" section ahead.

ALTERNATIVE OPTIONS:

- Feverfew (*Tanacetum parthenium*): Lignans in feverfew bind to estrogen receptors. The herb feverfew also contains flavonoids that are anti-inflammatory.[4] Feverfew can be taken daily to prevent migraines, but you might not need to take it every day. The dosage I recommend to my patients is 100 to 300 mg up to four times daily.[5] If you find that it works for you, after a few months you should experiment with only taking it in the days leading up to your period or, if applicable, ovulation. Because feverfew addresses both the estrogenic and inflammatory components of menstrual headaches, it's a good place to start.

- Black cohosh (*Cimicifuga racemosa*): Black cohosh is a phytoestrogen, so it acts similarly to estrogen in the body without creating the harmful effects of excess, inflammatory estrogen.[6] The dosage I recommend to my patients is 50 mg daily. Please note that you should not take this herbal medicine during your luteal phase if there is a chance you could be pregnant.
- Chaste tree (*Vitex agnus-castus*): Vitex binds to dopamine receptors in your brain to reduce pain. It also improves estrogen-progesterone balance.[7] The dosage I recommend to my patients is 40 to 100 mg daily.[8]
- Progesterone cream: Progesterone acts like the calming neurotransmitter GABA and also stimulates pain-relieving centers in the brain that mitigate the effect of fluctuating estrogen. It also directly relieves pain.[9] See the dosage instructions earlier in this chapter. Note that in a small percentage of users, progesterone use may paradoxically worsen headaches.

MIGRAINES CAUSED BY INFLAMMATION

If a menstrual migraine isn't caused by estrogen withdrawal it is likely related to inflammation in some capacity. Inflammatory chemicals called prostaglandins increase during the premenstrual phase, and this is enough to trigger a headache in susceptible women. In addition to laying a foundation to reduce inflammation as outlined in chapters 6 and 8, the following natural treatment strategies can be used to prevent or treat inflammatory menstrual migraines.

ALTERNATIVE OPTIONS:

- Feverfew: See "Feverfew" in the previous section: "Migraines Caused by Estrogen Withdrawal"
- Magnesium glycinate: Magnesium is involved in hundreds of chemical reactions in the body, including the regulation of blood flow to the brain, neurotransmitter release, and how pain signals are transmitted. Taken daily as a preventative, the dosage I recommend to my patients is 400 mg of magnesium glycinate daily with food. This dose should be continued for at least one month and, if no benefit is seen,

can be increased to 400 mg twice or up to three times daily with food. Note that while digestive symptoms are less common with this form of magnesium (glycinate), higher doses of magnesium may cause nausea, diarrhea, and/or bowel urgency.[10]
- Melatonin: Melatonin is a hormone that regulates sleep, and it should be used with caution. However, it also functions as an anti-inflammatory in many bodily systems and can be used to regulate cortisol balance. The dosage I recommend to my patients is 5 mg every evening before bed to prevent menstrual migraines.[11] If this strategy works for you, consider reducing your usage to just the phase in your cycle when you are most prone to migraines. You may prefer to use tart cherry juice, which is a natural source of melatonin. However, you should note that the levels of melatonin will vary, so it will be challenging to have a predictable, repeatable dose when using this form.
- Turmeric (*Curcuma longa*): Curcumin blocks the inflammatory chemical interleukin-6, making it a very effective and safe treatment for numerous inflammatory disorders, including migraines. The dosage I recommend to my patients in this instance is 1,000 mg twice daily.[12]

Breast Tenderness

When estrogen increases throughout the cycle, it stimulates the growth of milk-producing breast tissue in preparation for a possible pregnancy. Sometimes, this proliferation causes pain and depending on the woman's breasts as well as what else may be going on, like inflammation. (Note: this is often accompanied by swelling, typically attributed to the increase in progesterone that occurs after ovulation. This is a separate topic from pain and is not pathological. Some women even go up more than a cup size!)

PHARMACOLOGICAL TREATMENT

In many cases, patients are told that premenstrual breast tenderness is "normal" and not to worry about it. In some cases, this is true—many women experience breast tenderness, and, by that definition, it could therefore be considered "normal" because it is commonplace. However, menstrual cycles shouldn't be painful, even if pain is "the norm." Recognizing this, the birth control pill is a common prescription for premenstrual breast tenderness because it blocks ovarian production of estrogen. If estrogen levels flatline, it will suppress the normal, cyclic breast tissue changes. In severe cases, providers may also prescribe Tamoxifen, a pharmacological estrogen blocker often used to manage certain types of breast cancers. You should not take Tamoxifen if you are of childbearing age because it is not safe to take if you become pregnant. It also increases the risk of developing osteoporosis and other conditions associated with low estrogen.

BREAST TENDERNESS CAUSED BY FIBROCYSTIC BREAST DISEASE

Fibrocystic breast disease is a common and noncancerous condition in which a woman's breasts develop an irregular, bumpy consistency. These areas of increased density are different from the surrounding tissue and may be more likely to become painful during the premenstrual phase. Fortunately, there are numerous natural treatments available, so you don't have to completely shut down your hormones if you experience pain related to your fibrocystic breasts. (Note: although the overwhelming majority of breast lumps are benign, not all are. If you notice a change in your breasts, make an appointment with a breast specialist and ask for imaging tests to make sure that your lumps are truly a consequence of fibrocystic changes.)

ALTERNATIVE OPTIONS:

- Evening primrose oil: The active component of evening primrose oil, gamma-linolenic acid, reduces the sensitivity of breasts to prostaglandins during the menstrual cycle.[13] The dosage I recommend to my patients is 3,000 mg of evening primrose oil daily.[14]
- Vitamin E: The antioxidant effect of vitamin E reduces pain and sensitivity of breasts by improving detoxification of prostaglandins.[15] The dosage I recommend to my patients is 1,200 international units (IU) of vitamin E daily.[16]
- Chaste tree (*Vitex agnus-castus*): Vitex interacts with the brain's dopamine receptors, reducing the perception of pain. The dosage I recommend to my patients is 40 mg daily for at least three months.[17]

BREAST TENDERNESS CAUSED BY ESTROGEN DOMINANCE

Breast tissue is very sensitive to estrogen, and when excess estrogen is present, inflammation commonly results. When estrogen is high in relation to progesterone, breasts are more likely to become painful. If you don't have diagnosed fibrocystic breasts, cyclic mastalgia—the technical phrase for menstrual breast pain—usually is the result of estrogen dominance.

ALTERNATIVE OPTIONS:

- Iodine: Research shows that using up to 6 mg per day of iodine supplementation reduces the level of cyclic breast pain in patients who do not have a thyroid disorder because it reduces the response of breast tissue to estrogen signaling.[18] Interestingly, this was true even in patients who did not have an iodine deficiency.[19] In clinical practice, 6 mg of iodine is often far too much and poses the risk of toxicity. The dosage I recommend to my patients is to start with is 1 mg daily for at least three months, and slowly increase to 3 mg daily, if needed. It's a good idea to have your iodine levels monitored by a health care provider if you are supplementing with more than 1 mg. The molecular form of iodine, I2, is more efficiently used by breast tissue and less likely to have a negative effect on your thyroid. You should note that it is not safe to supplement with any form of iodine if you have Hashimoto's disease, and that iodine excess can damage your health.

Fatigue

Feeling tired and more lethargic before and during your period is normal due to the drop in estrogen levels. As we discussed in the section on cycle syncing in chapter 8, lifestyle strategies during the different phases of the menstrual cycle may be enough to eliminate symptoms of fatigue and prevent it from negatively impacting quality of life. However, fatigue that is more intense and debilitating may be a sign of another health problem such as anemia caused by heavy menstrual bleeding and subsequent iron deficiency, a stress response in the body (so-called hypothalamic-pituitary-adrenal [HPA] axis dysfunction or "adrenal fatigue"), or inflammation.

PHARMACOLOGICAL TREATMENT

In many cases, doctors don't offer a prescription for premenstrual fatigue apart from offering the birth control pill. The exception would be if there is an underlying problem with heavy bleeding or iron deficiency. In the case of heavy bleeding, jump ahead a few paragraphs to the section titled "Heavy Periods."

FATIGUE CAUSED BY IRON DEFICIENCY

Iron carries oxygen in the bloodstream, and oxygen directly translates to cellular energy. So, without enough iron, your cells won't be getting enough energy, and you will feel tired. If you already have iron deficiency anemia, monthly blood loss may compound that enough to make you feel extremely fatigued around your period. Iron deficiency anemia can be caused by your diet—not getting enough bioavailable iron from animal food—as well as from absorption problems resulting from gut inflammation. It may also be directly caused by heavy menstrual bleeding. If you have heavy periods, jump ahead to the "Heavy Periods" section to treat your iron deficiency at the root cause. If you don't have heavy periods, it might be a good idea to see a health care provider to have some tests run to make sure your stomach and intestines are functioning as they should. If all of those tests come back normal, this section is for you. (Note: some birth control pills, like Lo Loestrin Fe, have iron added to the placebo pills, which may cause constipation or iron toxicity if it is not needed.)

ALTERNATIVE OPTIONS:

- Consume iron-rich foods: The best way to boost your levels of any nutrient is from food. Iron, in particular, is best absorbed and utilized by your body when you eat meat because it's already in the ready-to-use animal form. (Humans are animals, after all!) Iron from plant foods is still a great option, but it needs to be converted into its usable form through a series of enzymatic steps that make the net return much lower. Some plant foods also contain other chemicals that prevent iron absorption, like the oxalates found in spinach, kale, beets, nuts, and wheat. Excellent animal sources of iron include beef or chicken liver, red meat, oysters, and eggs. Steer clear of "fortified" foods because these don't naturally contain iron but rather have had iron supplements added to them from the manufacturer. Food manufacturers often use the cheapest ingredients possible, which means that the form of iron added to these foods is often difficult to digest and harsh on the stomach, often causing constipation or nausea as side effects if you're even able to absorb it at all.

- Increase vitamin C intake (*ascorbic acid*): Vitamin C enhances iron absorption from foods when eaten at the same time. You can naturally boost your body's iron content by eating a vitamin-C-rich food such as a mandarin orange or handful of grape tomatoes with meals. I sometimes recommend that my patients take a vitamin C supplement, such as a 100 mg chewable tablet with meals. This is a great option, because vitamin C supplements are much better tolerated than iron supplements, which often cause constipation and nausea. Be mindful that high doses of vitamin C may cause diarrhea. This is unlikely to occur with a total daily supplementation of less than 1,000 mg, so that's why I recommend a 100 mg chewable tablet up to three times daily to my patients.
- Iron supplements (if necessary): With the exception of pregnancy, I try to refrain from prescribing iron supplements unless absolutely necessary, such as in cases when the iron deficiency is at a dangerously low level or following profound blood loss. That being said, such situations do occur. If iron supplementation is necessary, I recommend first using a heme-based iron supplement derived from bovine or porcine hemoglobin. You should note that rarely, allergic reactions can occur from these types of supplements. If a heme iron supplement is not preferred, consider using iron bisglycinate. Most over-the-counter iron supplements contain ferrous sulfate, which commonly causes side effects of constipation and nausea. Iron bisglycinate, on the other hand, is gentler and more easily absorbed.[20] The dosage I recommend to my patients is 27 mg iron bisglycinate daily on an empty stomach. If your iron deficiency is caused by blood loss such as is the case with heavy periods, I also recommend supplementation with vitamins B12 and folate. The best way to do this is with a prenatal vitamin containing methylcobalamin and methylfolate, even if you are not actively trying to conceive. Taking a combination multivitamin like this will reduce the number of capsules you need to take! Unlike stand-alone iron supplements, however, prenatal vitamins should be taken with food. Do not take iron supplements without first having a blood test that shows depleted levels of both ferritin and serum iron because supplementing with iron when you don't need it can be dangerous.

FATIGUE CAUSED BY HPA AXIS DYSFUNCTION

Chronic stress affects every system of the body, and almost always results in decreased energy levels and stamina. In fact, persistent fatigue in the absence of other known health issues (but often even with them) almost always signals adrenal dysfunction in some capacity. With an existing adrenal fatigue or tax on the body's stress regulation system, the natural dip in energy levels that occurs during the premenstrual period may exacerbate the adrenal response enough to become debilitating. This may occur with or without other symptoms, like mood changes.

ALTERNATIVE OPTIONS:

- Ashwagandha (*Withania somnifera*): Adaptogenic herbs like ashwagandha regulate the nervous system response. The dosage I recommend to my patients is 200 mg twice daily during the premenstrual and menstrual phases.[21]
- Maca (*Lepidium peruvianum*): Maca is another adaptogen well suited to reproductive health concerns. It benefits premenstrual fatigue by modulating cortisol and other components of the stress response in addition to regulating estrogen expression in cells. The dosage I recommend to my patients is 500 mg of pre-gelatinized maca powder three times daily.[22]

FATIGUE CAUSED BY INFLAMMATION

Early studies have demonstrated a relationship between reduced antioxidant status and premenstrual symptoms, such as fatigue, in women.[23] Oxidative stress and inflammation are primary drivers of fatigue in all contexts, and supporting this axis of the human body by supplementing with anti-inflammatory herbs during the premenstrual period is very effective at lowering blood markers of oxidative stress.

ALTERNATIVE OPTIONS:

- Omega-3s: Omega-3 fatty acids increase the anti-inflammatory division of the immune system and serve as building blocks for

healthy hormone production. They have been demonstrated in the research to directly reduce premenstrual symptoms.[24] The dosage I recommend to my patients is at least 3,000 mg of cod liver oil daily. For a more potent effect, take 5,000 mg daily during the premenstrual and menstrual phases and reduce to 1,000 mg daily during the other phases of your cycle.
- Turmeric (*Curcuma longa*): While we do not currently have robust literature demonstrating the effects of turmeric specifically in premenstrual conditions, understanding the mechanism of how inflammation creates fatigue makes this anti-inflammatory herb a logical choice and I find it to be very effective for my patients, when necessary. The dosage I recommend to my patients in this instance is 500 mg twice daily.

Mood Changes

Mood changes are common and normal during the premenstrual period. This is part of the reason that the cycle syncing method outlined in chapter 8 can be so beneficial, because it empowers you to understand how your mood and affect will naturally change due to fluctuating hormone levels. That being said, profound mood disturbances that manifest as anxiety or depression (or exacerbations of those conditions) are not normal. If you find yourself feeling particularly anxious, irritable, or down in the dumps before or during your period, this section is for you.

Keep in mind that in many cases, life circumstances influence the degree of severity of premenstrual mood changes. Please make sure that you have the support you need, whether from a therapist, counselor, or confidant to take care of your mental health.

PHARMACOLOGICAL TREATMENT

The pill is usually the first choice for premenstrual mood changes because it flatlines hormone production and shuts down the cyclical changes and their subsequent effect on mood. In more advanced cases, providers may recommend a continuous pill that limits the frequency of periods to once every three months or eliminates them altogether. The logic here is that if you have fewer "periods," you will subsequently also have fewer "premenstrual periods." Keep in mind that medically induced amenorrhea is not safe and affects your long-term health. In other instances, primary care providers may refer for comanagement with a psychiatrist or may prescribe antidepressant or anxiolytic medications (selective serotonin reuptake inhibitors) such as fluoxetine, sertraline, citalopram, or paroxetine specifically for premenstrual dysphoric disorder (PMDD). Paradoxically, PMDD symptoms are often worsened by the pill.

IRRITABILITY AND/OR ANXIETY

When it comes to mood balance, estrogen is like Goldilocks—she needs levels to be "just right" or else she is finicky and unsatisfied. Both estrogen dominance as well as low estrogen, such as what we see in perimenopause, can cause irritability and anxiety. These symptoms often also present with HPA axis dysfunction: sympathetic overdrive, high cortisol, and an overactive nervous system response. These symptoms of feeling "on edge," whether that be on the edge of anger or on the edge of anxiety, may be caused by a stress response, an estrogen imbalance, or both. To figure it out, we need to look at the bigger picture. Here's why: estrogen levels always decline toward the end of the cycle, right before your period starts. These dropping hormone levels precipitate menstrual bleeding. Whether estrogen is overall high during the cycle or overall low, it still decreases during the premenstrual phase. If you tend to have other symptoms of low estrogen throughout the month, then low estrogen is likely the cause of the mood changes. On the contrary, if you experience symptoms of high estrogen throughout the month, the irritability or anxiety in the premenstrual period is still likely the result of this overall estrogen-dominance pattern and you need to take steps to support estrogen-progesterone balance. If you don't experience a clear pattern of high-estrogen or low-estrogen symptoms elsewhere throughout the month, the mood symptoms are likely the result of HPA axis dysfunction and should be treated as such. In reality, many times there are multiple factors at play, so keep this in mind when you look at the big picture of your health.

ALTERNATIVE OPTIONS:

- Irritability/Anxiety Caused by Estrogen Deficiency
  - Maca (*Lepidium meyenii*): Studies show that this adaptogenic herb reduces psychological symptoms including anxiety and depression during the premenstrual period. The dosage used in the study is

3.5 grams per day for twelve weeks,[25] though you may find tremendous benefit from a much lower dose of 500 mg three times daily. This is the dose I prescribe to my patients to start. In many cultures, maca root is used as a food, so it is thought to be likely safe for use at much higher doses as well as for use in breastfeeding mothers.
- Ashwagandha (*Withania somnifera*): Adaptogenic herbs like ashwagandha regulate the nervous system response and facilitate activation of the parasympathetic nervous system. The dosage I recommend to my patients is 200 mg twice daily during the premenstrual and menstrual phases.[26]
- Black cohosh (*Cimifuga racemosa*): Due to its effectiveness in treating menopausal symptoms that are driven by low estrogen, this herb, which stimulates opiate receptors, also effectively mitigates mood symptoms driven by other low-estrogen conditions.[27] The dosage I recommend to my patients is 50 mg daily. Please note that you should not take this herbal medicine during the luteal phase if there is a chance you could be pregnant.
- Irritability/Anxiety Caused by Estrogen Dominance
  - Diindolylmethane (DIM): DIM modulates estrogen metabolism and supports clearance of estrogen and its metabolites. The dosage I recommend to my patients is 300 mg DIM as a dietary supplement daily, and consider increasing consumption of cruciferous vegetables, which are a natural source of DIM.[28]
  - Chaste tree (*Vitex agnus-castus*): Because vitex binds to estrogen receptors and modulates their expression in cells, it is an effective method for mitigating the effects of excess estrogen.[29] The dosage I recommend to my patients is 40 mg daily for at least three months.
  - Omega-3s: In a pilot trial, omega-3s reduced the severity of psychiatric symptoms of PMS including both depression and anxiety.[30] The dosage I recommend to my patients is at least 3,000 mg of cod liver oil daily. For a more potent effect, take 5,000 mg daily during the premenstrual and menstrual phases and reduce to 1,000 mg daily during the other phases of your cycle.
  - Natural progesterone: When the more conservative approaches listed above in combination with foundational lifestyle changes are not effective at significantly reducing estrogen-dominant premenstrual mood changes for my patients, I prescribe natural progesterone therapy.

- Irritability/Anxiety Caused by HPA Axis Dysfunction
    - Ashwagandha (*Withania somnifera*): Adaptogenic herbs like ashwagandha regulate the nervous system response and facilitate activation of the parasympathetic nervous system. The dosage I recommend to my patients is 200 mg twice daily during the premenstrual and menstrual phases.[31]
    - Rhodiola (*Rhodiola rosea*): An adaptogenic herb, rhodiola is particularly effective at treating cognitive symptoms of chronic stress reactions such as anxiety and anger. The dosage I recommend to my patients is 200 mg twice daily, once before breakfast and once before lunch.[32]
    - Valerian root: Commonly prescribed to combat anxiety symptoms of multiple origins, clinical trials have shown its effectiveness in addressing specifically premenstrual anxiety as well. I commonly prescribe 500 mg twice daily, but doses as low as 200 mg may be effective depending on the person.[33]
    - Maca (*Lepidium meyenii*): Studies show that this adaptogenic herb reduces psychological symptoms including anxiety and depression during the premenstrual period. The dosage used in the study is 3.5 grams per day for twelve weeks,[34] though you may find tremendous benefit from a much lower dose of 500 mg three times daily. This is the dose I prescribe to my patients to start. In many cultures, maca root is used as a food, so it is thought to be likely safe for use at much higher doses as well as for use in breastfeeding mothers.

DEPRESSION

Premenstrual depression is classically an estrogen dominant condition, occurring in the five to seven days prior to your period starting. Keep in mind that this should be distinguished from other types of depression that are noncyclic. If you feel depressed most of the time on most days, it is not likely to be related to your period and is outside the scope of this book. You should speak with your doctor about next steps. If you ever experience suicidal thoughts or thoughts of harming yourself or others, please seek immediate help by calling 911.

ALTERNATIVE OPTIONS:

- Omega-3s: In a pilot trial, omega-3s reduced the severity of psychiatric PMS symptoms including both depression and anxiety.[35] The dosage I recommend to my patients is at least 3,000 mg of cod liver oil daily. For a more potent effect, take 5,000 mg daily during the premenstrual and menstrual phases and reduce to 1,000 mg daily during the other phases of your cycle.
- Chaste tree (*Vitex agnus-castus*): Because vitex binds to estrogen receptors and modulates their expression in cells, it is an effective method for mitigating the effects of estrogen that is insufficiently opposed by progesterone.[36] The dosage I recommend to my patients is 40 mg daily for at least three months.
- 5-Hydroxytryptophan (5-HTP): 5-HTP is an amino acid derivative of tryptophan, found in many food products. This particular form is a direct precursor to the formation of serotonin, which is a powerful neurotransmitter that regulates mood, energy and cognition. In many contexts, supplementing with 5-HTP achieves an antidepressant effect[37] and early studies have shown that women dealing with premenstrual depression may actually exhibit a relative deficiency of 5-HTP in the left side of their brains compared to the right.[38] Because doses above 100 mg may cause gastrointestinal symptoms like vomiting, the dosage I recommend to my patients is starting with 50 mg twice daily for at least eight weeks (or two full menstrual cycles). It takes time for 5-HTP to influence serotonin levels, so the effects are much more delayed compared to some other strategies. Do not combine 5-HTP with psychiatric medications, especially SSRIs.
- S-adenosylmethionine (SAMe): SAMe is a methyl donor, which means it regulates other metabolic and chemical processes in the body. (Adding or removing a methyl molecule is akin to turning on or off a switch.) This is especially true of neurotransmitters and regulation of inflammation. Research has shown that SAMe effectively reduces symptoms of depression, including premenstrual and perinatal depression. The dosage I recommend to my patients is to start with 1,600 mg daily, though this can be increased to 3,200 mg daily if symptoms do not respond within three months.[39]
- Vitamin B6: Studies show that oral supplementation of up to 100 mg/day of vitamin B6 is beneficial in treating premenstrual depression.[40] The mechanism for how this works is yet unclear.

PREMENSTRUAL DYSPHORIC DISORDER (PMDD)

Premenstrual dysphoric disorder is a severe form of premenstrual depression characterized by mood changes, headaches, fatigue, and often an amalgamation of other premenstrual symptoms. Please consider the impact of these symptoms on your quality of life when choosing a treatment strategy. If you ever experience suicidal thoughts or thoughts of harming yourself or others, please seek immediate help by calling 911.

ALTERNATIVE OPTIONS:

- St. John's wort (*Hypericum perforatum*): St. John's wort influences neurotransmitter levels in the brain, which are responsible for regulating mood and cognitive function. This herb functions similarly to SSRIs, prescription medications used to treat anxiety and depression. The dosage I recommend to my patients is 900 mg per day of St. John's wort root (standardized to include 0.18 percent hypericin, 3.38 percent hyperforin) for at least two full cycles.[41] Note that it takes at least six weeks for levels to build up in your system high enough to see a change in mood, so you likely won't notice a difference in your first cycle. Do not combine St. John's wort with psychiatric medications, especially SSRIs or 5-HTP.
- GABA: GABA is a neurotransmitter in the brain that helps regulate sleep, mood, and energy levels. Hormones related to progesterone, secreted in the luteal phase, react with GABA receptors in the brain and subsequently exacerbate mood changes in the premenstrual period.[42] Dosage ranges from 100 mg to 300 mg. The dosage I recommend to my patients is 100 mg for at least four weeks before increasing to a higher dosage. GABA supplementation also strongly influences sleep and can be used to treat insomnia both in the premenstrual period and otherwise.[43] Do not combine GABA with psychiatric medications.

Painful Periods

Painful periods aren't normal. While some degree of pelvic tenderness and inflammation is to be expected as a result of prostaglandins released during this time, anything that debilitates you to where you can't function in your day-to-day life is a problem. You really shouldn't even need to take painkillers to manage the cramping despite the ubiquity of this practice. Heating pads, warm baths, and stretching are also helpful for managing period pain but again—period pain is not normal. Severe menstrual pain is called dysmenorrhea. It's a classified medical condition and should be treated as such. If menstrual pain is so bad that over-the-counter strategies don't work, it's dysmenorrhea, which is a category apart from the type of period pain that lasts a few days around the onset of your period.

PHARMACOLOGICAL TREATMENT

Ibuprofen and acetaminophen are the most common painkillers prescribed for management of period pain. Acetaminophen is more commonly recommended, but it doesn't work as well because it lacks the anti-inflammatory properties found in NSAIDs like ibuprofen and it also depletes glutathione, which damages your liver and lead to a buildup of toxins. When over-the-counter strategies don't work, physicians may prescribe high-dose NSAIDs, such as 800 mg tablets of ibuprofen or mefenamic acid. They also typically prescribe hormonal contraceptives. In severe cases of dysmenorrhea, extended cycle pills are recommended to reduce the number of bleeds. The idea here is that if you aren't having periods, then you can't have period pain.

You should note that although dysmenorrhea is its own diagnosed condition, it is sometimes driven by another underlying issue such as adenomyosis or endometriosis (see below). Ovarian cysts occasionally cause pain and tenderness in the pelvic area, and that pain can become severe if the cyst ruptures. Keep in mind that ovarian cysts are not the same thing as polycystic ovarian syndrome (PCOS), as the "cysts" seen on ultrasound in PCOS are not true cysts. Many women have ovarian cysts and most resolve on their own. However, some become very large and can cause pain (even separately from menstruation) and irregular bleeding. Others may be cancerous. If you think you have an ovarian cyst, it's important that you see a health care provider because you may need to have it surgically removed. Recurrent ovarian cysts may be caused by hypothyroidism, and likewise hypothyroidism has a strong clinical relationship with PCOS,[44] though PCOS is not typically understood to be a direct cause of period pain. If you have PCOS, treat that first. If you still have pain, then this section is for you.

ALTERNATIVE OPTIONS:

- Omega-3s: Omega-3 fatty acids increase the anti-inflammatory division of the immune system and reduce prostaglandins. They have been demonstrated in the research to directly reduce menstrual pain.[45] The dosage I recommend to my patients is at least 3,000 mg of cod liver oil daily. For a more potent effect, take 5,000 mg daily during the premenstrual and menstrual phases and reduce to 1,000 mg daily during the other phases of your cycle.
- Turmeric (*Curcuma cyminum*): Curcumin is an anti-inflammatory herb, reducing the prostaglandins associated with menstrual pain. This form of turmeric has been shown in clinical trials to have a comparable albeit lower-risk pain-relieving effect compared to prescription NSAIDs in treating dysmenorrhea. The dosage I recommend to my patients is 1,000 mg of curcumin twice daily, as needed.[46]
- Magnesium glycinate: Magnesium is involved in hundreds of chemical reactions in the body and has been shown in the research to be an effective treatment for dysmenorrhea. To take daily as a preventative, the dosage I recommend to my patients is 400 mg of magnesium glycinate daily with food. This dose should be continued for at least one month and if no benefit is seen, the dose can be increased to 400 mg twice or up to three times daily with food. Note that while digestive symptoms are less common with this form of magnesium (glycinate), higher doses of magnesium may cause nausea, diarrhea, and/or bowel urgency.[47]
- Ginger (*Zinziber officinale*): Ginger inhibits prostaglandins, the inflammatory chemicals released when your uterine lining starts to break down at the onset of your period.[48] The dosage I recommend to my patients is 300 mg three times daily during a period.
- Fennel (*Foeniculum vulgare*): Fennel has been shown to be as effective as prescription NSAIDs in treating period pain but with fewer risks.[49] Similar to ginger, fennel works by inhibiting prostaglandins. The dosage I recommend to my patients is 30 mg four times daily when cramping occurs.[50]
- Pycnogenol (French pine bark): Research shows that supplementing with 60 mg daily of pine bark for at least two full menstrual cycles significantly reduces the pain response. This pain-relieving effect increases the longer that the strategy is used, and the effect continues even after discontinuation of the pycnogenol, but we don't know

exactly how long this pain-relieving effect continues. (It probably depends on the person.)[51]
- Acupuncture: Research shows that acupuncture and techniques of Traditional Chinese Medicine (TCM) are also effective at reducing menstrual pain.[52] One common point used in acupuncture for relieving pain, including menstrual pain, is Large Intestine 4 (LI-4). You can stimulate this point with acupressure at home, as needed, by pinching or rubbing the webbing between your thumb and pointer finger on each hand for about ninety seconds.

IS IT YOUR MENSTRUAL PRODUCTS?

We've come a long way since the late 1800s when menstrual products first became commercially available to the average consumer. Today, options abound for keeping clean during your period, with everything from disposable pads and tampons to reusable ones, to the menstrual disc, menstrual cup, and even washable, absorbent bamboo period underwear that eliminates the need for other types of protection. Having options available is super empowering, but sometimes the specific options chosen may worsen period problems, like pain. There are two key ways that this can occur, one being with inflammatory chemicals and two being structural problems.

With regards to inflammation, some of the materials used to produce disposable menstrual products like bleach and preservatives cause irritation and immunoreactivity when they come into contact with your body. The tissue lining the vaginal walls is very sensitive and absorbent, and these chemicals can leach into the surrounding space and stimulate an inflammatory immune response. Compounding the already increased prostaglandin levels around onset of menstruation, the inflammatory problem multiplies and worsens pain. Consider choosing unbleached varieties of pads and tampons made with organic ingredients and see if that alone makes a difference for you.

If it doesn't, you might be experiencing a structural problem. During your period, the thick muscular walls of your uterus contract downward to expel blood and tissue. When this occurs, the cervix moves downward in the vaginal canal. When a tampon is inserted behind the cervix, sometimes the cervix itself pushes up against the tampon during uterine contraction, which can be really painful. The cervix is sensitive to touch as it is, but when contracting against a foreign object, this is akin to the difference between punching up into the air versus punching a wall. *Ouch!* If you notice that your pain is worse when using a tampon than it is when you use external menstrual products, first make sure that your tampon is inserted correctly: angled slightly backward and far enough up into your vagina. If you still experience pain, consider avoiding tampons altogether and instead choose a menstrual cup (which surrounds the cervix instead of abutting it) or avoiding internal methods in favor of pads or period underwear.

Sometimes painful periods are caused by an underlying problem with how the menstrual lining develops. If you recall from earlier chapters, the endometrial lining normally develops on the interior of the uterine walls, within the uterine body. This tissue thickens throughout the cycle and ultimately sheds as menstrual blood. However, sometimes this endometrial tissue develops incorrectly, such as outside the uterus, attached to the ovaries, bowel, or other pelvic structures as is the case with endometriosis, or within the muscular walls of the uterus itself, as in adenomyosis. Both conditions are accompanied by intense pain, inflammation, and bleeding. They may also affect fertility.

Adenomyosis

Adenomyosis is a condition in which the uterine lining grows into the muscular wall of the uterus. Because of this, it is often accompanied by uterine enlargement that leads to worsened bloating and pelvic inflammation in addition to heavy bleeding and severe pain. Adenomyosis is often identified through pelvic imaging, such as ultrasound or MRI but the only definitive diagnosis can be made if a hysterectomy is performed and the tissue is examined afterward. We understand adenomyosis to be an estrogen-dominant condition, though it is paradoxically more common in women who have taken the drug tamoxifen for treatment of breast cancer. Although tamoxifen is an estrogen blocker, it actually creates an exaggerated estrogen response in certain types of tissue such as the endometrial lining.[53]

PHARMACOLOGICAL TREATMENT

The usual treatment for adenomyosis is not classically pharmacological in nature but rather surgical. The hysterectomy is considered the only "cure" for adenomyosis. Given that adenomyosis symptoms typically resolve after menopause, a hysterectomy can cause significant concerns for women of child-bearing age, so some providers utilize endometrial ablation or excisional surgery in which the endometrium is the only tissue removed. This gives mixed results, and both of these procedures still affect fertility. Likewise, some women experience relief from using hormonal contraceptives such as the birth control pill or the Mirena intrauterine device (IUD) when they have adenomyosis. However, the downside of hormonal contraceptives is that they block the body's own, good hormones, especially progesterone, which natural has pain-relieving effects.

ALTERNATIVE OPTIONS:

- Proteolytic enzymes: Proteases are enzymes that help break down proteins such as muscle tissue, particularly when affected by inflammation. In medicine, these are classically used to heal and repair inflamed muscle tissue and restore blood flow.[54] Clinically, they can be applied to conditions like adenomyosis that are characterized by this type of inflammation. The dosage I recommend to my patients is between 500 and 1,000 mg three times daily at least one hour apart from food. Note that proteolytic enzymes have multiple applications in medicine, including for digestion. If you take these enzymes with food, they will exert their activity on breaking down the food rather than in repair of your own tissues. Taken this way, however, they may cause mild stomach upset or heartburn. Serrapeptase (serratiopeptidase) is one such proteolytic enzyme that works well in this context, but bromelain, papain, and other blends are also effective.
- Diindolylmethane (DIM): DIM modulates estrogen metabolism and supports clearance of estrogen and its metabolites through liver detoxification pathways. Because adenomyosis is an estrogen-dominant condition, proper estrogen metabolism is essential. The dosage I recommend to my patients is 300 mg DIM as a daily dietary supplement, and consider increasing consumption of cruciferous vegetables, which are a natural source of DIM.[55]
- Calcium-D-glucarate (CDG): Like DIM, CDG regulates estrogen metabolism and clearance through liver detoxification pathways.[56] With a condition like adenomyosis with extremely debilitating symptoms, often a multipronged approach for estrogen clearance is

warranted. In addition to DIM, I recommend that my patients with adenomyosis take 500 mg of CDG daily.
- Dong quai (*Angelica sinensis*): In TCM, the herb dong quai improves blood flow and tone of the uterus, with adenomyosis reflecting a condition of blood and qi stagnation. This herb helps relieve spasming and pain, and modulates estrogen levels,[57] though in some cases it may actually increase bleeding. For this reason, it is typically combined with other modulating herbs such as lady's mantle. The typical dose of dong quai is 500 mg to 1,000 mg three times daily.
- Lady's mantle (*Alchemilla vulgaris*): This herb is used in combination with dong quai from a TCM perspective to cool the uterus and release dampness and laxity, and to control menstrual flow. It has also been theorized to promote progesterone production, an essential hormone for controlling inflammation and balancing estrogen. Lady's mantle is typically dosed as a tincture of half a teaspoon two to three times daily.
- Omega-3s: Omega-3 fatty acids increase the anti-inflammatory division of the immune system and reduce prostaglandins. They have been demonstrated in the research to directly reduce menstrual pain.[58] The dosage I recommend to my patients is at least 3,000 mg of cod liver oil daily. For a more potent effect, take 5,000 mg daily during the premenstrual and menstrual phases and reduce to 1,000 mg daily during the other phases of your cycle.
- Progesterone cream: Given the estrogen-dominant nature of adenomyosis and the anti-inflammatory, pain-relieving effects of progesterone, progesterone therapy just makes sense. I recommend natural progesterone cream to my patients as a safer, healthier alternative to oral contraceptives.[59]

Endometriosis

Similar to adenomyosis, endometriosis is accompanied by severe pain and cramping, bleeding and bloating. Especially when the tissue affects the bowel, menstrual cycles with endometriosis are often accompanied by digestive pain and constipation. Scar tissue formation in the pelvic cavity resulting from this inflammation may significantly affect fertility outcomes—even more so than in adenomyosis. Endometriosis is officially diagnosed through laparoscopy surgery when the pelvic cavity can be clearly seen, though inflammatory changes related to endometriosis can also often be identified through imaging such as ultrasound and MRI. Like adenomyosis, we also understand endometriosis to be an estrogen-dominant condition, though it also shares links with autoimmunity and some physicians treat it as such.

PHARMACOLOGICAL TREATMENT

Birth control pills are often a first-line treatment for endometriosis, often utilizing an extended-cycle strategy to reduce the number of periods the woman has per year. The progestins in the birth control pill are considered the standard of care for endometriosis. Physicians may also prescribe aromatase inhibitors such as letrozole or anastrozole which reduce the concentration of estrogen in the body, as endometriosis is an estrogen-dominant condition. In severe cases, surgery may be recommended to remove the tissue growing in the pelvic cavity. This reduces the inflammatory response and pain because the inflammatory tissue itself is removed. Surgery often improves fertility for several months afterward. This is not a permanent solution, however, and some women end up having several surgeries throughout their life. Gynecologists also commonly prescribe pain medications or recommend high doses of over-the-counter ibuprofen and acetaminophen to manage the symptoms of endometriosis.

ALTERNATIVE OPTIONS:

If you have endometriosis, you know that it's another level of period pain—it affects your whole body. Treatment is not as simple as taking some enzymes or herbs, just like it's not as simple as taking the birth control pill. However, overhauling your lifestyle to be as foundationally healthy as possible and implementing some of the following strategies can be extremely helpful and hopefully reduce the need for surgery, or other types of high-level interventions.

- Proteolytic enzymes: Like adenomyosis, proteolytic enzymes can be useful in treatment of endometriosis which is characterized by scar tissue and inflammation. The dosage I recommend to my patients is between 500 and 1,000 mg three times daily at least one hour apart from food. Note that proteolytic enzymes have multiple applications in medicine, including for digestion. If you take these enzymes with food, they will exert their activity on breaking down the food rather than in repair of your own tissues. Taken this way, however, they may cause mild stomach upset or heartburn. Serrapeptase (serratiopeptidase) is one such proteolytic enzyme that works well in this context, but bromelain, papain, and other blends are also effective.

- Omega-3s: Omega-3 fatty acids are highly effective at reducing the prostaglandin-related inflammation seen in endometriosis and subsequent pelvic pain.[60] The dosage I recommend to my patients is at least 3,000 mg of cod liver oil daily. For a more potent effect, take 5,000 mg daily during the premenstrual and menstrual phases and reduce to 1,000 mg daily during the other phases of your cycle.
- Turmeric (*Curcuma longa*): Curcumin blocks the inflammatory chemical interleukin-6 making it a very effective and safe treatment for inflammatory disorders like endometriosis. The dosage I recommend to my patients is 1,000 mg twice daily.[61]
- Resveratrol: Resveratrol is an antioxidant, anti-inflammatory compound that helps modulate the immune system—an especially helpful effect in quasi-autoimmune conditions like endometriosis. Likewise, research has demonstrated that resveratrol decreases the formation of endometriomas, the term used to describe the menstrual tissue that develops outside of the uterus.[62] Studies show effectiveness at doses as low as 40 mg per day, but it is safe to take up to 200 mg daily.
- Pycnogenol (French pine bark): In addition to the studies demonstrating a pain-relieving effect of supplementation with 60 mg daily of pycnogenol in the context of dysmenorrhea, we also have data regarding pycnogenol's effectiveness in reducing the pathogenesis of endometriosis. Pycnogenol reduces inflammatory markers, estrogen levels and pain symptoms, and has a more potent effect in cases where the endometrial growth is smaller.[63] For this reason, I especially recommend using pycnogenol following surgery if a woman utilizes this form of treatment.
- Progesterone cream: Given the estrogen-dominant nature of endometriosis, a high-level progesterone support just makes sense. Progesterone therapy is the standard of treatment in endometriosis, and I recommend natural progesterone cream to my patients as a safer, healthier alternative to oral contraceptives.[64]

Heavy Periods

If you lose more than 80 milliliters (mL) of blood during your period, this is considered heavy menstrual bleeding. This can occur through periods that involve a very heavy flow, or through periods that last more than seven days. The medical term for this is "menorrhagia" and you need to have an idea of how to measure your flow to figure out if your bleeding is normal. (Refer back to chapter 5 if you need help with this.) Even if your periods don't meet the criteria for menorrhagia, your bleeding still might be too much *for you* if you develop iron deficiency or anemia as a result. Refer back to the section on fatigue and iron deficiency if that applies to you. Here are a few other things to note about heavy periods:

- Menorrhagia characterized by very long periods (more than seven days) often are a sign of anovulatory cycles. Confirm this by tracking your cycle through the methods we outlined in chapter 7.
- Heavy periods are an estrogen-dominant condition. (Anovulatory cycles are progesterone-deficient cycles.)
- During puberty, heavy bleeding can be more common because the body's estrogen receptors haven't figured out how to regulate yet. They sometimes have an overactive response, leading to heavy bleeding and more estrogen-dominant symptoms even if hormone levels are normal. This should resolve within a few years, but you still may benefit from some of the strategies outlined in this section if this applies to you.
- Hypothyroidism is another potential cause of menorrhagia. Ask your doctor to include this screen in your labs.
- Uterine fibroids and polyps are also notorious for causing heavy menstrual flow. Particularly if your periods are accompanied by irregular bleeding, such as bleeding mid-cycle, after sex, with exercise, or otherwise, it's important to find out if you have one of these structural problems with your uterus. Make an appointment with your health care provider and ask for both internal and external pelvic ultrasounds. If you know you are dealing with one of these conditions, jump ahead to the section titled "Fibroids and Polyps."

IS IT YOUR GENES?

Sometimes a genetically related clotting disorder is the culprit behind menorrhagia. Whenever you experience bleeding (such as through a cut in your skin,) your body has to clot the blood flow to slow it down and stop it. Inability to do this correctly can lead to excessive blood loss. One such clotting disorder called hemophilia is typically diagnosed in early childhood, so you'd likely know if you have it by the time you start menstruating. Von Willebrand disease, however, can exist in a milder form and not show signs until the time of your first period. Heavy bleeding is often the first sign of this clotting disorder.[65] Both hemophilia and Von Willebrand disease can be diagnosed by a blood test. Ask your doctor to test you for these conditions if you've had heavy periods your whole life.

Pharmacological Treatment

Hormonal IUDs are commonly recommended for heavy periods because they lighten or completely eliminate menstrual bleeding. Hormonal birth control is another common strategy, though it's less likely than an IUD to reduce menstrual flow. In addition to their uses in pain-management, anti-inflammatory medications like ibuprofen are often commonly recommended during your period because they have a secondary effect of reducing menstrual bleeding by as much as 36 mLs, which is nearly half of a "normal" period.[66]

ALTERNATIVE OPTIONS:

- Pomegranate flower (*Punica granatum*, Persian Golnar): Research demonstrates that supplementing with 500 mg of this herb for five days starting on the first day of your period reduces menstrual flow and increases hemoglobin concentration.[67]
- Ginger (*Zinziber officinale*): Taking 300 mg of ginger three times daily for seven days beginning on the first day of your period significantly reduces menstrual bleeding, with a comparable effect to ibuprofen.[68]
- Frankincense (*Olibanum*): Taking 300 mg of frankincense three times daily for seven days beginning on the first day of your period significantly reduces menstrual bleeding, comparably to ibuprofen.[69]
- Chaste tree (*Vitex agnus-castus*): In addition to its progesterone-boosting effects, research shows that vitex is effective in controlling abnormal uterine bleeding, including both menorrhagia as well as other forms of abnormal bleeding and spotting.[70] The dosage I recommend to my patients is 40 to 100 mg daily throughout the cycle.
- Diindolylmethane (DIM): DIM modulates estrogen metabolism and can reduce menstrual bleeding. The dosage I recommend to my

patients is 300 mg DIM as a dietary supplement daily, and consider increasing consumption of cruciferous vegetables, which are a natural source of DIM.
- Iron supplementation: Iron deficiency commonly results from heavy menstrual bleeding due to blood loss, but iron supplementation itself has been shown in the research to decrease menstrual blood flow. The mechanisms for this effect are not totally clear, though researchers currently understand the iron supplements to affect the growth of the endometrial lining that ultimately sheds as menstrual blood loss.[71] I recommend that my patients start with 27 mg of an easy-to-digest form of iron such as iron bisglycinate and closely monitor levels via blood work.
- Progesterone is a common first-line treatment for heavy menstrual bleeding, and I recommend natural progesterone cream to my patients as a safer, healthier alternative to oral contraceptives.[72]

Fibroids and Polyps

Although fibroids and polyps are separate conditions, they have similar causes and similar treatments. Both fibroids and polyps are abnormal growths within the uterus. However, while polyps are made up of endometrial tissue, fibroids derive from the muscular walls of the uterus. Because fibroids are made of muscle tissue, they may cause abnormal cramping or pain with intercourse. Sometimes they are very large and cause a bloated or distended abdomen. Polyps are less likely to cause pain, but both polyps and fibroids are known for causing abnormal menstrual bleeding. This includes bleeding between periods, very heavy periods, bleeding after sex, with exercise, or other types of abdominal pressure. Sometimes, fibroids and polyps may get in the way of a fertilized egg implanting in the uterus and cause fertility problems. Fibroids and polyps are both estrogen-dominant conditions, classically caused by estrogen excess.

PHARMACOLOGICAL TREATMENT

Particularly in cases where severe pain or bleeding result from polyps or fibroids, or if they are particularly large, health care providers recommend their removal. This is often a good idea because the tissue can be biopsied to make sure it isn't cancerous. Small fibroids or polyps may not need to be removed. Severe cases are often followed up with estrogen-blocking medications after surgery.

Whether you have surgery or not, it's a good idea to use some natural strategies to prevent them from growing, or to prevent them from coming back if you've had them removed. Fibroids and polyps are both considered estrogen-dominant, inflammatory conditions and are more common in women with PCOS.[73] If you have PCOS, make sure you take steps to address this in order to help manage your polyps and/or fibroids.

ALTERNATIVE OPTIONS:

- Diindolylmethane (DIM): DIM modulates estrogen metabolism and supports clearance of estrogen and its metabolites. The dosage I recommend to my patients is 300 mg DIM as a dietary supplement daily, and consider increasing consumption of cruciferous vegetables, which are a natural source of DIM.[74]
- Calcium-D-Glucarate (CDG): Like DIM, CDG regulates estrogen metabolism and clearance through liver detoxification pathways.[75] With conditions like uterine polyps and fibroids, a multipronged approach for estrogen clearance is often warranted. In addition to DIM, I recommend that my patients take 500 mg of CDG daily.
- Indole-3-carbinol (I3C): Another estrogen regulator, I3C functions similarly to CDG and DIM.[76] With fibroids and polyps typically resulting from estrogen excess, I recommend a high-level anti-estrogen therapy involving all three compounds. The dosage I recommend to my patients is 200 to 400 mg of I3C daily in addition to DIM and CDG.
- Gui Zhi Fu Ling Wan: This blend of Chinese herbs is commonly prescribed to treat the imbalance between qi and blood that is understood from a TCM perspective to contribute to uterine fibroids. This herbal blend consists of five different Chinese herbs in predetermined proportions. Research shows that treatment with Guizhi Fuling increases the efficacy of pharmacological strategies in treatment of fibroids and is a promising treatment of its own.[77] The recommended dosage is 1,500 mg twice daily of a 10:1 concentrated herbal extract.

Irregular Periods

Recall from chapter 5 that irregular periods are periods that deviate from the normal interval of twenty-one to thirty-five days, the *ideal* interval of twenty-seven to thirty-three days, or that deviate more than three days from each other from cycle to cycle. Keep in mind that most women experience irregular cycles every now and then, as bouts of illness, stress, and changes in routine can all affect reproductive health. But three or more irregular cycles in a given year should catch your attention, as you may be dealing with a more significant health concern.

The classic protocol for irregular periods from a pharmacological perspective is a prescription for the birth control pill. Using a twenty-eight-day pill pack—*poof!*—the problem is solved: bleeding occurs every four weeks, like clockwork. In this sense, the birth control pill really does solve the problem of irregular periods. Previously unpredictable cycles arrive perfectly on time with hormonal contraceptives. But the pill does nothing to address (or correct) the underlying cause of irregular periods. That's where this section of this book becomes essential.

There are three main hormonal reasons for irregular periods: PCOS, hypothalamic amenorrhea, and perimenopause, all of which are described in this section. Thyroid disorders are another cause of irregular periods and can coexist with the above conditions, so make sure that you ask your provider to run a complete thyroid panel. Please also keep in mind that the condition of irregular periods is different from abnormal bleeding, such as spotting or bleeding *between* periods. That section is further along in this chapter.

Polycystic Ovarian Syndrome (PCOS)

Polycystic ovarian syndrome is a reproductive health disorder characterized by elevated androgen levels. These androgens create symptoms like facial hair growth, hair loss on the scalp, abdominal weight gain, irregular periods, cystic acne, blood sugar imbalances and more. A woman need not have all of these symptoms in order to have PCOS and she really doesn't even need to have any of them. The current most widely accepted diagnostic criteria for PCOS derive from the Rotterdam criteria that include three markers, at least two of which need to be present: elevated androgens on blood work, the polycystic appearance of ovaries on ultrasound, and ovulatory dysfunction (aka irregular periods, anovulatory cycles, or both). Remember that there are two types of androgens, dehydroepiandrosterone (DHEA) and testosterone, and at least one but not both needs to be elevated in order to diagnose PCOS, though some women indeed have elevations of both.

Because there are three different criteria that don't all need to be met in order for a PCOS diagnosis to be made, the clinical symptoms and laboratory features can look very different among different women with PCOS. In fact, in the realm of functional medicine, we have identified four different subtypes of PCOS, each with different root causes and, subsequently, different treatment plans. This is quite different from the traditional model of care that has the same pharmacological protocol for all cases: you guessed it, the pill! This is obviously counterintuitive in the context of fertility, so unfortunately fertility medications often follow birth control use in women with PCOS if they never had the chance to address the underlying root cause of their symptoms. Susceptibility to developing PCOS has genetic origins, but the factors that trigger the disorder may differ. These triggers are how we classify the four different types of PCOS: (1) insulin-resistant, (2) adrenal, (3) post-pill, and (4) inflammatory.[78]

PHARMACOLOGICAL TREATMENT

If you have irregular periods, the pill is most commonly prescribed. Ironically, three of the four possible types of progestin available in birth control pills increase androgenic side effects, often worsening PCOS symptoms. The fourth generation of progesterone blocks androgens but significantly elevates risks of cancers and potentially deadly blood clots. This is why I strongly recommend *against* birth control for PCOS. Some health care providers recommend spironolactone as an androgen blocker, or metformin to address the blood sugar and weight gain problems that often accompany PCOS. These make a little more sense to me, but they both come with side effects and there are better options available.

ALTERNATIVE OPTIONS FOR INSULIN-RESISTANT PCOS

Insulin-resistant PCOS is the most common type of PCOS, making up about 70 percent of cases.[79] With insulin-resistant PCOS, the main driver of androgen production is elevated insulin. This can be identified on a blood test and is commonly seen when a woman has high levels of abdominal body fat. It is also often (but not always) accompanied by elevated fasting glucose and/or glycated hemoglobin levels, which may indicate prediabetes or diabetes. In PCOS, the cells that produce testosterone are sensitive to insulin, so insulin in the blood leads to a higher-than-normal production of testosterone by the ovaries. In turn, the higher levels of testosterone feed forward into poor blood sugar control and decreased insulin sensitivity (i.e., causing insulin resistance), leading to even more insulin production. This insulin then stimulates fat cell growth, and those fat cells produce even more insulin. It becomes a feed-forward cycle, which is why addressing insulin as the root cause is essential for treating the PCOS.

- Inositol: Inositol is a special type of sugar that hormones and neurons use to signal to each other. It's not like dietary sugar, though, and isn't processed by the body the way that typical carbohydrates are. The research shows that inositol is very effective in controlling blood sugar in PCOS[80] and it also serves as an anti-inflammatory.[81] Moreover, its use has been shown to improve all symptoms, signs, and diagnostic lab markers in PCOS regardless of the underlying cause,[82] which is why I include it as a treatment for all four types of PCOS. Inositol is sold as a powder that can be taken with or without food, at 2,000 mg twice daily. Look for a product that contains a 40:1 ratio of myo-inositol to D-chiro inositol.
- Magnesium glycinate: This essential mineral is commonly depleted, and supplementation has been shown to improve blood sugar elevations, elevated insulin, and insulin resistance.[83] The dosage I recommend to my patients is 300 to 450 mg daily with food.
- Berberine: This plant-derived compound improves insulin sensitivity and glucose metabolism. It also serves as an anti-inflammatory.[84] The dosage I recommend to my patients is 500 mg with each meal. Note that berberine also is commonly used as an antimicrobial agent and affects your microbiome. For this reason, I do not recommend using berberine for longer than three months at a time without monitoring your gut microbiome.
- Alpha lipoic acid (ALA): ALA improves ovulation rates and shortens cycles in women with PCOS.[85] It also acts as an anti-inflammatory[86] and regulates insulin responsiveness and glucose metabolism.[87] The dosage I recommend to my patients is 600 mg twice daily with food.

- Zinc: Zinc is an essential mineral, commonly deficient in the Western world due to soil-degenerating farming practices. Beyond zinc deficiency, however, zinc supplementation has been shown in the research to improve insulin sensitivity and fasting glucose levels in women with PCOS.[88] The dosage I recommend to my patients is 30 to 50 mg daily with food. Note that zinc taken on an empty stomach is likely to cause nausea, so I recommend taking it with your largest meal of the day.
- Diindolylmethane (DIM): Because PCOS (especially insulin-resistant PCOS) leads to estrogen excess, utilizing strategies to control estrogen is a good idea in the early stages of treatment. DIM modulates estrogen metabolism and limits estrogen excess. The dosage I recommend to my patients is 300 mg DIM as a dietary supplement daily, and consider increasing consumption of cruciferous vegetables, which are a natural source of DIM.[89]
- Spearmint tea: Clinical trials have demonstrated that consuming spearmint tea twice daily significantly reduces testosterone levels in women with PCOS. It also modulates blood sugar and improves the relationship of FSH and LH in blood.[90]

ALTERNATIVE OPTIONS FOR ADRENAL PCOS

The term "androgens" encompasses both testosterone and DHEA, and DHEA itself can be made by both ovaries and adrenal glands. DHEA is also converted into testosterone, so increased production of DHEA alone can itself produce the effects of elevated testosterone in addition to the other androgenic symptoms it causes on its own. If DHEA is the only elevated androgen, we consider this an adrenal cause of PCOS. The adrenal glands classically produce DHEA as a component of the stress response, so in this way chronic stress becomes a driver of increased androgen production and perpetuates the PCOS process. I also consider adrenal PCOS if a patient did not recently discontinue the pill, has relatively low levels of hs-CRP on blood work, and does not have insulin resistance, even if testosterone is also elevated in addition to DHEA. In other words, if we can rule out the other causes of PCOS *and* DHEA is elevated, it's adrenal PCOS.

CONGENITAL ADRENAL HYPERPLASIA

Because both the ovaries and the adrenal glands make DHEA, sometimes a genetic disorder that increases adrenal production of DHEA is the culprit behind elevated androgen levels. This disorder can be identified through a blood test for 17-hydroxyprogesterone. If your DHEA is elevated on blood work, ask your doctor to run this additional test. (If cortisol is also elevated, you may also ask about having a clinical workup for Cushing's syndrome.)

- Inositol: Inositol is a special type of sugar that hormones and neurons use to signal to each other. It's not like dietary sugar, though, and isn't processed by the body the way that typical carbohydrates are. The research shows that inositol is very effective in controlling blood sugar in PCOS[91] and it also serves as an anti-inflammatory.[92] Moreover, its use has been shown to improve all symptoms, signs, and diagnostic lab markers in PCOS regardless of the underlying cause,[93] which is why I include it as a treatment for all four types of PCOS. Inositol is sold as a powder that can be taken with or without food, at 2,000 mg twice daily. Look for a product that contains a 40:1 ratio of myo-inositol to D-chiro inositol.
- Vitamin C (ascorbic acid): Vitamin C is utilized in high amounts by the adrenal glands, and depletion can lead to adrenal dysfunction. Supplementing with vitamin C lowers adrenal production of both cortisol and DHEA and can improve the fatigue that often accompanies adrenal PCOS.[94] The dosage I recommend to my patients is 1,000 mg daily in divided doses, with food. Note that vitamin C taken on an empty stomach, or large doses taken all at once, may cause diarrhea.
- White peony (*Paeonia lactiflora*): In addition to correcting the androgen excess seen in PCOS,[95] this herb modulates the hypothalamic-pituitary-adrenal axis[96] making it an excellent choice for adrenal PCOS. The dosage I recommend to my patients is 250 mg of paeoniflorin, the active component in white peony, twice daily.
- Ashwagandha (*Withania somnifera*): In addition to the numerous other benefits of this powerful herb, ashwagandha improves insulin sensitivity and adrenal production of hormones. This effect is so potent that it even can be used in the treatment of congenital adrenal hyperplasia and may improve adrenal causes of scalp hair loss.[97] The dosage I recommend to my patients is 200 mg twice daily every day of the cycle.

Alternative Options for Post-Pill PCOS

The pill blocks ovarian function and interrupts the signaling between the brain and ovaries. (This is the whole point.) Coming off the pill (or other hormonal contraceptives, like an IUD) sometimes leads to rebound androgen production that returns with a vengeance. Post-pill PCOS is diagnosed when you never had symptoms or lab markers of PCOS prior to using birth control but developed them afterward. The good news about post-pill PCOS is that it almost always resolves completely, though this can take several years if you aren't actively managing it through the strategies outlined below. Keep in mind that this is different from PCOS that was present prior to using hormonal contraceptives and returned after discontinuing their use.

- Inositol: Inositol is a special type of sugar that hormones and neurons use to signal to each other. It's not like dietary sugar, though, and isn't processed by the body the way that typical carbohydrates are. The research shows that inositol is very effective in controlling blood sugar in PCOS[98] and it also serves as an anti-inflammatory.[99] Moreover, its use has been shown to improve all symptoms, signs, and diagnostic lab markers in PCOS regardless of the underlying cause, which is why I include it as a treatment for all four[100] types of PCOS. Inositol is sold as a powder that can be taken with or without food, at 2,000 mg twice daily. Look for a product that contains a 40:1 ratio of myo-inositol to D-chiro inositol.
- Post-pill support: In addition to inositol, which has such robust scientific support in all forms of PCOS, you will benefit tremendously from taking some targeted steps to help your body heal from the excess hormone exposure from birth control use. Refer back to the section "Coming Off the Pill: Other Ways to Support Your Body" in chapter 10.

ALTERNATIVE OPTIONS FOR INFLAMMATORY PCOS

Inflammation directly stimulates ovarian androgen production. However, as we have referenced many times[101] already, inflammation doesn't just come from one place. Insulin resistance, chronic stress, and using hormonal contraceptives all create inflammation and drive androgen production. So, if those three factors are not present and you still are experiencing PCOS and elevated inflammatory markers on blood work (including but not limited to hs-CRP and ESR), we call it inflammatory PCOS. The best treatment, of course, is to identify the driver of inflammation and treat it there. Doing so isn't always easy and ultimately goes beyond the scope of this book. That being said, you sometimes need to address the most glaringly obvious health issue and if PCOS is that for you, please see the following:

- Inositol: Inositol is a special type of sugar that hormones and neurons use to signal to each other. It's not like dietary sugar, though, and isn't processed by the body the way that typical carbohydrates are. The research shows that inositol is very effective in controlling blood sugar in PCOS[102] and it also serves as an anti-inflammatory.[103] Moreover, its use has been shown to improve all symptoms, signs, and diagnostic lab markers in PCOS regardless of the underlying cause,[104] which is why I include it as a treatment for all four types of PCOS. Inositol is sold as a powder that can be taken with or without food, at 2,000 mg twice daily. Look for a product that contains a 40:1 ratio of myo-inositol to D-chiro inositol.
- Turmeric (*Curcuma longa*): Curcumin blocks the inflammatory chemical interleukin-6 making it a very effective and safe treatment for inflammatory disorders. The dosage I recommend to my patients is 1,000 mg twice daily.[105]
- Alpha lipoic acid (ALA): ALA improves ovulation rates and shortens cycles in women with PCOS.[106] It also acts as an anti-inflammatory[107] and regulates insulin responsiveness and glucose metabolism.[108] The dosage I recommend to my patients is 600 mg twice daily with food.
- N-acetyl-cysteine (NAC): This anti-inflammatory amino acid is great for PCOS because it not only fights inflammation but also improves insulin sensitivity.[109] The dosage I recommend to my patients is 500 to 600 mg twice daily.
- Melatonin: Commonly thought of as a natural sleep treatment, melatonin is a hormone that interacts with other hormonal pathways in the body. In PCOS specifically, it improves ovulatory outcomes and suppresses inflammation and oxidative stress.[110] I recommend that my patients take 5 mg melatonin every night around bedtime. Note that sometimes melatonin use can cause morning grogginess. If this occurs for you, cut your dosage in half.

Hypothalamic Amenorrhea

Unlike PCOS in which the ovaries fail to respond to signaling from the brain, in hypothalamic amenorrhea, the brain does not send signals to the ovaries to trigger ovulation at all. In hypothalamic amenorrhea, irregular or missing periods are the result of stress suppressing the brain's ovarian signaling. As a result of this, the ovaries never get the message to ripen follicles, the uterine lining never starts to grow and thicken, and subsequently neither ovulation nor periods occur. Although hypothalamic amenorrhea (HA) can be a complicating factor in PCOS or other reproductive disorders, worsening those existing problems, we diagnose it only after ruling out other causes. Because HA involves lack of brain signaling to the ovaries, we see low levels of both brain hormones and ovarian hormones on blood work. These levels include FSH, LH, estrogen, and progesterone. Classically, DHEA and testosterone are also low, but this is not always the case, especially if intense exercise is the cause—because exercise can increase DHEA and testosterone.

PHARMACOLOGICAL TREATMENT

The classic treatment for HA is hormone replacement therapy through oral contraceptive use. The artificial estrogen in the pill thickens the uterine lining and results in eventual bleeding during the placebo pack. However, since the root cause of HA is suppression of brain hormones LH and FSH, the pill does not truly treat the problem because FSH and LH remain low when the pill is used. However, users of the pill usually experience the return of monthly bleeding, which merely masks the underlying problem. Periods typically disappear again as soon as the pill is stopped.

ALTERNATIVE OPTIONS:

The number one way to treat HA naturally is to remove the stressor that suppressed brain hormones in the first place—that is, when doing so is possible. Sometimes, psychological stressors and traumas are not so easily solved, and in those cases I strongly recommend psychotherapy and social support as needed. Hypothalamic amenorrhea is also very common in eating disorders, so if you are struggling in your relationship with food, please seek help. HA is also common in those who engage in intense exercise without sufficient caloric intake. There is a common misconception that low weight and/or low body fat percentage are necessary for HA to result from exercise, but this is not true. Women of all shapes and sizes experience biological stress from excessive exercise and insufficient calorie intake, and the risks of HA are equally dangerous for all: loss of bone mineral density, infertility, heart disease, hair loss, and all the other risks associated with low estrogen and progesterone. As a complement to the necessary lifestyle changes, the following natural treatments can help calm the body's stress response and support a faster return to fertility.

- Ashwagandha (*Withania somnifera*): Adaptogenic herbs like ashwagandha regulate the nervous system response and facilitate activation of the parasympathetic nervous system. The dosage I recommend to my patients is 200 mg twice daily.[111]
- Black Cohosh (*Cimifuga racemosa*): Similar to the fertility drug Clomid, 20 mg daily doses of black cohosh trigger an LH surge (notoriously missing in HA) and results in higher progesterone levels (also absent in HA) during the luteal phase.[112]
- Maca (*Lepidium peruvianum*): Maca is another adaptogen well suited to reproductive health concerns. It benefits hypothalamic amenorrhea by lowering cortisol and other components of the stress response in addition to regulating estrogen expression in cells. The dosage I recommend to my patients is 500 mg of pre-gelatinized maca powder three times daily.[113]
- Acupuncture: In TCM, amenorrhea is understood to result from a deficiency of qi and blood. In the case of HA, the specific obstructions to the flow of qi and blood influence treatment. Despite its highly individualized nature, acupuncture treatment has been demonstrated to improve brain-ovarian signaling in hypothalamic amenorrhea.[114]

Perimenopause

A third common cause of irregular or missing periods is perimenopause. Perimenopause refers to the time when ovarian function declines due to age, until full menopause (absence of a menstrual period for twelve consecutive months due to age) has been achieved. During perimenopause, the ovaries respond inconsistently to LH and FSH signals from the brain causing estrogen and progesterone levels to likewise rise and fall irregularly. These dramatic changes in estrogen and progesterone levels are responsible for symptoms like irregular periods, mood changes, and mid-cycle spotting. We diagnose perimenopause when a woman is above forty and her LH level is normal, but FSH is above 30 IU/L. Sometimes perimenopause can occur between ages thirty-five and forty, but if it occurs prior to this we consider it to be premature.

PHARMACOLOGICAL TREATMENT

Hormone replacement therapy. Oral contraceptives override the natural rise and fall of hormones in the body and essentially flatlines them. The result is a chemically controlled albeit highly predictable bleed. Other times, a Mirena IUD is recommended, which bridges the gap between perimenopause and menopause while overriding ovarian hormones and suppressing brain hormones. It also classically eliminates the problem of irregular and unpredictable bleeding during this time due to its thinning effect on the uterine lining. Compared to hormonal contraceptives, the Mirena IUD is a lower dose and consequently safer form of hormonal intervention.

ALTERNATIVE OPTIONS:

- Cyclic therapy: Utilizing techniques that mimic a natural cycle, I recommend alternating between black cohosh during the follicular phase and natural progesterone during the luteal phase to facilitate the normal rise and fall of estrogen and progesterone. Take 50 mg daily of black cohosh for fourteen days beginning on the first day of a period. Then, on day fourteen, discontinue the black cohosh and instead utilize natural progesterone therapy, dosed either at quarter teaspoon or half teaspoon daily until the next period arrives. Repeat monthly, or according to your own cycle if you are tracking it.
- Melatonin: Researchers have long identified the relationship between circadian rhythms and menstrual cycles.[115] Melatonin has specifically been implicated for use in perimenopausal and menopausal disorders[116] through this circadian interrelationship. I recommend that my patients take 5 mg every night at bedtime while ensuring adequate natural light exposure during the day (at least fifteen minutes of natural sunlight first thing in the morning and mid-afternoon or using a full-spectrum light therapy lamp of at least 10,000 lux as a light replacement in the winter or when sunlight is unavailable).

Abnormal Bleeding (Spotting)

Unlike irregular periods, which involve bleeding at otherwise irregular intervals, there are other forms of abnormal bleeding that can occur, such as spotting between periods or even full, bright red blood despite true periods that arrive right on time. We outlined a few of these potential causes earlier, like fibroids, polyps, and ovarian cysts, but sometimes this abnormal bleeding can occur without these diagnosed problems. Cervical irritation from bacterial vaginosis, yeast infections, and sexually transmitted infections (STIs) may also result in bloody discharge or spotting, and more severe concerns such as malignant cervical changes or pelvic inflammatory disease may also be the culprit (though these are comparatively rare). Beyond this, spotting almost always results from a hormone imbalance, provided that other causes have been ruled out. Sometimes these hormonal imbalances directly arise from perimenopause. If that's the case for you, refer back to the previous section for treatment strategies.

PHARMACOLOGICAL TREATMENT

Often, a hormonal IUD is recommended for abnormal spotting provided that other causes such as fibroids, polyps, and ovarian cysts (see below) have been ruled out. This is because IUDs thin the uterine lining to reduce bleeding. Birth control pills are also commonly recommended, but they are a bit of a catch-22 because depending on the type of progestin in the given pill, it may actually worsen the problem of mid-cycle spotting. This is especially true of the mini pill.

Estrogen Dominance (Low Progesterone)
ALTERNATIVE OPTIONS:

Progesterone deficiency is almost always related to either a hypothalamic suppression of progesterone due to stress or to aging ovaries that produce insufficient progesterone after ovulation. Estrogen dominance involving low progesterone is often an early-stage precursor to hypothalamic amenorrhea in which both estrogen and progesterone are deficient. For this reason, the treatment strategy would be the same as is outlined in the "Hypothalamic Amenorrhea" section above, because both problems have the same root cause: stress. If the mid-cycle spotting is due instead to aging ovaries that produce insufficient progesterone, the treatment would involve addressing the underlying perimenopausal hormone irregularities. If this is the case for you, refer back to the section titled "Perimenopause."

Estrogen Dominance (Excess Estrogen)
ALTERNATIVE OPTIONS:

Excess estrogen is what it sounds like: too much of an otherwise good thing. However, this excess can have many different root causes. For example, estrogen excess may result from high androgens in PCOS, because enzymes called aromatases transform these androgens into estrogen. If this is the case for you, treat your PCOS first. Metabolically active abdominal fat cells are another source of excess estrogen production. Other times, excess estrogen accumulates in the body because it can't be cleared away properly through the liver or gastrointestinal tract. If you have a healthy foundation in place to support your body's detox pathways and are still dealing with excess estrogen, utilizing the three classic estrogen-detox herbs may help you:

- Diindolylmethane (DIM): DIM modulates estrogen metabolism and supports clearance of estrogen and its metabolites. The dosage I recommend to my patients is 300 mg DIM as a dietary supplement daily, and consider increasing consumption of cruciferous vegetables, which are a natural source of DIM.[117]
- Calcium-D-glucarate (CDG): Like DIM, CDG regulates estrogen metabolism and clearance through liver detoxification pathways.[118] In addition to DIM, I recommend that my patients take 500 mg of CDG daily.
- Indole-3-carbinol (I3C): Another estrogen regulator, I3C functions similarly to CDG and DIM.[119] I recommend that my patients take 200 to 400 mg of I3C daily in addition to DIM and CDG.

Ovarian Cysts

Normally each month, one ovarian follicle develops and ruptures, releasing an egg. Sometimes this process occurs incompletely and instead of rupturing to release a mature egg, the follicle continues to grow. We typically refer to these as "functional" ovarian cysts and the vast majority of them remain relatively small and don't cause problems. Rarely, they can grow to several centimeters in diameter, causing pelvic pain, fullness, or bloating. They may also rupture or cause the ovary to twist ("ovarian torsion"). Both of these situations are accompanied by sudden, severe abdominal pain and are a medical emergency. Ovarian cysts commonly cause mid-cycle spotting whether or not other symptoms, like pain, are present.

You should know that these cysts are different from the ovarian changes seen in PCOS, which result from many follicles failing to reach maturity. In contrast to functional ovarian cysts, the cystic changes in PCOS are the result of elevated androgens. While women with PCOS may also develop functional ovarian cysts, they are not the same thing. Most ovarian cysts are identified by accident on ultrasound and don't require treatment, but if they reach between 5 and 10 centimeters in diameter, surgery may be recommended.[120] Ovarian cysts are common after using fertility drugs like Clomid.

You should note that there is limited research regarding treatments for ovarian cysts—pharmacological, surgical, or otherwise. That being said, ovarian cysts are classically understood to be an estrogen-dominant condition, so utilizing the strategies outlined above will be helpful in prevention.

PHARMACOLOGICAL TREATMENT

Using hormonal birth control prevents follicular ripening, so this is usually the first-line treatment to prevent the formation of new ovarian cysts in women who are prone to them. On the other hand, IUDs increase the risk of developing ovarian cysts.[121]

ALTERNATIVE OPTIONS:

- Triphaladi kayasha: Preliminary research of the ayurvedic herb triphala was shown to reduce the size of ovarian cysts or, in 26 percent of cases, eliminate them completely. When I use triphala with my patients, it is dosed as a 50 mL decoction processed with guggulu (1 mg) and taken twice daily.[122]
- Sanjie zhentong: This herbal blend from TCM has promise in a pilot study evaluating its benefit in treating ovarian cysts which formed in women following fertility treatments. Although the trigger in this study was known medication use, this medicinal herbal blend may have a similar benefit in other cases of ovarian cysts.[123] Note that

this herbal blend is very difficult to obtain apart from a TMC practitioner. In this case, it is best used in combination with acupuncture.

Hormonal Acne

While acne has many potential causes, including microbial dysbiosis and food reactivity, skin lesions that fluctuate cyclically always have a hormonal influence.

PHARMACOLOGICAL TREATMENT

Birth control pills are not a predictable or typical way to manage hormonal acne because the progestogens in many of them cause acne as a side effect. However, some health care providers recommend the birth control pill to manage acne anyway. Alternatively, acne may be managed with a prescription drug called spironolactone, which blocks androgen production and can be highly effective for androgenic acne. Other prescription topical and oral medications are also available for acne treatment with mixed results.

ALTERNATIVE OPTIONS FOR ANDROGENIC ACNE

If you experience deep, cystic acne in combination with other androgenic symptoms such as irregular periods, facial hair growth, difficulty losing weight, and loss of hair on your head, you may be dealing with PCOS. In this case, addressing your acne begins with addressing your PCOS. Please refer back to the PCOS section.

ALTERNATIVE OPTIONS FOR ESTROGENIC ACNE

If you do not have PCOS or elevated androgens and you notice that your acne is worse around ovulation and the week after, you are likely experiencing estrogenic acne as these are the times in your cycle when estrogen rises. If this is the case for you, please refer back to the strategies for "Estrogen Dominance: Excess Estrogen" in the previous section.

OTHER ALTERNATIVES:

- Manage your blood sugar: In addition to its influence over androgen levels, blood sugar profoundly influences estrogen and acne. Researchers identified that up to 81 percent of acne patients have insulin resistance.[124] Additionally, there is strong research supporting reduction of glycemic index and glycemic load to manage acne, as well as increasing dietary intake of omega-3 fatty acids.[125] Note that ensuring the proper balance of blood sugars and omega-3 fatty acids is extremely difficult with a plant-based diet.
- Oil-based cleanser: Anecdotally, many acne cleansers lead to drying of skin, which perpetuates sebum production and inflammation. Transitioning to an oil-based cleanser may be very effective in these cases of acne.
- Ozonated oil: Ozonated oil is produced by bubbling ozone through oil until it solidifies. The ozone reactants in this product inhibit bacterial growth and reduce inflammation in skin. Due to the inflammatory nature of acne lesion and the microbial component involved, there is some implication for the topical use of ozonated oils in treatment of acne vulgaris.[126] I recommend that my patients apply a thin layer to the affected area each night until it heals. Note that this is not a root-cause solution but is a natural way to manage symptoms that may otherwise be slow to respond.

Hyperprolactinemia

Prolactin is a hormone produced by the pituitary gland during pregnancy to stimulate milk production. In some women, prolactin levels remain elevated after pregnancy, childbirth, breastfeeding, and weaning. In some cases, it is elevated on blood work even if a woman has never before been pregnant. Prolactin directly inhibits the HPG axis by preventing LH and FSH stimulation of the ovaries and subsequent ovulation. (See "Lactational Amenorrhea" in chapter 9 for more details.) When prolactin is elevated outside of pregnancy and breastfeeding, we call it hyperprolactinemia and it can cause missing or irregular periods and fertility problems (even if periods are regular). For unknown reasons, prolactin levels may also be high in women with PCOS. Rarely, a benign tumor on the pituitary gland called a prolactinoma may be the culprit behind elevated prolactin levels.

PHARMACOLOGICAL TREATMENT

Hyperprolactinemia is classically treated with a medication called Cabergoline. Even if prolactinoma is the reason for elevated prolactin levels, surgery is rarely recommended, and medication is the usual first choice. This is because the risks of surgery outweigh the benefit of having the tumor resected.

ALTERNATIVE OPTIONS:

- Chaste tree (*Vitex agnus-castus*): Vitex binds to dopamine receptors in the area of the brain responsible for producing prolactin. It is an effective means for reducing prolactin levels in women who have hyperprolactinemia for some reason other than prolactinoma.[127] The dosage I recommend to my patients is 40 to 100 mg daily, though I sometimes recommend even higher doses if blood levels are slow to respond to a lower level.[128]

Luteal Phase Defect

Luteal phase defect (or "luteal phase deficiency") refers to a luteal phase that is shorter than ten days long. This can cause fertility problems because the uterine lining sheds before a fertilized egg has the chance to implant. It also may lead to early miscarriage for the same reason. It is a common culprit for short menstrual cycles but should be differentiated from a short follicular phase which does not classically cause the same degree of fertility impairment that luteal phase defect does (though it is more likely to impact egg quality). Luteal phase defect is defined by low progesterone and low progesterone response, so treating the root cause naturally necessitates identifying the cause of low progesterone. This is therefore an estrogen-dominant, progesterone-deficient condition. In most cases, it relates to stress.

PHARMACOLOGICAL TREATMENT

If the patient is trying to conceive, she is treated with oral progesterone therapy. Otherwise, there is usually no treatment.

ALTERNATIVE OPTIONS:

The most important thing you can do for your health and for your fertility if you are dealing with luteal phase defect is identify and address the underlying root cause of your stress. You should note that thyroid disorders are also commonly associated with luteal phase defect, so make sure that you speak with your health care provider about comprehensively testing your thyroid labs and providing treatment as necessary.

- Vitamin B6: Double-blind studies show that oral supplementation of vitamin B6 between 200 to 800 mg daily increases progesterone levels.[129] However, there is risk of toxicity with vitamin B6, so I recommend not exceeding 100 mg, on average, daily. Instead, I recommend that my patients take 200 mg per day during the luteal phase only, or 100 mg every day.
- Natural progesterone: As an alternative to oral progesterone, natural progesterone therapy can be used to support the endometrial lining, delaying onset of menstruation and prolonging the luteal phase.
- Vitamin C: Higher levels of vitamin C are associated in the research with higher progesterone production because of its antioxidant activity.[130] The dosage I recommend to my patients is 500 mg daily with food to maximize absorption.

CLOSING THOUGHTS

Period problems are no joke. Whether they involve pain and cramping, fertility struggles, mood changes, or whatever else, the suffering they cause impacts every area of life. Likewise, mainstream medical "treatments" often don't help much at all and usually create as many problems as they cause. But it doesn't have to be that way. Your periods don't need to be painful; they really can be an incredible and empowering monthly experience! Moreover, you have options readily available at your fingertips to get you there (literally, if you're reading a physical copy of this book). You don't need to accept "no" for an answer, you don't need to keep on suffering, and you don't need to shut down your hormones if you don't want to.

I wanted to leave you with a few other reminders as we wrap up this book:

- You are the expert of your health! Remember this when you hire others for the important purpose of giving you medical advice.
- The more you know about yourself, the better! That means getting up close and personal with tracking your health, including your menstrual cycle. You can't advocate for what you don't know.
- Your fertility matters for more than just baby-making. Protect it.
- You have the right to safe and effective health care. If your doctor doesn't take you seriously or doesn't offer you options that align with your values, you can find a new one. That being said, most

doctors are trying to help you to the best of their ability. They just might not be trained in the modalities you're looking for.
- Your body is good. I promise, it's not out to get you. Even if you're dealing with debilitating symptoms, your body is on your side and is trying just as hard as you are to heal. Be gentle with yourself, and take care.

In health,
Dr. Alexandra MacKillop

ACKNOWLEDGMENTS

As a physician, I could never do what I do without my colleagues, mentors, and teachers who have lifted me up, taught me all I know, and continue to support me in my learning. Thank you to my patients, who have entrusted me with their health and allowed me to see the real-life effects of integrative and functional medicine.

Thank you to Dr. Gersh for your support of this project and the work you do to help women everywhere.

Personally, I also want to thank Kenzie, my incredible husband who lifts me up in every way imaginable. Your love and friendship mean everything to me. Thank you to my sister and to Jeanie, who always encourage me to chase my dreams even if it means doing crazy things like writing a book with toddlers at home. Thank you to Keely, my awesome agent, my editors Victoria and Jacquie, and all the other wonderful staff at Bloomsbury.

And I thank God—the creator of the female body—for His daily grace and mercies, and for making me new.

APPENDIX

Hormone Imbalances

THYROID IMBALANCES

Primary Hypothyroidism

- Symptoms
  - Fatigue
  - Sensitivity to cold
  - Weight gain
  - Constipation
  - Depression
  - Brain fog
  - Dizziness
  - Low blood pressure
  - Low heart rate
  - Menstrual changes
- Lab Test Results
  - TSH: high
  - Total T4: low
  - T4, free: low
  - Total T3: normal or low
  - T3, free: normal or low

Hypothalamic Hypothyroidism

- Symptoms
  - Fatigue
  - Sensitivity to cold
  - Weight gain
  - Constipation
  - Depression
  - Brain fog
  - Dizziness
  - Low blood pressure
  - Low heart rate
  - Light, irregular, or absent periods
- Lab Test Results
  - TSH: low
  - Total T4: low or normal
  - T4, free: low or normal
  - Total T3: normal or low
  - T3, free: normal or low

Hashimoto's Hypothyroidism

- Symptoms
  - Fatigue
  - Sensitivity to cold
  - Weight gain
  - Constipation
  - Depression
  - Brain fog
  - Dizziness
  - Low blood pressure
  - Low heart rate
  - Intermittent fevers
  - Muscle aches
  - Joint pain
  - Abdominal pain
  - Menstrual changes
- Lab Test Results
  - TSH: high or normal
  - Total T4: low or normal

- T4, free: low or normal
- Total T3: normal or low
- T3, free: normal or low
- Anti-TPO Antibodies: high
- Anti-Tg antibodies: high or normal

Peripheral Conversion Defect Hypothyroidism

- Symptoms
  - Fatigue
  - Sensitivity to cold
  - Weight gain
  - Constipation
  - Depression
  - Brain fog
  - Dizziness
  - Low blood pressure
  - Low heart rate
  - Intermittent fevers
  - Muscle aches
  - Joint pain
  - Abdominal pain
- Lab Test Results
  - TSH: high or normal
  - Total T4: normal
  - T4, free: normal
  - Total T3: normal or low
  - T3, free: normal or low

Hormone Receptor Competition Hypothyroidism

- Symptoms
  - Fatigue
  - Sensitivity to cold
  - Weight gain
  - Constipation
  - Depression
  - Brain fog
  - Dizziness
  - Low blood pressure

- Low heart rate
    - Intermittent fevers
    - Muscle aches
    - Joint pain
    - Abdominal pain
- Lab Test Results
    - TSH: high or normal
    - Total T4: normal
    - T4, free: normal
    - Total T3: normal
    - T3, free: normal

Binding Globulin Availability Hypothyroidism

- Symptoms
    - Fatigue
    - Sensitivity to cold
    - Weight gain
    - Constipation
    - Depression
    - Brain fog
    - Dizziness
    - Low blood pressure
    - Low heart rate
    - GI problems
- Lab Test Results
    - TSH: high
    - Total T4: normal or high
    - T4, free: low
    - Total T3: normal or high
    - T3, free: low
    - Thyroid-binding globulin: high

Nutrient Deficiency Hypothyroidism

- Symptoms
    - Fatigue
    - Sensitivity to cold
    - Weight gain
    - Constipation

- Depression
- Brain fog
- Dizziness
- Low blood pressure
- Low heart rate
- Lab Test Results
  - TSH: high or normal
  - Total T4: low or normal
  - T4, free: low or normal
  - Total T3: normal or low
  - T3, free: normal or low
  - Iodine, serum: may be low
  - Zinc, RBC: may be low
  - Selenium, RBC: may be low

SEX HORMONE IMBALANCES

Estrogen Excess (Estrogen Dominance)

- Symptoms
  - Low libido
  - Increased PMS symptoms
  - Weight gain
  - Fatigue
  - Muscle aches and joint pain
  - Irregular periods
  - Anxiety and irritability
  - Difficulty concentrating
  - Bloating
  - Breast tenderness
  - Heat intolerance
  - Heavy periods
  - Clotting in periods
  - Painful periods
  - Insomnia
  - Acne on face, chest, or back
- Lab Test Results
  - Estradiol (day 3 or 21): high
  - Progesterone (day 21): low or normal

Progesterone Deficiency (Estrogen Dominance)

- Symptoms
  - Low libido
  - Increased PMS symptoms
  - Weight changes
  - Fatigue
  - Muscle aches and joint pain
  - Irregular periods
  - Anxiety, depression, or irritability
  - Difficulty concentrating
  - Bloating
  - Breast tenderness
  - Heat intolerance
  - Short menstrual cycles
  - Heavy bleeding with clotting
  - Hot flashes
- Lab Test Results
  - Estradiol (day 3): high or normal
  - Progesterone (day 21): low

Other Estrogen Dominance

- Symptoms
  - Low libido
  - Increased PMS symptoms
  - Weight gain
  - Fatigue
  - Muscle aches and joint pain
  - Irregular periods
  - Anxiety and irritability
  - Difficulty concentrating
  - Bloating
  - Breast tenderness
  - Heat intolerance
  - Heavy periods
  - Insomnia
  - Acne on face, chest or back
- Lab Test Results
  - Estradiol (day 3 or 21): high
  - Progesterone: low or normal

PCOS

- Symptoms
  - Weight gain
  - High blood sugar
  - Increased abdominal fat
  - Cystic acne
  - Hirsutism
  - Thinning of hair on head
  - Irregular periods
  - Very light periods
  - Fertility problems
  - Stretch marks
  - Skin tags
  - Dark patches of skin
  - Recurrent yeast infections
- Lab Test Results
  - DHEA: high or normal; can be normal if testosterone is high
  - Testosterone: high or normal; can be normal if DHEA is high
  - Estradiol (day 3): usually high
  - Progesterone (day 21): normal or low
  - LH: usually high

Low Androgens

- Symptoms
  - Low libido
  - Depression
  - Decreased breast size
  - Depression
  - Fatigue
  - Reduced muscle mass and strength
  - Increased abdominal fat
- Lab Test Results
  - Testosterone: low
  - DHEA: low
  - LH/FSH: often low

Sex Hormone Deficiency

- Symptoms
  - Low libido
  - Dry skin
  - Breast tenderness
  - Difficulty concentrating
  - Irritability
  - Vaginal dryness
  - Hot flashes and night sweats
  - Irregular or absent periods
  - Fatigue
- Lab Test Results
  - Estradiol (day 3 or 21): low
  - Progesterone (day 21): low
  - Testosterone (day 3): low
  - DHEA (day 3): low
  - LH and FSH: low
  - TSH: often low

ADRENAL HORMONE IMBALANCES

Chronic Stress Response

- Symptoms
  - Increased abdominal fat
  - Thinning of arms and legs
  - Facial flushing and redness
  - Increased blood pressure
  - Insomnia
  - Anxiety or irritability, mood swings
  - Stretch marks
  - Weight gain or loss
  - Hot flashes
- Lab Test Results
  - Cortisol: high
  - DHEA: high or normal

Adrenal Dysfunction

- Symptoms
  - Increased abdominal fat
  - Thinning of arms and legs
  - Facial flushing and redness
  - Increased blood pressure
  - Insomnia
  - Anxiety or irritability, mood swings
  - Stretch marks
  - Weight gain or loss
  - Difficulty regulating temperature
  - Irregular periods
- Lab Test Results
  - Cortisol: high or low
  - DHEA: high or low
  - TSH: usually low, unless in the case of primary hypothyroidism
  - LH/FSH: usually low

Adrenal Fatigue aka "Burnout Syndrome"

- Symptoms
  - Irregular periods
  - Weight changes
  - Fatigue
  - Low blood pressure
  - Insomnia or excess sleepiness
  - Anxiety and depression, mood swings
  - Body aches
  - Dizziness
  - Cravings for sweet or salty food
- Lab Test Results
  - Cortisol: low
  - DHEA: low
  - TSH: low
  - TSH: usually low, unless in the case of primary hypothyroidism
  - LH/FSH: usually low

NOTES

CHAPTER 1

1. "Yaz (drospirenone and ethinyl estradiol) Tablets." Accessed June 25, 2024. https://www.accessdata.fda.gov/drugsatfda_docs/label/2010/021676s009lbl.pdf.
2. Berkey, Jennifer. "Staying Active Increases Your Long-Term Happiness." Michigan State University Extension, March 8, 2013. https://www.canr.msu.edu/news/staying_active_increases_your_long-term_happiness#:~:text=Recent%20research%20published%20in%20the,activity%20tend%20to%20be%20unhappier.
3. "Healthy Habits Can Lengthen Life." National Institutes of Health (NIH), May 7, 2018. https://www.nih.gov/news-events/nih-research-matters/healthy-habits-can-lengthen-life.

CHAPTER 2

1. Taşkaldıran, Işılay, Emre Vuraloğlu, Yusuf Bozkuş, Özlem Turhan İyidir, Aslı Nar, and Neslihan Başçıl Tütüncü. "Menstrual Changes after COVID-19 Infection and COVID-19 Vaccination." *International Journal of Clinical Practice* (2022): 3199758. doi: 10.1155/2022/3199758.
2. Awwad, Johnny, Ghina Ghazeeri, Thomas Toth, Antoine Hannoun, Miche Abou Abdallah, and Chantal Farra. "Fever in Women May Interfere with Follicular

Development during Controlled Ovarian Stimulation." *International Journal of Hyperthermia* 28, no. 8 (2012): 742–46. doi: 10.3109/02656736.2012.724516.

3. Li, Quan-Zhen, David R. Karp, Jiexia Quan, Valerie K. Branch, Jinchun Zhou, Yun Lian, Benjamin F. Chong, Edward K. Wakeland, and Nancy J. Olsen. "Risk Factors for Ana Positivity in Healthy Persons." *Arthritis Research and Therapy* 13, no. 2 (2011): R38. doi: 10.1186/ar3271.

4. Ogunrinola, Grace A., John O. Oyewale, Oyewumi O. Oshamika, and Grace I. Olasehinde. "The Human Microbiome and Its Impacts on Health." *International Journal of Microbiology* (2020): 8045646. doi: 10.1155/2020/8045646.

5. Yan, Han, Yi Chen, Hong Zhu, Wei-Hua Huang, Xin-He Cai, Dan Li, Ya-Juan Lv, Si-Zhao, Hong-Hao Zhou, Fan-Yan Luo, Wei Zhang, and Xi Li. "The Relationship among Intestinal Bacteria, Vitamin K, and Response of Vitamin K Antagonist: A Review of Evidence and Potential Mechanism." *Frontiers in Medicine* 9 (2022): 829304. doi: 10.3389/fmed.2022.829304.

6. Baker, James M., Layla Al-Nakkash, and Melissa Herbst-Kralovets. "Estrogen-Gut Microbiome Axis: Physiological and Clinical Implications." *Maturitas* 103 (2017): 45–53. doi: 10.1016/j.maturitas.2017.06.025.

7. Travis, Ruth C., and Timothy J. Key. "Oestrogen Exposure and Breast Cancer Risk." *Breast Cancer Research (BCR)* 5, no. 5 (2003): 239–47. doi: 10.1186/bcr628.

8. Ciarambino, Tiziana, Pietro Crispino, Gloria Guarisco, and Mauro Giordano. "Gender Differences in Insulin Resistance: New Knowledge and Perspectives." *Current Issues in Molecular Biology* 45, no. 10 (2023): 7845–61. https://doi.org/10.3390/cimb45100496.

CHAPTER 3

1. Loukas, Marios, Michael Hanna, Nada Alsaiegh, Mohammadali Shoja, and Shane Tubbs. "Clinical Anatomy as Practiced by Ancient Egyptians." *Clinical Anatomy* 24, no. 4 (2011): 409–15. doi: 10.1002/ca.21155.

2. Underwood, E. Ashworth, and Robert Richardson. "History of Medicine." *Encyclopædia Britannica*, last updated December 13, 2024. https://www.britannica.com/science/history-of-medicine.

3. Hilton, Robin. "The History of the Clitoris." University of Regina Students Union, October 1, 2021. https://www.ursu.ca/2021/10/01/the-history-of-the-clitoris/.

4. Nguyen, John D. "Anatomy, Abdomen and Pelvis: Female External Genitalia." *StatPearls* (online). Treasure Island, FL: StatPearls Publishing, 2023. https://www.ncbi.nlm.nih.gov/books/NBK547703/.

5. Verhaeghe, J., R. Gheysen, and P. Enzlin. "Pheromones and Their Effect on Women's Mood and Sexuality." *Facts, Views, and Vision in ObGyn* 5, no. 3 (2013): 189–95. https://pubmed.ncbi.nlm.nih.gov/24753944/.

6. Lanfranchi, Angela. "A Scientific Basis for Humanae Vitae and Natural Law: The Role of Human Pheromones on Human Sexual Behavior Preferences by Oral Contraceptives and the Abortifacient Effects of Oral Contraceptives." *Linacre Quarterly* 85, no. 2 (2018): 148–54. doi: 10.1177/0024363918756191.

7. Nguyen, "Anatomy, Abdomen and Pelvis: Female External Genitalia."

8. Gross, Rachel E. "The Clitoris, Uncovered: An Intimate History." *Scientific American*, March 4, 2020. https://www.scientificamerican.com/article/the-clitoris-uncovered-an-intimate-history/.

9. Oriji, P. C., D. O. Allagoa, A. E. Ubom, and V. K. Oriji. "A 5-Year Review of Incidence, Presentation and Management of Bartholin Gland Cysts and Abscesses in a Tertiary Hospital, Yenagoa, South-South Nigeria." *medRxiv* (2022). doi: 10.1101/2022.05.01.22274551.

10. Rivard, Allyson B., Laura Galarza-Paez, and Diana C. Peterson. "Anatomy, Thorax, Breast." *StatPearls* (online). Treasure Island, FL: StatPearls Publishing, 2023.

11. Bowman, Katy. "Thanks for the Mammaries." *Nutritious Movement*, June 1, 2017. https://www.nutritiousmovement.com/thanks-for-the-mammaries/.

12. Rivard et al. "Anatomy, Thorax, Breast."

13. Kikuchi, K., H. Tagami, R. Akaraphanth, and S. Aiba. "Functional Analyses of the Skin Surface of the Areola Mammae: Comparison between Healthy Adult Male and Female Subjects and between Healthy Individuals and Patients with Atopic Dermatitis." *British Journal of Dermatology* 164, no. 1 (2011): 97–102. doi: 10.1111/j.1365-2133.2010.10076.x.

14. Zucca-Matthes, Gustavo, Cícero Urban, and André Vallejo. "Anatomy of the Nipple and Breast Ducts." *Gland Surgery* 5, no. 1 (2016): 32–36. doi: 10.3978/j.issn.2227-684X.2015.05.10.

15. Wilcox, A. J., D. D. Baird, and C. R. Weinberg. "Time of Implantation of the Conceptus and Loss of Pregnancy." *New England Journal of Medicine* 340, no. 23 (1999): 1796–99. doi: 10.1056/NEJM199906103402304.

16. Han, Joan, and Nazia Sadiq. "Anatomy, Abdomen and Pelvis: Fallopian Tube." *StatPearls* (online). Treasure Island, FL: StatPearls Publishing, 2023. https://www.ncbi.nlm.nih.gov/books/NBK547660/.

17. Farwell, Alan, ed. "Volume 7 Issue 1." *Clinical Thyroidology for the Public*, 2014. https://www.thyroid.org/patient-thyroid-information/ct-for-patients/vol-7-issue-1/.

CHAPTER 4

1. Mckellar, Kerry, and Elizabeth Sillence. "Menstrual Cycle." In *Teenagers, Sexual Health Information and the Digital* Age. Cambridge, MA: Academic Press, 2020. https://doi.org/10.1016/C2018-0-01310-9.

2. Sharma, Medhavi. "Ovulation Induction Techniques." *StatPearls* (online). Treasure Island, FL: StatPearls Publishing, 2023. https://www.ncbi.nlm.nih.gov/books/NBK574564/.

3. Sharma, "Ovulation Induction Techniques."

4. Thiyagarajan, Dhanalakshmi K. "Physiology, Menstrual Cycle." *StatPearls* (online). Treasure Island, FL: StatPearls Publishing, 2023. https://www.ncbi.nlm.nih.gov/books/NBK500020/.

5. Bouma, E. M. C., H. Riese, J. Ormel, F. C. Verhulst, and A. J. Oldehinkl. "Adolescents' Cortisol Responses to Awakening and Social Stress; Effects of Gender, Menstrual Phase and Oral Contraceptives. The TRAILS Study." *Psychoneuroendocrinology* 34, no. 6 (2009): 884–93. https://doi.org/10.1016/j.psyneuen.2009.01.003.

6. Torre F., A. E. Calogero, R. A. Condorelli, R. Cannarella, A. Aversa, and S. La Vignera. "Effects of Oral Contraceptives on Thyroid Function and Vice Versa." *Journal of Endocrinological Investigation* 43, no. 9 (2020): 1181–88. doi: 10.1007/s40618-020-01230-8.

7. Hill, Sarah. "What Does the Pill's Effect on the Human Stress Response Mean?" Sarah E. Hill, March 31, 2021. https://www.sarahehill.com/pill_and_stress/.

CHAPTER 5

1. Mayo Clinic Staff. "Period Irregularities to Get Checked Out." Mayo Clinic, April 22, 2023. https://www.mayoclinic.org/healthy-lifestyle/womens-health/in-depth/menstrual-cycle/art-20047186.

2. McLaughlin, Jessica E. "Menstrual Cycle." *Merck Manual Consumer Version*, September 2022. https://www.merckmanuals.com/home/women-s-health-issues/biology-of-the-female-reproductive-system/menstrual-cycle.

3. Mihm, M., S. Gangooly, and S. Muttukrishna. "The Normal Menstrual Cycle in Women." *Animal Reproduction Science* 124, no. 3–4 (2011): 229–36. doi: 10.1016/j.anireprosci.2010.08.030.

4. Mckellar, Kerry, and Elizabeth Sillence. "Menstrual Cycle." In *Teenagers, Sexual Health Information and the Digital Age*. Cambridge, MA: Academic Press, 2020. https://doi.org/10.1016/C2018-0-01310-9.

5. Grieger, Jessica A., and Robert J. Norman. "Menstrual Cycle Length and Patterns in a Global Cohort of Women Using a Mobile Phone App: Retrospective Cohort Study." *Journal of Medical Internet Research* 22, no. 6 (2020): e17109. doi: 10.2196/17109.

6. Jacobson, Melanie H., Penelope P. Howards, James S. Kesner, Juliana W. Meadows, Celia E. Dominguez, Jessica B. Spencer, Lyndsey A. Darrow, Metrecia L. Terrell, and Michele Marcus. "Hormonal Profiles of Menstrual Bleeding

Patterns during the Luteal-Follicular Transition." *Journal of Clinical Endocrinology and Metabolism* 105, no. 5 (2020): e2024–31. doi: 10.1210/clinem/dgaa099.

7. Mckellar and Sillence. "Menstrual Cycle."

8. Munro, Malcom, Hillary Critchley, and Ian Fraser. "The Figo Classification of Causes of Abnormal Uterine Bleeding in the Reproductive Years." *Fertility and Sterility* 95, no. 7 (2011): 2024–8. doi: 10.1016/j.fertnstert.2011.03.079.

9. Dasharathy, Sonya S., Sunni L. Mumford, Anna Z. Pollack, Neil J. Perkins, Donald R. Mattison, Jean Wactawski-Wende, and Enrique F Schisterman. "Menstrual Bleeding Patterns among Regularly Menstruating Women." *American Journal of Epidemiology* 175, no. 6 (2012): 536–45. doi: 10.1093/aje/kwr356.

10. Heitmann, Ryan, Kelly Langan, Raywin Huang, Gregory Chow, and Richard Burney. "Premenstrual Spotting of ≥2 Days Is Strongly Associated with Histologically Confirmed Endometriosis in Women with Infertility." *American Journal of Obstetrics and Gynecology* 211, no. 4 (2014): 358.e–6. doi: 10.1016/j.ajog.2014.04.041.

11. Xiping, Liu, W. U. Xiaqiu, Bao Lirong, Peng Jin, and Ka-Kit Hui. "Menstrual Cycle Characteristics as an Indicator of Fertility Outcomes: Evidence from Prospective Birth Cohort Study in China." *Journal of Traditional Chinese Medicine* 42, no. 2 (2022): 272–78. doi: 10.19852/j.cnki.jtcm.2022.02.010.

12. Xiping et al. "Menstrual Cycle Characteristics as an Indicator of Fertility Outcomes."

13. Eske, Jamie. "Period Blood Chart: What Does the Blood Color Mean?" *Medical News Today*, November 23, 2023. https://www.medicalnewstoday.com/articles/324848#black.

14. Ginsen, ed. "Period Colour Meaning According to Chinese Medicine." *TCM Blog*, August 16, 2023. https://tcmblog.co.uk/what-can-we-learn-from-period-colour/#:~:text=If%20the%20blood%20is%20slimy,fever%20and%20other%20inflammatory%20conditions.

15. Manley, Hannah, James Sprinks, and Phillip Breedon. "Menstrual Blood-Derived Mesenchymal Stem Cells: Women's Attitudes, Willingness, and Barriers to Donation of Menstrual Blood." *Journal of Women's Health* 28, no. 12 (2019): doi: 10.1089/jwh.2019.7745.

16. Malanchuk, Larysa, Mariia Riabokon, Artem Malanchuk, Svitlana Riabokon, Serhiy Malanchuk, Viktoriia Martyniuk, Tetiana Grabchak, and Inna Pitsyk. "Relationship between Pathological Menstrual Symptoms and the Development of Extragenital Forms of Local Inflammation." *Wiadomosci lekarskie* 74, no. 1 (2021): 64–67. PMID: 33851589.

17. Xiping et al. "Menstrual Cycle Characteristics as an Indicator of Fertility Outcomes."

18. Malik, Mokerrum, Henry Adekola, William Porter, and Janet Poulik. "Passage of Decidual Cast Following Poor Compliance with Oral Contraceptive Pill." *Fetal and Pediatric Pathology* 34, no. 2 (2014): 103–7. doi: 10.3109/15513815.2014.970263.

19. "Overview: Heavy Periods." InformedHealth.org. Last updated June 17, 2021. https://www.ncbi.nlm.nih.gov/books/NBK279294/#:~:text=Although%20it%20can%20feel%20like,pad%20to%20become%20fully%20soaked.

20. Dasharathy et al. "Menstrual Bleeding Patterns among Regularly Menstruating Women."

21. Hapangama, Dharani K., and Judith N. Bulmer. "Pathophysiology of Heavy Menstrual Bleeding." *Women's Health* 12, no. 1 (2016): 3–13. doi: 10.2217/whe.15.81.

22. Adnane, Mounir, Kieran G. Meade, and Cliona O'Farrelly. "Cervico-Vaginal Mucus (CVM)—an Accessible Source of Immunologically Informative Biomolecules." *Veterinary Research Communications* 42, no. 4 (2018): 255–63. https://www.ncbi.nlm.nih.gov/pmc/articles/PMC6244541/.

23. Najmabadi, Shahpar, Karen C. Schliep, Sara E. Simonsen, Christina A. Porucznik, Marlene J. Egger, and Joseph B. Stanford. "Cervical Mucus Patterns and the Fertile Window in Women without Known Subfertility: A Pooled Analysis of Three Cohorts." *Human Reproduction* 36, no. 7 (2021): 1784–95. doi: 10.1093/humrep/deab049.

24. Lewis, Radha, Deshawn Taylor, Melissa Natavio, Alexander Melamed, Juan Felix, and Daniel Mishell. "Effects of the Levonorgestrel-Releasing Intrauterine System on Cervical Mucus Quality and Sperm Penetrability." *Contraception* 82, no. 6 (2010): 491–96. doi: 10.1016/j.contraception.2010.06.006.

25. D'Arrigo, Terri. "Risk of Depression May Increase during First Two Years of Oral Contraceptive Use." *Psychiatric News* 58, no. 9 (2023). doi: 10.1176/appi.pn.2023.09.9.6.

26. Weisz, George, and Loes Knaapen. "Diagnosing and Treating Premenstrual Syndrome in Five Western Nations." *Social Science & Medicine* 68, no. 8 (2009): 1498–1505. doi: 10.1016/j.socscimed.2009.01.036.

CHAPTER 6

1. Halmos, Gabor, and Andrew Schally. "Thyrotropin Release." In *Hormonal Signaling in Biology and Medicine*, edited by Gerald Litwack, 43–68. Cambridge, MA: Academic Press, 2020. doi: 10.1016/B978-0-12-813814-4.00003-1.

2. Adam, Emma K., Meghan E. Quinn, Royette Tavernier, Mollie T. McQuillan, Katie A. Dahlke, and Kirsten E. Gilbert. "Diurnal Cortisol Slopes and Mental and Physical Health Outcomes: A Systematic Review and Meta-Analysis." *Psychoneuroendocrinology* 24, no. 83 (2017): 25–41. doi: 10.1016/j.psyneuen.2017.05.018.

3. Cahill, David J., Peter G. Wardle, Christopher R. Harlow, and M. G. R. Hull. "Onset of the Preovulatory Luteinizing Hormone Surge: Diurnal Timing and Critical Follicular Prerequisites." *Fertility and Sterility* 70, no. 1 (1998): 56–59. doi: 10.1016/S0015-0282(98)00113-7.

4. Butler, Karyn Geralyn. "Relationship between the Cortisol-Estradiol Phase Difference and Affect in Women." *Journal of Circadian Rhythms* 16, no. 3 (2018): article 3. doi: 10.5334/jcr.154.

5. Chaput, Jean-Philippe, Caroline Dutil, and Hugues Sampasa-Kanyinga. "Sleeping Hours: What Is the Ideal Number and How Does Age Impact This?" *Nature and Science of Sleep* 10 (2018): 421–30. doi: 10.2147/NSS.S163071.

6. "Low Blood Glucose (Hypoglycemia)." National Institute of Diabetes and Digestive and Kidney Diseases (NIH). Accessed June 25, 2024. https://www.niddk.nih.gov/health-information/diabetes/overview/preventing-problems/low-blood-glucose-hypoglycemia#:~:text=Although%20you%20may%20not%20wake,blood%20glucose%20during%20the%20day.

7. Hartley, Sarah, Sylvie Royant-Parola, Ayla Zayoud, Isabelle Gremy, and Bobette Matulonga. "Do Both Timing and Duration of Screen Use Affect Sleep Patterns in Adolescents?" *PloS One* 17, no. 10 (2022): e0276226. doi: 10.1371/journal.pone.0276226.

8. Mindell, Jodi, and Ariel Williamson. "Benefits of a Bedtime Routine in Young Children: Sleep, Development, and Beyond." *Sleep Medicine Reviews* 40 (2018): 93–108. doi: 10.1016/j.smrv.2017.10.007.

9. Komori, Teruhisa. "The Effects of Phosphatidylserine and Omega-3 Fatty Acid–Containing Supplement on Late Life Depression." *Mental Illness* 7, no. 1 (2015): 5647. doi: 10.4081/mi.2015.5647.

10. Pistollato, Francesca, Sandra Sumalla Cano, Iñaki Elio, Manuel Masias Vergara, Francesca Giampieri, and Maurizio Battino. "Associations between Sleep, Cortisol Regulation, and Diet: Possible Implications for the Risk of Alzheimer Disease." *Advances in Nutrition* 7, no. 4 (2016): 679–89. doi: 10.3945/an.115.011775.

11. Abbasi, Behnood, Masud Kimiagar, Khosro Sadeghniiat, Minoo M Shirazi, Mehdi Hedayati, and Bahram Rashidkhani. "The Effect of Magnesium Supplementation on Primary Insomnia in Elderly: A Double-Blind Placebo-Controlled Clinical Trial." *Journal of Research in Medical Sciences* 17, no. 12 (2012): 1161–69. https://www.ncbi.nlm.nih.gov/pmc/articles/PMC3703169/.

12. Abbasi et al. "The Effect of Magnesium Supplementation on Primary Insomnia in Elderly: A Double-Blind Placebo-Controlled Clinical Trial."

13. Abbasi et al. "The Effect of Magnesium Supplementation on Primary Insomnia in Elderly: A Double-Blind Placebo-Controlled Clinical Trial."

14. Emet, Mucahit, Halil Ozcan, Lutfu Ozel, Muhammed Yayla, Zekai Halici, and Ahmet Hacimuftuoglu. "A Review of Melatonin, Its Receptors and Drugs." *Eurasian Journal of Medicine* 48, no. 2 (2016): 135–41. https://www.ncbi.nlm.nih.gov/pmc/articles/PMC4970552/.

15. Reiter, R. J., J. R. Calvo, M. Karbownik, W. Qi, and X. Tan. "Melatonin and Its Relation to the Immune System and Inflammation." *Annals of the New York Academy of Sciences* 917 (2000): 376–86. https://pubmed.ncbi.nlm.nih.gov/11268363/.

16. Qu, Jingwen, Huiru Hu, Haoyuan Niu, Xiaomei Sun, and Yongjun Li. "Melatonin Restores the Declining Maturation Quality and Early Embryonic Development of Oocytes in Aged Mice." *Theriogenology* 210 (2023): 110–18. doi: 10.1016/j.theriogenology.2023.07.021.

17. Venkatasamy, Vighnesh Vetrivel, Sandeep Pericherla, Sachin Manthuruthil, Shikha Mishra, and Ram Hanno. "Effect of Physical Activity on Insulin Resistance, Inflammation and Oxidative Stress in Diabetes Mellitus." *Journal of Clinical and Diagnostic Research (JCDR)* 7, no. 8 (2013): 1764–66. doi: 10.7860/JCDR/2013/6518.3306.

18. Duclos, Martine, and Antoine Tabarin. "Exercise and the Hypothalamo-Pituitary-Adrenal Axis." *Frontiers of Hormone Research* 47 (2016): 12–26. doi: 10.1159/000445149.

19. Smith, R. L., K. L. Vernon, D. E. Kelley, J. R. Gibbons, and C. J. Mortensen. "Impact of Moderate Exercise on Ovarian Blood Flow and Early Embryonic Outcomes in Mares." *Journal of Animal Science* 90, no. 11 (2012): 3770–77. doi: 10.2527/jas.2011-4713.

20. "Adult Activity: An Overview." Physical Activity Basics, December 20, 2023. Centers for Disease Control and Prevention. https://www.cdc.gov/physical-activity-basics/guidelines/adults.html?CDC_AAref_Val=https%3A%2F%2Fwww.cdc.gov%2Fphysicalactivity%2Fbasics%2Fadults%2Findex.htm.

21. Hertel, Johannes, Johanna König, Georg Homuth, Sandra Van der Auwera, Katharina Wittfeld, Maik Pietzner, Tim Kacprowski, et al. "Evidence for Stress-like Alterations in the Hpa-Axis in Women Taking Oral Contraceptives." *Scientific Reports* 7 (2017): 14111. doi: 10.1038/s41598-017-13927-7.

22. Fern, M., D. P. Rose, and E. B. Fern. "Effect of Oral Contraceptives on Plasma Androgenic Steroids and Their Precursors." *Obstetrics and Gynecology* 51, no. 5 (1978): 541–44. doi: 10.1097/00006250-197805000-00005.

23. Whitehead, Brenda R., and C. S. Bergeman. "Daily Religious Coping Buffers the Stress-Affect Relationship and Benefits Overall Metabolic Health in Older Adults." *Psychology of Religion and Spirituality* 12, no. 4 (2019): 393–99. doi: 10.1037/rel0000251.

24. Goyal, Madhav, Sonal Singh, Erica M. S. Sibinga, Neda F. Gould, Anastasia Rowland-Seymour, Ritu Sharma, Zackary Berger, et al. "Meditation Programs for Psychological Stress and Well-Being: A Systematic Review and Meta-Analysis." *JAMA Internal Medicine* 174, no. 3 (2014): 357–68. doi: 10.1001/jamainternmed.2013.13018.

25. Zaccaro, Andrea, Andrea Piarulli, Marco Laurino, Erika Garbella, Danilo Menicucci, Bruno Neri, and Angelo Gemignani. "How Breath-Control Can Change Your Life: A Systematic Review on Psycho-Physiological Correlates of Slow Breathing." *Frontiers in Human Neuroscience* 12 (2018): 353. doi: 10.3389/fnhum.2018.00353.

26. Madore, Kevin P., and Anthony D. Wagner. "Multicosts of Multitasking." *Cerebrum* (2019): cer-04-19. https://www.ncbi.nlm.nih.gov/pmc/articles/PMC7075496/.

27. Ewert, Alan, and Yun Chang. "Levels of Nature and Stress Response." *Behavioral Sciences* 8, no. 5 (2018): doi: 10.3390/bs8050049.

28. Beyer, Kirsten M. M., Aniko Szabo, Kelly Hoormann, and Melinda Stolley. "Time Spent Outdoors, Activity Levels, and Chronic Disease among American Adults." *Journal of Behavioral Medicine* 41, no. 4 (2018): 494–503. doi: 10.1007/s10865-018-9911-1.

29. Zhu, Zhanhui, Yang Lei, and Zheng Lin. "Effects of Crohn's Disease Exclusion Diet on Remission: A Systematic Review." *Therapeutic Advances in Gastroenterology* 16 (2023): doi: 10.1177/17562848231184056.

30. Chandrasekaran, Anita, Bhuvan Molparia, Ehsaan Akhtar, Xiaoyun Wang, James D. Lewis, John T Chang, Glenn Oliveira, Ali Torkamani, and Gauree Gupta Konijeti. "The Autoimmune Protocol Diet Modifies Intestinal RNA Expression in Inflammatory Bowel Disease." *Crohn's & Colitis* 1, no. 3 (2019): otz016. doi: 10.1093/crocol/otz016.

31. Ułamek-Kozioł, Marzena, Stanisław J. Czuczwar, Sławomir Januszewski, and Ryszard Pluta. "Ketogenic Diet and Epilepsy." *Nutrients* 11, no. 10 (2019): 2510. doi: 10.3390/nu11102510.

32. Wartella, E. A., A. H. Lichenstein, and C. S. Boon, eds. "History of Nutrition Labeling." In *Front-of-Package Nutrition Rating Systems and Symbols: Phase I Report*. Washington, DC: National Academies Press, 2010. https://www.ncbi.nlm.nih.gov/books/NBK209859/.

33. Loeffelholz, Christian von, and Andreas L. Birkenfeld. "Non-Exercise Activity Thermogenesis in Human Energy Homeostasis." In *Endotext* (online) edited by Kenneth R. Feingold et al. South Dartmouth, MA: MDText.com, Inc., 2000 November 25, 2022. https://www.ncbi.nlm.nih.gov/books/NBK279077/.

34. McEvedy, Samantha, Gillian Sullivan-Mort, Sian McLean, and Michaela Pascoe. "Ineffectiveness of Commercial Weight-Loss Programs for Achieving Modest but Meaningful Weight Loss: Systematic Review and Meta-Analysis." *Journal of Health Psychology* 22, no. 12 (2017): 1614–27. doi: 10.1177/1359105317705983.

35. Jurczewska, Justyna, and Dorota Szostak-Węgierek. "The Influence of Diet on Ovulation Disorders in Women: A Narrative Review." *Nutrients* 14, no. 8 (2022): 1556. doi: 10.3390/nu14081556.

36. Manthou, Eirini, Maria Kanaki, Kalliopi Georgakouli, Chariklia K. Deli, Dimitrios Kouretas, Yiannis Koutedakis, and Athanasios Z. Jamurtas. "Glycemic Response of a Carbohydrate-Protein Bar with Ewe-Goat Whey." *Nutrients* 6, no. 6 (2014): 2240–50. doi: 10.3390/nu6062240.

37. Jurczewska and Szostak-Węgierek. "The Influence of Diet on Ovulation Disorders in Women-A Narrative Review."

38. "NIH Study Shows How Insulin Stimulates Fat Cells to Take in Glucose." News Releases. National Institutes of Health (NIH). September 7, 2010. https://

www.nih.gov/news-events/news-releases/nih-study-shows-how-insulin-stimulates-fat-cells-take-glucose#:~:text=September%207%2C%202010-,NIH%20study%20shows%20how%20insulin%20stimulates%20fat%20cells%20to%20take,glucose%20in%20a%20rat%20model.

39. Baptiste, Catherine G., Marie-Claude Battista, Andréanne Trottier, and Jean-Patrice Baillargeon. "Insulin and Hyperandrogenism in Women with Polycystic Ovary Syndrome." *Journal of Steroid Biochemistry and Molecular Biology* 122, nos. 1–3 (2009): 42–52. doi: 10.1016/j.jsbmb.2009.12.010.

40. Wang, Xiaoxia, Tongzhang Xian, Xiaofan Jia, Lina Zhang, Li Liu, Fuli Man, Xianbo Zhang, Jie Zhang, Qi Pan, and Lixin Guo. "A Cross-Sectional Study on the Associations of Insulin Resistance with Sex Hormone, Abnormal Lipid Metabolism in T2DM and IGT Patients." *Medicine* 96, no. 26 (2017): doi: 10.1097/MD.0000000000007378.

41. Chen, Li, Rui Chen, Hua Wang, and Fengxia Liang. "Mechanisms Linking Inflammation to Insulin Resistance." *International Journal of Endocrinology* 2015, no. 1 (2015): 50/8409. doi: 10.1155/2015/508409.

42. Rytz, Andreas, Dorothée Adeline, Kim-Anne Lê, Denise Tan, Lisa Lamothe, Olivier Roger, and Katherine Macé. "Predicting Glycemic Index and Glycemic Load from Macronutrients to Accelerate Development of Foods and Beverages with Lower Glucose Responses." *Nutrients* 11, no. 5 (2019): 1172. doi: 10.3390/nu11051172.

43. Hall, Marianna, Magdalena Walicka, and Iwona Traczyk. "[Reactive Hypoglycemia: An Interdisciplinary Approach of the Disease of XXI Century]." *Wiadomosci lekarskie* 73, no. 2 (2020): 384–89. Polish. PMID: 32248180.

44. Xiao, Keyi, Akiko Furutani, Hiroyuki Sasaki, Masaki Takahashi, and Shigenobu Shibata. "Effect of a High Protein Diet at Breakfast on Postprandial Glucose Level at Dinner Time in Healthy Adults." *Nutrients* 15, no. 1 (2022): 85. doi: 10.3390/nu15010085.

45. LeWine, Howard. "How Much Protein Do You Need Every Day?" *Harvard Health*, June 22, 2023. https://www.health.harvard.edu/blog/how-much-protein-do-you-need-every-day-201506188096.

46. Lim, Meng Thiam, Bernice Jiaqi Pan, Darel Wee Kiat Toh, Clarinda Nataria Sutanto, and Jung Eun Kim. "Animal Protein versus Plant Protein in Supporting Lean Mass and Muscle Strength: A Systematic Review and Meta-Analysis of Randomized Controlled Trials." *Nutrients* 13, no. 2 (2021): 661. doi: 10.3390/nu13020661.

47. Biro, Frank, Suzanne Summer, Bin Huang, Chen Chen, Janie Benoit, and Susan Pinney. "The Impact of Macronutrient Intake on Sex Steroids during Onset of Puberty." *Journal of Adolescent Health* 70, no. 3 (2022): 483–87. doi: 10.1016/j.jadohealth.2021.10.011.

48. Aoun, Antoine, Veronique El Khoury, and Roubina Malakieh. "Can Nutrition Help in the Treatment of Infertility?" *Preventive Nutrition and Food*

Science 26, no. 2 (2021): 109–20. https://www.ncbi.nlm.nih.gov/pmc/articles/PMC8276703/.

49. Wu, Guoyao. "Dietary Protein Intake and Human Health." *Food & Function* 7, no. 3 (2016): 1251–65. doi: 10.1039/c5fo01530h.

50. Ryterska, Karina, Agnieszka Kordek, and Patrycja Załęska. "Has Menstruation Disappeared? Functional Hypothalamic Amenorrhea—What Is This Story About?" *Nutrients* 13, no. 8 (2021): 2827. doi: 10.3390/nu13082827.

51. Mergenthaler, Philipp, Ute Lindauer, Gerald A Dienel, and Andreas Meisel. "Sugar for the Brain: The Role of Glucose in Physiological and Pathological Brain Function." *Trends in Neurosciences* 36, no. 10 (2013): 587–97. doi: 10.1016/j.tins.2013.07.001.

52. Sun, Jiayi, Xin Shen, Hui Liu, Siying Lu, Jing Peng, and Haibin Kuang. "Caloric Restriction in Female Reproduction: Is It Beneficial or Detrimental?" *Reproductive Biology and Endocrinology* 19, no. 1 (2021): 1. doi: 10.1186/s12958-020-00681-1.

53. Wise, Lauren A., Amelia K. Wesselink, Katherine L. Tucker, Shilpa Saklani, Ellen M. Mikkelsen, Heidi Cueto, Anders H. Riis, Ellen Trolle, Craig J. McKinnon, Kristen A. Hahn, Kenneth J. Rothman, Henrik Toft Sørensen, and Elizabeth E. Hatch. "Dietary Fat Intake and Fecundability in 2 Preconception Cohort Studies." *American Journal of Epidemiology* 187, no. 1 (2018): 60–74. doi: 10.1093/aje/kwx204.

54. Wang, Ruohan, Ying Feng, Jiahe Chen, Yingjiao Chen, and Fang Ma. "Association between Polyunsaturated Fatty Acid Intake and Infertility among American Women Aged 20–44 Years." *Frontiers in Public Health* 10 (2022): 938343. doi: 10.3389/fpubh.2022.938343.

55. "Omega-3 Fatty Acids: Fact Sheet for Health Professionals." National Institutes of Health, Office of Dietary Supplements. Accessed June 26, 2024. https://ods.od.nih.gov/factsheets/Omega3FattyAcids-HealthProfessional/.

56. Arterburn, Linda, Eileen Hall, and Harry Oken. "Distribution, Interconversion, and Dose Response of N-3 Fatty Acids in Humans." *American Journal of Clinical Nutrition* 83, no. 6 (2006): 1467S–1476S. https://pubmed.ncbi.nlm.nih.gov/16841856/.

57. "Fish: Friend or Foe?" *The Nutrition Source*. Harvard T.H. Chan School of Public Health, May 9, 2024. https://nutritionsource.hsph.harvard.edu/fish/.

58. Teicholz, Nina. "A Short History of Saturated Fat: The Making and Unmaking of a Scientific Consensus." *Current Opinion in Endocrinology, Diabetes, and Obesity* 30, no. 1 (2022): 65–71. doi: 10.1097/MED.0000000000000791.

59. Lambert, Charles P. "Saturated Fat Ingestion Regulates Androgen Concentrations and May Influence Lean Body Mass Accrual." *Journals of Gerontology* 63, no. 11 (2008): 1260–61. doi: 10.1093/gerona/63.11.1260.

60. Kozimor, Amanda, Hui Chang, and Jamie Cooper. "Effects of Dietary Fatty Acid Composition from a High Fat Meal on Satiety." *Appetite* 69 (2013): 39–45. doi: 10.1016/j.appet.2013.05.006.

61. McDonald, Daniel, et al. "American Gut: An Open Platform for Citizen Science Microbiome Research" *mSystems*, May 15, 2018. doi: 10.1128/msystems.00031-18.

62. Ko, Jade Heejae, and Seung-Nam Kim. "A Literature Review of Women's Sex Hormone Changes by Acupuncture Treatment: Analysis of Human and Animal Studies." *Evidence-Based Complementary and Alternative Medicine*, no. 1 (2018): doi: 10.1155/2018/3752723.

63. Liu, Zhan-Wen, Jin Shu, Jia-Ying Tu, Cui-Hong Zhang, and Jue Hong. "Liver in the Chinese and Western Medicine." *Integrative Medicine International* 4, nos. 1–2 (2017): 39–45. doi: 10.1159/000466694.

64. Bondi, Cara A. M., Julia L. Marks, Lauren B. Wroblewski, Heidi S. Raatikainen, Shannon R. Lenox, and Kay E. Gebhardt. "Human and Environmental Toxicity of Sodium Lauryl Sulfate (SLS): Evidence for Safe Use in Household Cleaning Products." *Environmental Health Insights* 9 (2015): 27–32. doi: 10.4137/EHI.S31765.

65. Patel, S. "Fragrance Compounds: The Wolves in Sheep's Clothings." *Medical Hypotheses* 102 (2017): 106–11. doi: 10.1016/j.mehy.2017.03.025.

66. Vom Saal, Frederick S., and Laura N. Vandenberg. "Update on the Health Effects of Bisphenol A: Overwhelming Evidence of Harm." *Endocrinology* 162, no. 3 (2020): bqaa171. doi: 10.7860/JCDR/2013/6518.3306.

67. Wise, Amber, Kacie O'Brien, and Tracey Woodruff. "Are Oral Contraceptives a Significant Contributor to the Estrogenicity of Drinking Water?" *Environmental Science and Technology* 45, no. 1 (2011): 51–60. doi: 10.1021/es1014482.

68. Bretveld, Reini W., Chris M. G. Thomas, Paul T. J. Scheepers, Gerhard A. Zielhuis, and Nel Roeleveld. "Pesticide Exposure: The Hormonal Function of the Female Reproductive System Disrupted?" *Reproductive Biology and Endocrinology* 4, no. 30 (2006). doi: 10.1186/1477-7827-4-30.

69. Ong, Hooi-Theng, Hayati Samsudin, and Herlinda Soto-Valdez. "Migration of Endocrine-Disrupting Chemicals into Food from Plastic Packaging Materials: An Overview of Chemical Risk Assessment, Techniques to Monitor Migration, and International Regulations." *Critical Reviews in Food Science and Nutrition* 62, no. 4 (2022): 957–79. doi: 10.1080/10408398.2020.1830747.

70. Mokra, Katarzyna. "Endocrine Disruptor Potential of Short- and Long-Chain Perfluoroalkyl Substances (PFASs)—a Synthesis of Current Knowledge with Proposal of Molecular Mechanism." *International Journal of Molecular Sciences* 22, no. 4 (2021): 2148. doi: 10.3390/ijms22042148.

71. Hlisníková, Henrieta, Ida Petrovičová, Branislav Kolena, Miroslava Šidlovská, and Alexander Sirotkin. "Effects and Mechanisms of Phthalates' Action on Reproductive Processes and Reproductive Health: A Literature Review." *International Journal of Environmental Research and Public Health* 17, no. 18 (2020):6811. doi: 10.3390/ijerph17186811.

72. Boberg, Julie, Camilla Taxvig, Sofie Christiansen, and Ulla Hass. "Possible Endocrine Disrupting Effects of Parabens and Their Metabolites." *Reproductive Toxicology* 30 no. 2 (2010): 301–12. doi: 10.1016/j.reprotox.2010.03.011.

73. Pacyga, Diana C., Catheryne Chiang, Zhong Li, Rita S. Strakovsky, and Ayelet Ziv-Gal. "Parabens and Menopause-Related Health Outcomes in Midlife Women: A Pilot Study." *Journal of Women's Health* 31, no. 11 (2022): 1645–54. doi: 10.1089/jwh.2022.0004.

74. "EWG Skin Deep®: Your Guide to Safer Personal Care Products." Skin Deep (online database). Accessed June 26, 2024. https://www.ewg.org/skindeep/.

75. "BPA and BPS in Thermal Paper." Minnesota Pollution Control Agency. Accessed June 26, 2024. https://www.pca.state.mn.us/business-with-us/bpa-and-bps-in-thermal-paper#:~:text=Studies%20have%20found%20that%20individual,in%20a%20can%20of%20food.

CHAPTER 7

1. "How to Take a Basal Body Temperature." Pedagogy Education. Accessed June 26, 2024. https://pedagogyeducation.com/getmedia/f6b6c1a6-d4ca-40ca-b119-a4b06cfbc3a2/Basal-Temperature.pdf.

2. Casey, Frances E. "Fertility Awareness-Based Methods of Contraception." *Merck Manual Consumer Version*, August 2023. https://www.merckmanuals.com/home/women-s-health-issues/family-planning/fertility-awareness-based-methods-of-contraception#:~:text=Thus%2C%20of%20the%20fertility%20awareness,she%20gets%20out%20of%20bed.

3. Dunne, F. P., D. G. Barry, J. B. Ferriss, Ginsen Grealy, and D. Murphy. "Changes in Blood Pressure during the Normal Menstrual Cycle." *Clinical Science* 81, no. 4 (1991): 515–18. doi: 10.1042/cs0810515.

4. McKinley, Paula S., Arlene R. King, Peter A. Shapiro, Iordan Slavov, Yixin Fang, Ivy S. Chen, Larry D. Jamner, and Richard P. Sloan. "The Impact of Menstrual Cycle Phase on Cardiac Autonomic Regulation." *Psychophysiology* 46, no. 4 (2009): 904–11. doi: 10.1111/j.1469-8986.2009.00811.x.

5. Fehring, Richard J., Donna Lawrence, and Connie Philpot. "Use Effectiveness of the Creighton Model Ovulation Method of Natural Family Planning." *Journal of Obstetric, Gynecologic, and Neonatal Nursing* 23, no. 4 (2015): 303–9. doi: 10.1111/j.1552-6909.1994.tb01881.x.

6. Hemmatzadeh, Shahla, Sakineh Mohammad Alizadeh Charandabi, Afsaneh Veisy, and Mojgan Mirghafourvand. "Evening Primrose Oil for Cervical Ripening in Term Pregnancies: A Systematic Review and Meta-Analysis." *Journal of Complementary and Integrative Medicine* 20, no. 2 (2021): 328–37. doi: 10.1515/jcim-2020-0314.

7. Palacios, S., C. Mustata, J. M. Rizo, and P. A. Regidor. "Improvement in Menopausal Symptoms with a Nutritional Product Containing Evening Primrose

Oil, Hop Extract, Saffron, Tryptophan, Vitamins B6, D3, K2, B12, and B9." *European Review for Medical and Pharmacological Sciences* 27, no. 17 (2023): 8180–89. doi: 10.26355/eurrev_202309_33578.

8. Kazemi, Farideh, Seyedeh Zahra Masoumi, Arezoo Shayan, and Khodayar Oshvandi. "The Effect of Evening Primrose Oil Capsule on Hot Flashes and Night Sweats in Postmenopausal Women: A Single-Blind Randomized Controlled Trial." *Journal of Menopausal Medicine* 27, no. 1 (2021): 8–14. doi: 10.6118/jmm.20033.

9. Keefe, Catherine E., Renee Mirkes, and Patrick Yeung. "The Evaluation and Treatment of Cervical Factor Infertility a Medical-Moral Analysis." *Linacre Quarterly* 79, no. 4 (2012): 409–25. doi: 10.1179/002436312804827127.

10. Keefe et al. "The Evaluation and Treatment of Cervical Factor Infertility a Medical-Moral Analysis."

11. Kerin, J. "Ovulation Detection in the Human." *Clinical Reproduction and Fertility* 1, no. 1 (1982): 27–54. PMID: 6821195.

CHAPTER 8

1. Mauvais-Jarvis, Franck, Deborah J. Clegg, and Andrea L. Hevener. "The Role of Estrogens in Control of Energy Balance and Glucose Homeostasis." *Endocrine Reviews* 34, no. 3 (2013): 309–38. doi: 10.1210/er.2012-1055.

CHAPTER 9

1. Delgado, Benjamin J., and Wilfredo Lopez-Ojeda. "Estrogen." *StatPearls* (online). Treasure Island, FL: StatPearls Publishing, 2023. https://www.ncbi.nlm.nih.gov/books/NBK538260/.

2. "Sterilization as Birth Control: Types, Cost, Side Effects & Benefits." *Bedsider*. Accessed June 26, 2024. https://www.bedsider.org/birth-control/sterilization.

3. "Levonorgestrel IUDs: Mirena, Kyleena, and Skyla." University Health Services (clinical handout), January 2023. https://uhs.berkeley.edu/sites/default/files/iud_hormonal.pdf.

4. "Levonorgestrel IUDs: Mirena, Kyleena and Skyla."

5. "Levonorgestrel IUDs: Mirena, Kyleena and Skyla."

6. Bayer Healthcare. Mirena (levonorgestrel-releasing intrauterine system), August 2022. https://labeling.bayerhealthcare.com/html/products/pi/Mirena_PI.pdf.

7. "Label: Liletta—Levonorgestrel Intrauterine Device." DailyMed (online database). US National Library of Medicine. Last updated June 9, 2023. https://dailymed.nlm.nih.gov/dailymed/lookup.cfm?setid=aaf0eb2a-f88a-4f26-a445-0fd30176c326.

8. Xiao, Bryan, Tianna Zeng, S. Wu, H. Sun, and N. Xiao. "Effect of Levonorgestrel-Releasing Intrauterine Device on Hormonal Profile and Menstrual Pattern after Long-Term Use." *Contraception* 51, no. 6 (1995): 359–65. doi: 10.1016/0010-7824(95)00102-g.

9. "Copper IUD Contraception." Sexual Health Victoria. Accessed June 26, 2024. https://shvic.org.au/for-you/contraception/iud-intrauterine-device/copper-iud#how-does-the-copper-iud-work.

10. Copper IUD Contraception."

11. "Nexplanon (Etonogestrel Implant): Side Effects, Uses, Dosage, Interactions, Warnings." *RxList*. Last updated October 17, 2023. https://www.rxlist.com/nexplanon-drug.htm.

12. "Birth Control Implant (Nexplanon): Costs, Benefits, and Side Effects." *Bedsider*. Accessed June 26, 2024. https://www.bedsider.org/birth-control/implant.

13. "Side Effects of NEXPLANON." Risks and Side Effects of NEXPLANON® (etonogestrel implant) 68 mg Radiopaque. Organon. Accessed June 26, 2024. https://www.nexplanon.com/side-effects/.

14. "Birth Control Shot (Depo-Provera): Costs, Benefits, and Side Effects." *Bedsider*. Accessed June 26, 2024. https://www.bedsider.org/birth-control/the_shot.

15. Depo-Provera Contraceptive Injection. "Highlights of Prescribing Information." October 2010. https://www.accessdata.fda.gov/drugsatfda_docs/label/2010/020246s036lbl.pdf.

16. Sharts-Hopko, N. C. "Depo–Provera." *American Journal of Maternal/Child Nursing (MCN)* 18, no. 2 (1993): 128. doi: 10.1097/00005721-199303000-00015.

17. Depo-Provera Contraceptive Injection. "Highlights of Prescribing Information."

18. Depo-Provera Contraceptive Injection. "Highlights of Prescribing Information."

19. Cooper, Danielle B., and Preeti Patel. "Oral Contraceptive Pills." *StatPearls* (online). Treasure Island, FL: StatPearls Publishing, 2024. https://www.ncbi.nlm.nih.gov/books/NBK430882/.

20. National Health Service. (NHS). "How Well Contraception Works at Preventing Pregnancy." Last updated January 31, 2024. https://www.nhs.uk/contraception/choosing-contraception/how-well-it-works-at-preventing-pregnancy/#:~:text=Contraceptive%20pill&text=than%2099%25%20effective.-,Fewer%20than%201%20in%20100%20women%20will%20get%20pregnant%20in, get%20pregnant%20in%20a%20year.

21. Cooper and Patel. "Oral Contraceptive Pills."

22. Davtyan, Camelia. "Four Generations of Progestins in Oral Contraceptives." *Clinical Vignette*, Proceedings of UCLA Healthcare 16 (2012). https://www.proceedings.med.ucla.edu/wp-content/uploads/2017/01/Four-generations-of.pdf.

23. Edwards, Michael. "Progestins." *StatPearls* (online). Treasure Island, FL: StatPearls Publishing, 2024. https://www.ncbi.nlm.nih.gov/books/

NBK563211/#:~:text=Each%20of%20the%20progestin%20drugs,levonorgestrel%2C%20desogestrel%2C%20norgestimate%2C%20gestodene.

24. Shoupe, Donna. "The Progestin Revolution 2: Progestins Are Now a Dominant Player in the Tight Interlink between Contraceptive Protection and Bleeding Control-plus More: Contraception and Reproductive Medicine." *Contraceptive and Reproductive Medicine* 8, no. 48 (2023). doi: 10.1186/s40834-023-00249-5.

25. Shoupe. "The Progestin Revolution 2."

26. Shoupe. "The Progestin Revolution 2."

27. Leblanc, Erin S., and Ami Laws. "Benefits and Risks of Third-Generation Oral Contraceptives." *Journal of General Internal Medicine* 14, no. 10 (1999): 625–32. doi: 10.1046/j.1525-1497.1999.08108.x.

28. Shoupe. "The Progestin Revolution 2."

29. Van Vliet, H., D. A. Grimes, F. M. Helmerhorst, and K. F. Schulz. "Biphasic versus Monophasic Oral Contraceptives for Contraception." *Cochrane Database of Systematic Reviews* 2006, no. 3 (2006): CD0022032. doi: 10.1002/14651858.CD002032.pub2.

30. Van Vliet, Hubertus, and Kenneth Schultz. "Triphasic Contraceptive Agent." *Contraception* 65, no. 5 (2002): 321–24. doi: 10.1016/S0010-7824(01)00314-6.

31. Zabin, L. S., P. W. Scher, R. H. DuRant, J. D. Forrest, S. K. Henshaw, and S. J. Emans. "Contraceptive Compliance with a Triphasic and a Monophasic Norethindrone-Containing Oral Contraceptive Pill in a Private Adolescent Practice." *Adolescent and Pediatric Gynecology* 7, no. 1 (1994). https://www.sciencedirect.com/science/article/abs/pii/S0932861012801757.

32. Cohen, J. "Clinical Use of Biphasic and Triphasic Pills." *International Planned Parenthood Federation (IPPF) Medical Bulletin* 19, no. 4 (1985): 1–2. PMID: 12280230.

33. Van Vliet and Schulz. "Triphasic Contraceptive Agent."

34. Berdah, J. "[Pros and Cons of Triphasic Oral Contraception]." *Contraception, fertilite, sexualite* 13, no. 12 (1985): 1205–10. https://pubmed.ncbi.nlm.nih.gov/12267512/.

35. Van Vliet et al. "Biphasic versus Monophasic Oral Contraceptives for Contraception: A Cochrane Review."

36. American College of Obstetricians and Gynecologists (ACOG). "Progestin-Only Hormonal Birth Control: Pill and Injection." *Frequently Asked Questions.* ACOG. Accessed June 27, 2024. https://www.acog.org/womens-health/faqs/progestin-only-hormonal-birth-control-pill-and-injection#:~:text=About%204%20in%2010%20women,the%20lining%20of%20the%20uterus.

37. Cornell. "Progestin-Only Oral Contraceptives (Minipills)." Cornell Health. Accessed June 27, 2024. https://health.cornell.edu/sites/health/files/pdf-library/MiniPills.pdf.

38. "XULANE-Norelgestromin and Ethinyl Estradiol Patch." Xulane. Accessed June 27, 2024. https://dailymed.nlm.nih.gov/dailymed/fda/fdaDrugXsl.cfm?setid=f7848550-086a-43d8-8ae5-047f4b9e4382&type=display.

39. "XULANE-Norelgestromin and Ethinyl Estradiol Patch."

40. Wooltorton, Eric. "The Evra (Ethinyl Estradiol/Norelgestromin) Contraceptive Patch: Estrogen Exposure Concerns." *Canadian Medical Association Journal (CMAJ)* 174, no. 2 (2006): 164–65. doi: 10.1503/cmaj.051623.

41. "Internal Condoms: How to Use an Internal Condom (Insertion ad Removal)." *Bedsider.* Accessed June 27, 2024. https://www.bedsider.org/birth-control/internal_condom.

42. Glasier, A., and A. Gebbie. "Spermicide." *International Encyclopedia of Public Health.* Cambridge, MA: Academic Press, 2008. https://www.sciencedirect.com/topics/agricultural-and-biological-sciences/spermicide#:~:text=Use%20of%20a%20spermicide%20more,urinary%20tract%20infections%20to%20thrive.

43. "Cervical Cap: Birth Control: How It Works and Effectiveness." *Bedsider.* Accessed June 27, 2024. https://www.bedsider.org/birth-control/cervical_cap.

44. "All Birth Control Options: Types of Birth Control: Learn More." *Bedsider.* Accessed June 27, 2024. https://www.bedsider.org/birth-control.

45. "Birth Control Sponges?" Planned Parenthood. Accessed June 27, 2024. https://www.plannedparenthood.org/learn/birth-control/birth-control-sponge.

46. "How Effective Is Pulling Out?" Planned Parenthood. Accessed June 27, 2024. https://www.plannedparenthood.org/learn/birth-control/withdrawal-pull-out-method/how-effective-is-withdrawal-method-pulling-out#:~:text=What%20we%20do%20know%20is,or%20not%20you're%20ovulating.

47. Vekemans, M. "Postpartum Contraception: The Lactational Amenorrhea Method." *European Journal of Contraception and Reproductive Health Care* 2, no. 2 (1997): 105–11. doi: 10.3109/13625189709167463.

48. "Sympto-Thermal Method." Fertility Appreciation Collaborative to Teach the Science (FACTS), 2014. https://www.factsaboutfertility.org/wp-content/uploads/2014/09/SymptoThermalPEH.pdf.

CHAPTER 10

1. Taylor, Alison. "ABC of Subfertility: Extent of the Problem." *British Medical Journal (BMJ)* 327, no. 7412 (2003): 434–36. doi: 10.1136/bmj.327.7412.434.

2. Carson, Sandra Ann, and Amanda N. Kallen. "Diagnosis and Management of Infertility: A Review." *Journal of the American Medical Association (JAMA)* 326, no. 1 (2021): 65–76. doi: 10.1001/jama.2021.4788.

3. Walker, Matthew H., and Kyle Tobler. "Female Infertility." *StatPearls* (online). Treasure Island, FL: StatPearls Publishing, 2023. https://www.ncbi.nlm.nih.gov/books/NBK556033/#:~:text=Ovulatory%20disorders%20make%20up%2025,opportunity%20for%20fertilization%20and%20pregnancy.

4. Samuels, Michelle. "When Does Fertility Return after Stopping Contraceptive Use?" *Birth Control*, November 16, 2020. https://www.bu.edu/sph/news/articles/2020/when-does-fertility-return-after-stopping-contraceptive-use/#:~:text=Earlier%20research%20has%20focused%20mainly,after%20women%20stopped%20taking%20them.

5. Hodges, Romilly E., and Deanna M. Minich. "Modulation of Metabolic Detoxification Pathways Using Foods and Food-Derived Components: A Scientific Review with Clinical Application." *Journal of Nutrition and Metabolism* 1 (2015): doi: 10.1155/2015/760689.

6. Reyes-Hernández, Octavio Daniel, Gabriela Figueroa-González, Laura Itzel Quintas-Granados, Stephany Celeste Gutiérrez-Ruíz, Hector Hernández-Parra, Alejandra Romero-Montero, María Luisa Del Prado-Audelo, Sergio Alberto Bernal-Chavez, Hernán Cortés, Sheila I. Peña-Corona, Lashyn Kiyekbayeva, Dilek Arslan Atessahin, Tamar Goloshvili, Gerardo Leyva-Gómez, and Javad Sharifi-Rad. "3,3′-Diindolylmethane and Indole-3-Carbinol: Potential Therapeutic Molecules for Cancer Chemoprevention and Treatment via Regulating Cellular Signaling Pathways." *Cancer Cell International* 23 (2023): 180. doi: 10.1186/s12935-023-03031-4.

7. Rajoria, Shilpi, Robert Suriano, Perminder Singh Parmar, Yushan Lisa Wilson, Uchechukwu Megwalu, Augustine Moscatello, H Leon Bradlow, Daniel W. Sepkovic, Jan Geliebter, Stimson P. Schantz, and Raj K. Tiwari. "3,3′-Diindolylmethane Modulates Estrogen Metabolism in Patients with Thyroid Proliferative Disease: A Pilot Study." *Thyroid* 21 no. 3 (2011): 299–304. doi: 10.1089/thy.2010.0245.

8. Gupta, K., and M. K. Rana. "Brussels Sprout." *Encyclopedia of Food Sciences and Nutrition*. Cambridge, MA: Academic Press, 2003. https://www.sciencedirect.com/topics/pharmacology-toxicology-and-pharmaceutical-science/brussels-sprout.

9. "Drug-Nutrient Check." Integrative Therapeutics®. Accessed June 27, 2024. https://integrativepro.com/pages/drug-nutrient-interaction-checker.

10. Garner, Tyler, James Malcolm Hester, Allison Carothers, and Francisco J. Diaz. "Role of Zinc in Female Reproduction." *Biology of Reproduction* 104, no. 5 (2021): 976–94. doi: 10.1093/biolre/ioab023.

11. Agbalalah, Tarimoboere, Faith Owabhel Robert, and Emmanuel Amabebe. "Impact of Vitamin B12 on the Reproductive Health of Women with Sickle Cell Disease: A Narrative Review." *Reproduction & Fertility* 4, no. 3 (2023): e230015. https://www.ncbi.nlm.nih.gov/pmc/articles/PMC10388680/.

12. Zhan, Xiaoshu, Lauren Fletcher, Serena Dingle, Enzo Baracuhy, Bingyun Wang, Lee-Anne Huber, and Julang Li. "Choline Supplementation Influences Ovarian Follicular Development." *Frontiers in Bioscience* 26, no. 12 (2021): 1525–36. doi: 10.52586/5046.

13. Rodríguez-Varela, Cristina, and Elena Labarta. "Does Coenzyme Q10 Supplementation Improve Human Oocyte Quality?" *International Journal of Molecular Sciences* 22, no. 17 (2021): 9541. doi: 10.3390/ijms22179541.

14. Sergin, Selin, Vijayashree Jambunathan, Esha Garg, Jason E. Rowntree, and Jenifer I. Fenton. "Fatty Acid and Antioxidant Profile of Eggs from Pasture-Raised Hens Fed a Corn- and Soy-Free Diet and Supplemented with Grass-Fed Beef Suet and Liver." *Foods* 11, no. 21 (2022): 3404. doi: 10.3390/foods11213404.

15. Bentov, Yaakov, Thomas Hannam, Andrea Jurisicova, Navid Esfandiari, and Robert F. Casper. "Coenzyme Q10 Supplementation and Oocyte Aneuploidy in Women Undergoing IVF-ICSI Treatment." *Clinical Medicine Insights: Reproductive Health* 8 (2014): 31–36. doi: 10.4137/CMRH.S14681.

16. Langsjoen, Peter, and Alena Langsjoen. "Comparison Study of Plasma Coenzyme Q10 Levels in Healthy Subjects Supplemented with Ubiquinol Versus Ubiquinone." *Clinical Pharmacology in Drug Development* 3, no. 1 (2014): 13–17. doi: 10.1002/cpdd.73.

17. Nasiadek, Marzenna, Joanna Stragierowicz, Michał Klimczak, and Anna Kilanowicz. "The Role of Zinc in Selected Female Reproductive System Disorders." *Nutrients* 12, no. 8 (2020): 2464. doi: 10.3390/nu12082464.

18. Jamilian, Mehri, Fatemeh Foroozanfard, Fereshteh Bahmani, Rezvan Talee, Mahshid Monavari, and Zatollah Asemi. "Effects of Zinc Supplementation on Endocrine Outcomes in Women with Polycystic Ovary Syndrome: A Randomized, Double-Blind, Placebo-Controlled Trial." *Biological Trace Element Research* 170, no. 2 (2015): 271–78. doi: 10.1007/s12011-015-0480-7.

19. Ośko, Justyna, Wiktoria Pierlejewska, and Małgorzata Grembecka. "Comparison of the Potential Relative Bioaccessibility of Zinc Supplements-in Vitro Studies." *Nutrients* 15, no. 12 (2023): 2813. doi: 10.3390/nu15122813.

20. Cirillo, Michela, Rossella Fucci, Sara Rubini, Maria Elisabetta Coccia, and Cinzia Fatini. "5-Methyltetrahydrofolate and Vitamin B12 Supplementation Is Associated with Clinical Pregnancy and Live Birth in Women Undergoing Assisted Reproductive Technology." *International Journal of Environmental Research and Public Health* 18, no. 23 (2021): 12280. doi: 10.3390/ijerph182312280.

21. D'souza, Naomi, Rishikesh V Behere, Bindu Patni, Madhavi Deshpande, Dattatray Bhat, Aboli Bhalerao, Swapnali Sonawane, Rohan Shah, Rasika Ladkat, Pallavi Yajnik, Souvik K. Bandyopadhyay, Kalyanaraman Kumaran, Caroline Fall, and Chittaranjan S. Yajnik. "Pre-Conceptional Maternal Vitamin B12 Supplementation Improves Offspring Neurodevelopment at 2 Years of Age: Priya Trial." *Frontiers in Pediatrics* 9 (2021): 755977. doi: 10.3389/fped.2021.755977

22. Graydon, James S., Karla Claudio, Seth Baker, Mohan Kocherla, Mark Ferreira, Abiel Roche-Lima, Jovaniel Rodríguez-Maldonado, Jorge Duconge, and Gualberto Ruaño. "Ethnogeographic Prevalence and Implications of the 677C>T and 1298A>C *MTHFR* Polymorphisms in US Primary Care Populations." *Biomarkers in Medicine* 13, no. 8 (2019): 649–61. doi: 10.2217/bmm-2018-0392.

23. Cirillo et al. "5-Methyltetrahydrofolate and Vitamin B12 Supplementation Is Associated with Clinical Pregnancy and Live Birth in Women Undergoing Assisted Reproductive Technology."

24. "Vitamin B12: Fact Sheet for Health Professionals." National Institutes of Health, Office of Dietary Supplements. Accessed June 27, 2024. https://ods.od.nih.gov/factsheets/VitaminB12-HealthProfessional/#:~:text=Even%20at%20large%20doses%2C%20vitamin,does%20not%20store%20excess%20amounts.

25. Korsmo, Hunter W., Xinyin Jiang, and Marie A. Caudill. "Choline: Exploring the Growing Science on Its Benefits for Moms and Babies." *Nutrients* 11, no. 8 (2019): https://www.ncbi.nlm.nih.gov/pmc/articles/PMC6722688/.

26. Stanhiser, J., A. M. Z. Jukic, D. R. McConnaughey, and A. Z. Steiner. "Omega-3 Fatty Acid Supplementation and Fecundability." *Human Reproduction* 37, no. 5 (2022): 1037–46. doi: 10.1093/humrep/deac027.

27. Carlson, Susan E., John Colombo, Byron J. Gajewski, Kathleen M. Gustafson, David Mundy, John Yeast, Michael K. Georgieff, Lisa A. Markley, Elizabeth H. Kerling, and D. Jill Shaddy. "DHA Supplementation and Pregnancy Outcomes." *American Journal of Clinical Nutrition* 97, no. 4 (2013): 808–15. doi: 10.3945/ajcn.112.050021.

28. Bumrungpert, Akkarach, Patcharanee Pavadhgul, Theera Piromsawasdi, and M. R. Mozafari. "Efficacy and Safety of Ferrous Bisglycinate and Folinic Acid in the Control of Iron Deficiency in Pregnant Women: A Randomized, Controlled Trial." *Nutrients* 14, no. 3 (2022): 452. doi: 10.3390/nu14030452.

29. Robinson, Janet, Melanie Wakelin, and Jayne Ellis. "Increased Pregnancy Rate with Use of the Clearblue Easy Fertility Monitor." *Fertility and Sterility* 87, no. 2 (2007): 329–34. doi: 10.1016/j.fertnstert.2006.05.054.

30. "Intercourse Timing and Frequency." Fertility Friend. Accessed June 28, 2024. https://www.fertilityfriend.com/Faqs/Intercourse-Timing-and-Frequency.html.

31. Johnson, Sarah, Lorrae Marriott, and Michael Zinaman. "Increased Likelihood of Pregnancy from Sex on the Two Days Before Ovulation." *Obstetrics & Gynecology* 131 (2018): 20S. doi: 10.1097/01.AOG.0000532907.57204.dd.

32. "Pre-Seed™ Fertility Lubricant." First Response™. Accessed June 27, 2024. https://www.firstresponse.com/en/product-listings/fertility-lubricant.

33. Li, De-Kun, Liyan Liu, and Roxana Odouli. "Exposure to Non-Steroidal Anti-Inflammatory Drugs during Pregnancy and Risk of Miscarriage: Population Based Cohort Study." *BMJ* (*British Medical Journal*) 327, no. 7411 (2003): 368. doi: 10.1136/bmj.327.7411.368.

34. Martinez, LaQuita. "Cell Division" *MedlinePlus Medical Encyclopedia* (video). August 23, 2023. https://medlineplus.gov/ency/anatomyvideos/000025.htm#:~:text=For%20the%20first%2012%20hours,made%20up%20of%2016%20cells.

35. Sharma, Alok, and Pratap Kumar. "Understanding Implantation Window, a Crucial Phenomenon." *Journal of Human Reproductive Sciences* 5, no. 1 (2012): 2–6. doi: 10.4103/0974-1208.97777.

36. Wilcox, A. J., D. D. Baird, and C. R. Weinberg. "Time of Implantation of the Conceptus and Loss of Pregnancy." *New England Journal of Medicine* 340, no. 23 (1999): 1796–99. doi: 10.1056/NEJM199906103402304.

37. Editor. "What Is Implantation Bleeding?" American Pregnancy Association, September 20, 2023. https://americanpregnancy.org/pregnancy-symptoms/what-is-implantation-bleeding/#:~:text=Generally%2C%20around%20a%20third%20of,is%20lighter%20than%20menstrual%20bleeding.

38. Coad, Felicity, and Charlotte Frise. "Tachycardia in Pregnancy: When to Worry?" *Clinical Medicine* 21, no. 5 (2021): e434–37. doi: 10.7861/clinmed.2021-0495.

39. Cole, Laurence A., Jaime M. Sutton-Riley, Sarah A. Khanlian, Marianna Borkovskaya, Brittany B. Rayburn, and William F. Rayburn. "Sensitivity of Over-the-Counter Pregnancy Tests: Comparison of Utility and Marketing Messages." *Journal of the American Pharmacists Association (JAPhA)* 45, no. 5 (2005): 608–15. doi: 10.1331/1544345055001391.

40. "When Can I Expect a Positive HPT If I Am Pregnant?" Fertility Friend. Accessed June 28, 2024. https://www.fertilityfriend.com/Faqs/When-can-I-expect-a-positive-HPT-if-I-am-pregnant.html.

CHAPTER 11

1. Asi, Noor, Khaled Mohammed, Qusay Haydour, Michael R. Gionfriddo, Oscar L. Morey Vargas, Larry J. Prokop, Stephanie S. Faubion, and Mohammad Hassan Murad. "Progesterone vs. Synthetic Progestins and the Risk of Breast Cancer: A Systematic Review and Meta-Analysis." *Systematic Reviews* 5, no. 121 (2016): doi: 10.1186/s13643-016-0294-5.

2. Hermann, Anne, Anne Nafziger, Jennifer Victory, Robert Kulaway, Mario Rocci, and Joseph Bertino. "Over-the-Counter Progesterone Cream Produces Significant Drug Exposure Compared to a Food and Drug Administration-Approved Oral Progesterone Product." *Journal of Clinical Pharmacology* 45, no. 6 (2005): 614–19. https://doi.org/10.1177/0091270005276621.

3. "Headaches." Headaches & Migraines, Menopause Information & Articles | The North American Menopause Society, NAMS. Accessed June 29, 2024. https://www.menopause.org/for-women/menopauseflashes/women's-health-and-menopause/headaches#:~:text=The%20fluctuation%20in%20estrogen%20levels,to%20have%20headaches%20after%20menopause.

4. Doyle, Brian J., Jonna Frasor, Lauren E. Bellows, Tracie D. Locklear, Alice Perez, Jorge Gomez-Laurito, and Gail B. Mahady. "Estrogenic Effects of Herbal Medicines from Costa Rica Used for the Management of Menopausal Symptoms." *Menopause* 16, no. 4 (2009): 748–55. doi: 10.1097/gme.0b013e3181a4c76a.

5. Pareek, Anil, Manish Suthar, Garvendra S. Rathore, and Vijay Bansal. "Feverfew (Tanacetum Parthenium L.): A Systematic Review." *Pharmacognosy Reviews* 5, no. 9 (2011): 103–10. doi: 10.4103/0973-7847.79105.

6. Pareek et al. "Feverfew (Tanacetum Parthenium L.): A Systematic Review."

7. Shaw, Sarah, Katrina Wyatt, John Campbell, Edzard Ernst, and Joanna Thompson-Coon. "Vitex Agnus Castus for Premenstrual Syndrome." *Cochrane Database of Systematic Reviews* 2018, no. 3 (2018): CD004632. doi: 10.1002/14651858.CD004632.pub2.

8. Ambrosini, Anna, Cherubino Lorenzo, Gianluca Coppola, and Francesco Pierelli. "Use of Vitex Agnus-Castus in Migrainous Women with Premenstrual Syndrome: An Open-Label Clinical Observation." *Acta Neurologica Belgica* 113, no. 1 (2013): 25–29. https://pubmed.ncbi.nlm.nih.gov/22791378/.

9. Priyanto, Bambang, Rohadi Rosyidi, Andi Islam, Agus Turchan, and Tusra Pintaningrum. "The Effect of Progesteron for Expression Delta (δ) Opioid Receptor Spinal Cord through Peripheral Nerve Injury." *Annals of Medicine and Surgery* 75 (2022): 103376. doi: 10.1016/j.amsu.2022.103376.

10. Patel, Palak S., and Mia T. Minen. "Complementary and Integrative Health Treatments for Migraine." *Journal of Neuroophthalmology* 39, no. 3 (2019): 360–69. doi: 10.1097/WNO.0000000000000841.

11. Zduńska, Anna, Joanna Cegielska, and Izabela Domitrz. "The Pathogenetic Role of Melatonin in Migraine and Its Theoretic Implications for Pharmacotherapy: A Brief Overview of the Research." *Nutrients* 14, no. 16 (2022): 3335. doi: 10.3390/nu14163335.

12. Rezaie, Sheyda, Gholamreza Askari, Fariborz Khorvash, Mohammad Javad Tarrahi, and Reza Amani. "Effects of Curcumin Supplementation on Clinical Features and Inflammation, in Migraine Patients: A Double-Blind Controlled, Placebo Randomized Clinical Trial." *International Journal of Preventive Medicine* 12 (2021): 161. doi: 10.4103/ijpvm.IJPVM_405_20.

13. Malherbe, Kathryn. "Fibrocystic Breast Disease." *StatPearls* (online). Treasure Island, FL: StatsPearls Publishing, 2023. https://www.ncbi.nlm.nih.gov/books/NBK551609/.

14. Pruthi, Sandhya, Dietlind Wahner-Roedler, Carolyn Torkelson, Stephen Cha, Lori Thicke, Jennifer Hazelton, and Brent Bauer. "Vitamin E and Evening Primrose Oil for Management of Cyclical Mastalgia: A Randomized Pilot Study." *Alternative Medicine Review* 15, no. 1 (2010): 59–67. https://pubmed.ncbi.nlm.nih.gov/20359269/.

15. Hajizadeh, Khadije, Sakineh Mohammad Alizadeh Charandabi, Robab Hazanzade, and Mojgan Mirghafourvand. "Effect of Vitamin E on Severity and Duration of Cyclic Mastalgia: A Systematic Review and Meta-Analysis." *Complementary Therapies in Medicine* 44 (2019): 1–8. https://doi.org/10.1016/j.ctim.2019.03.014.

16. Pruthi et al. "Vitamin E and Evening Primrose Oil for Management of Cyclical Mastalgia: A Randomized Pilot Study."

17. Liang Ooi, Soo, Stephanie Watts, Rhett McClean, and Sok Cheon Pak. "Vitex Agnus-Castus for the Treatment of Cyclic Mastalgia: A Systematic Review and Meta-Analysis." *Journal of Women's Health* 29, no. 2 (2020): 262–78. doi: 10.1089/jwh.2019.7770.

18. Rösner, Harald, Wolfgang Möller, Sabine Groebner, and Pompilio Torremante. "Antiproliferative/Cytotoxic Effects of Molecular Iodine, Povidone-Iodine and Lugol's Solution in Different Human Carcinoma Cell Lines." *Oncology Letters* 12, no. 3 (2016): 2159–62. doi: 10.3892/ol.2016.4811.

19. Kessler, Jack. "The Effect of Supraphysiologic Levels of Iodine on Patients with Cyclic Mastalgia." *Breast Journal* 10, no. 4 (2004): 328–36. https://onlinelibrary.wiley.com/.

20. Bumrungpert, Akkarach, Patcharanee Pavadhgul, Theera Piromsawasdi, and M. R. Mozafari. "Efficacy and Safety of Ferrous Bisglycinate and Folinic Acid in the Control of Iron Deficiency in Pregnant Women: A Randomized, Controlled Trial." *Nutrients* 14, no. 3 (2022): 452. doi: 10.3390/nu14030452.

21. Smith, Stephen J., Adrian L. Lopresti, and Timothy J. Fairchild. "Exploring the Efficacy and Safety of a Novel Standardized Ashwagandha (*Withania Somnifera*) Root Extract (Witholytin®) in Adults Experiencing High Stress and Fatigue in a Randomized, Double-Blind, Placebo-Controlled Trial." *Journal of Psychopharmacology* 37, no. 11 (2023): 1091–104. doi: 10.1177/02698811231200023.

22. Meissner, H. O., A. Mscisz, H. Reich-Bilinska, W. Kapczynski, P. Mrozikiewicz, T. Bobkiewicz-Kozlowska, B. Kedzia, A. Lowicka, and I. Barchia. "Hormone-Balancing Effect of Pre-Gelatinized Organic Maca (Lepidium Peruvianum Chacon): (II) Physiological and Symptomatic Responses of Early-Postmenopausal Women to Standardized Doses of Maca in Double Blind, Randomized, Placebo-Controlled, Multi-Centre Clinical Study." *International Journal of Biomedical Science (IJBS)* 2, no. 4 (2006): 360–74. https://www.ncbi.nlm.nih.gov/pmc/articles/PMC3614647/.

23. Granda, Dominika, Maria Karolina Szmidt, and Joanna Kaluza. "Is Premenstrual Syndrome Associated with Inflammation, Oxidative Stress and Antioxidant Status? A Systematic Review of Case-Control and Cross-Sectional Studies." Antioxidants (Basel, Switzerland), April 14, 2021. https://www.ncbi.nlm.nih.gov/pmc/articles/PMC8070917/.

24. Mohammadi, Mohammad, Nahid Nayeri, Monireh Mashhadi, and Shokoh Varei. "Effect of Omega-3 Fatty Acids on Premenstrual Syndrome: A Systematic Review and Meta-Analysis." *Journal of Obstetrics and Gynaecology Research* 48, no. 6 (2022): 1293–305. doi: 10.1111/jog.15217.

25. Brooks, Nicole, Gisela Wilcox, Karen Walker, John Ashton, Marc Cox, and Lily Stojanovska. "Beneficial Effects of Lepidium Meyenii (MACA) on Psychological Symptoms and Measures of Sexual Dysfunction in Postmenopausal Women Are Not Related to Estrogen or Androgen Content." *Menopause* 15, no. 6 (2008): 1157–62. doi: 10.1097/gme.0b013e3181732953.

26. Smith, Stephen J., Adrian L. Lopresti, and Timothy J. Fairchild. "Exploring the Efficacy and Safety of a Novel Standardized Ashwagandha (*Withania Somnifera*) Root Extract (Witholytin®) in Adults Experiencing High Stress and Fatigue in a Randomized, Double-Blind, Placebo-Controlled Trial." *Journal of Psychopharmacology* 37, no. 11 (2023): 1091–104. doi: 10.1177/02698811231200023.

27. Rhyu, Mee-Ra, Jian Lu, Donna E. Webster, Daniel S. Fabricant, Norman R. Farnsworth, and Z. Jim Wang. "Black Cohosh (Actaea Racemosa, CIMICIFUGA Racemosa) Behaves as a Mixed Competitive Ligand and Partial Agonist at the Human MU Opiate Receptor." *Journal of Agricultural and Food Chemistry* 54, no. 26 (2006): 9852–57. doi: 10.1021/jf062808u.

28. Rajoria, Shilpi, Robert Suriano, Perminder Singh Parmar, Yushan Lisa Wilson, Uchechukwu Megwalu, Augustine Moscatello, H. Leon Bradlow, Daniel W. Sepkovic, Jan Geliebter, Stimson P. Schantz, and Raj K. Tiwari. "3,3'-Diindolylmethane Modulates Estrogen Metabolism in Patients with Thyroid Proliferative Disease: A Pilot Study." *Thyroid* 21, no. 3 (2011): 299–304. doi: 10.1089/thy.2010.0245.

29. Rafieian-Kopaei, Mahmoud, and Mino Movahedi. "Systematic Review of Premenstrual, Postmenstrual and Infertility Disorders of Vitex Agnus Castus." *Electronic Physician* 9, no. 1 (2017): 3685–89. doi: 10.19082/3685.

30. Sohrabi, Nahid, Maryam Kashanian, Sima Ghafoori, and Seyed Malakouti. "Evaluation of the Effect of Omega-3 Fatty Acids in the Treatment of Premenstrual Syndrome: 'A Pilot Trial.'" *Complementary Therapies in Medicine* 21, no. 3 (2013): 141–46. doi: 10.1016/j.ctim.2012.12.008.

31. Smith et al. "Exploring the Efficacy and Safety of a Novel Standardized Ashwagandha (*Withania Somnifera*) Root Extract (Witholytin®) in Adults Experiencing High Stress and Fatigue in a Randomized, Double-Blind, Placebo-Controlled Trial."

32. Cropley, Mark, Adrian Banks, and Julia Boyle. "The Effects of Rhodiola Rosea L. Extract on Anxiety, Stress, Cognition and Other Mood Symptoms." *Phytotherapy Research* 29, no. 12 (2015): 1934–39. doi: 10.1002/ptr.5486.

33. Behboodi Moghadam, Zahra, Elham Rezaei, Roghaieh Shirood Gholami, Masomeh Kheirkhah, and Hamid Haghani. "The Effect of Valerian Root Extract on the Severity of Pre-Menstrual Syndrome Symptoms." *Journal of Traditional and Complementary Medicine* 6, no. 3 (2016): 309–15. doi: 10.1016/j.jtcme.2015.09.001.

34. Brooks, Nicole, Gisela Wilcox, Karen Walker, John Ashton, Marc Cox, and Lily Stojanovska. "Beneficial Effects of Lepidium Meyenii (MACA) on Psychological Symptoms and Measures of Sexual Dysfunction in Postmenopausal Women Are Not Related to Estrogen or Androgen Content." *Menopause* 15, no. 6 (2008): 1157–62. doi: 10.1097/gme.0b013e3181732953.

35. Sohrabi et al. "Evaluation of the Effect of Omega-3 Fatty Acids in the Treatment of Premenstrual Syndrome: 'A Pilot Trial.'"

36. Rafieian-Kopaei, Mahmoud, and Mino Movahedi. "Systematic Review of Premenstrual, Postmenstrual and Infertility Disorders of Vitex Agnus Castus." *Electronic Physician* 9, no. 1 (2017): 3685–89. doi: 10.19082/3685.

37. Maffei, Massimo E. "5-Hydroxytryptophan (5-HTP): Natural Occurrence, Analysis, Biosynthesis, Biotechnology, Physiology and Toxicology." *International Journal of Molecular Sciences* 22, no. 1 (2020): 181. doi: 10.3390/ijms22010181.

38. Eriksson, Olle, Anders Wall, Ulf Olsson, Ina Marteinsdottir, Maria Holstad, Hans Ågren, Per Hartvig, Bengt Långström, and Tord Naessén. "Women with Premenstrual Dysphoria Lack the Seemingly Normal Premenstrual Right-Sided Relative Dominance of 5-HTP-Derived Serotonergic Activity in the Dorsolateral Prefrontal Cortices: A Possible Cause of Disabling Mood Symptoms." *PloS One* 11, no. 9 (2016): e01595838. doi: 10.1371/journal.pone.0159538.

39. Sharma, Anup, Patricia Gerbarg, Teodoro Bottiglieri, Lila Massoumi, Linda L. Carpenter, Helen Lavretsky, Philip R. Muskin, Richard P. Brown, David Mischoulon, and Work Group of the American Psychiatric Association Council on Research. "S-Adenosylmethionine (Same) for Neuropsychiatric Disorders: A Clinician-Oriented Review of Research." *Journal of Clinical Psychiatry* 78, no. 6 (2017): e656–67. doi: 10.4088/JCP.16r11113.

40. Wyatt, K. M., P. W. Dimmock, P. W. Jones, and P. M. Shaughn O'Brien. "Efficacy of Vitamin B-6 in the Treatment of Premenstrual Syndrome: Systematic Review." *British Medical Journal (BMJ)* 318, no. 7195 (1999): 1375–81. doi: 10.1136/bmj.318.7195.1375.

41. Canning, Sarah, Mitch Waterman, Nic Orsi, Julie Ayres, Nigel Simpson, and Louise Dye. "The Efficacy of Hypericum Perforatum (St John's Wort) for the Treatment of Premenstrual Syndrome: A Randomized, Double-Blind, Placebo-Controlled Trial." *CNS Drugs* 24, no. 3 (2010): 207–25. doi: 10.2165/11530120-000000000-00000.

42. Bixo, M., M. Johansson, E. Timby, L. Michalski, and T. Backstrom. "Effects of GABA Active Steroids in the Female Brain with a Focus on the Premenstrual Dysphoric Disorder." *Journal of Neuroendocrinology* 30, no. 2 (2018). doi: 10.1111/jne.12553.

43. Yoon, Seonmin, Jung-Ick Byun, and Won Chul Shin. "Efficacy and Safety of Low-Dose Gamma-Aminobutyric Acid from Unpolished Rice Germ as a Health Functional Food for Promoting Sleep: A Randomized, Double-Blind, Placebo-Controlled Trial." *Journal of Clinical Neurology* 18, no. 4 (2022): 478–80. doi: 10.3988/jcn.2022.18.4.478.

44. Singla, Rajiv, Yashdeep Gupta, Manju Khemani, and Sameer Aggarwal. "Thyroid Disorders and Polycystic Ovary Syndrome: An Emerging Relationship." *Indian Journal of Endocrinology and Metabolism* 19, no. 1 (2015): 25–29. doi: 10.4103/2230-8210.146860.

45. Mohammadi, Mohammad, Roghayeh Mirjalili, and Azam Faraji. "The Impact of Omega-3 Polyunsaturated Fatty Acids on Primary Dysmenorrhea: A Systematic Review and Meta-Analysis of Randomized Controlled Trials." *Journal*

of Obstetrics and Gynaecology Research 48, no. 6 (2022): 1293–305. doi: 10.1111/jog.15217.

46. Mirabi, Parvaneh, Seideh Hanieh Alamolhoda, Seddigheh Esmaeilzadeh, and Faraz Mojab. "Effect of Medicinal Herbs on Primary Dysmenorrhoea: A Systematic Review." *Iranian Journal of Pharmaceutical Research* 13, no. 3 (2014): 757–67. https://www.ncbi.nlm.nih.gov/pmc/articles/PMC4177637/.

47. Parazzini, Fabio, Mirella Martino, and Paolo Pellegrino. "Magnesium in the Gynecological Practice: A Literature Review." *Magnesium Research* 30, no. 1 (2017): 1–7. doi: 10.1684/mrh.2017.0419.

48. Mirabi et al. "Effect of Medicinal Herbs on Primary Dysmenorrhoea."

49. Mirabi et al. "Effect of Medicinal Herbs on Primary Dysmenorrhoea."

50. Omidvar, Shabnam, Sedighe Esmailzadeh, Mahmood Baradaran, and Zahra Basirat. "Effect of Fennel on Pain Intensity in Dysmenorrhoea: A Placebo-Controlled Trial." *Ayu* 33, no. 2 (2012): 311–13. doi: 10.4103/0974-8520.105259.

51. Suzuki, Nobutaka, Kazuo Uebaba, Takafumi Kohama, Nobuhiko Moniwa, Naohiro Kanayama, and Koji Koike. "French Maritime Pine Bark Extract Significantly Lowers the Requirement for Analgesic Medication in Dysmenorrhea: A Multicenter, Randomized, Double-Blind, Placebo-Controlled Study." *Journal of Reproductive Medicine* 53, no. 5 (2008): 338–46. PMID: 18567279.

52. Woo, Hye Lin, Hae Ri Ji, Yeon Kyoung Pak, Hojung Lee, Su Jeong Heo, Jin Moo Lee, and Kyoung Sun Park. "The Efficacy and Safety of Acupuncture in Women with Primary Dysmenorrhea: A Systematic Review and Meta-Analysis." *Medicine* 97, no 23 (2018): e11007. doi: 10.1097/MD.0000000000011007.

53. Taran, F. A., E. A. Stewart, and S. Brucker. "Adenomyosis: Epidemiology, Risk Factors, Clinical Phenotype and Surgical and Interventional Alternatives to Hysterectomy." *Geburtshilfe und Frauenheilkunde* 73, no. 9 (2013): 924–31. doi: 10.1055/s-0033-1350840.

54. Buford, Thomas W., Matthew B. Cooke, Liz L. Redd, Geoffrey M. Hudson, Brian D. Shelmadine, and Darryn S. Willoughby. "Protease Supplementation Improves Muscle Function after Eccentric Exercise." *Medicine and Science in Sports and Exercise* 41, no. 10 (2009): 1908–14. doi: 10.1249/MSS.0b013e3181a518f0.

55. Rajoria et al. "3,3'-Diindolylmethane Modulates Estrogen Metabolism in Patients with Thyroid Proliferative Disease: A Pilot Study."

56. "Calcium-D-Glucarate." *Alternative Medicine Review: A Journal of Clinical Therapeutic* 7, no. 4 (2002): 336–39. https://pubmed.ncbi.nlm.nih.gov/12197785/.

57. Dietz, Birgit M., Atieh Hajirahimkhan, Tareisha L. Dunlap, and Judy L. Bolton. "Botanicals and Their Bioactive Phytochemicals for Women's Health." *Pharmacological Reviews* 68, no. 4 (2016): 1026–73. doi: 10.1124/pr.115.010843.

58. Mohammadi et al. "The Impact of Omega-3 Polyunsaturated Fatty Acids on Primary Dysmenorrhea: A Systematic Review and Meta-Analysis of Randomized Controlled Trials."

59. Mitchell, Jon-Benay, Sarentha Chetty, and Fatima Kathrada. "Progestins in the Symptomatic Management of Endometriosis: A Meta-Analysis on Their Effectiveness and Safety." *BioMed Central Women's Health* 22 (2022): 526. doi: 10.1186/s12905-022-02122-0.

60. Mohammadi et al. "The Impact of Omega-3 Polyunsaturated Fatty Acids on Primary Dysmenorrhea: A Systematic Review and Meta-Analysis of Randomized Controlled Trials."

61. Rezaie et al. "Effects of Curcumin Supplementation on Clinical Features and Inflammation, in Migraine Patients."

62. Dull, Ana-Maria, Marius Alexandru Moga, Oana Gabriela Dimienescu, Gabriela Sechel, Victoria Burtea, and Costin Vlad Anastasiu. "Therapeutic Approaches of Resveratrol on Endometriosis via Anti-Inflammatory and Anti-Angiogenic Pathways." *Molecules* 24, no. 4 (2019): 667. doi: 10.3390/molecules24040667.

63. Kohama, Takafumi, Kotaro Herai, and Masaki Inoue. "Effect of French Maritime Pine Bark Extract on Endometriosis as Compared with Leuprorelin Acetate." *Journal of Reproductive Medicine* 52, no. 8 (2007): 703–8. doi: 10.1155/2018/3752723.

64. Mitchell et al. "Progestins in the Symptomatic Management of Endometriosis: A Meta-Analysis on Their Effectiveness and Safety."

65. Jacobson, Amanda, Sara Vesely, Terah Koch, Janis Campbell, and Sarah O'Brien. "Patterns of von Willebrand Disease Screening in Girls and Adolescents with Heavy Menstrual Bleeding." *Obstetrics & Gynecology* 131, no. 6 (2018): 1121–29. doi: 10.1097/AOG.0000000000002620.

66. Mounsey, Anne, and Rita M. Lahlou. "Heavy Menstrual Bleeding in Premenopausal Patients and the Role of NSAIDs." *American Family Physician* 102, no. 3 (2020): 147–48. https://www.aafp.org/pubs/afp/issues/2020/0801/p147.html.

67. Goshtasebi, Azita, Ziba Mazari, Samira Behboudi Gandevani, and Mohsen Naseri. "Anti-Hemorrhagic Activity of Punica Granatum L. Flower (Persian Golnar) against Heavy Menstrual Bleeding of Endometrial Origin: A Double-Blind, Randomized Controlled Trial." *Medical Journal of the Islamic Republic of Iran* 29 (2015): 199. https://www.ncbi.nlm.nih.gov/pmc/articles/PMC4476216/.

68. Eshaghian, Razieh, Mohammad Mazaheri, Mustafa Ghanadian, Safoura Rouholamin, Awat Feizi, and Mahmoud Babaeian. "The Effect of Frankincense (Boswellia Serrata, Oleoresin) and Ginger (Zingiber Officinale, Rhizoma) on Heavy Menstrual Bleeding: A Randomized, Placebo-Controlled, Clinical Trial." *Complementary Therapies in Medicine* 42 (2018): 42–47. https://pubmed.ncbi.nlm.nih.gov/30670277/.

69. Eshaghian et al. "The Effect of Frankincense (Boswellia Serrata, Oleoresin) and Ginger (Zingiber Officinale, Rhizoma) on Heavy Menstrual Bleeding."

70. Yavarikia, Parisa, Mahnaz Shahnazi, Samira Hadavand Mirzaie, Yousef Javadzadeh, and Razieh Lutfi. "Comparing the Effect of Mefenamic Acid and Vitex

Agnus on Intrauterine Device Induced Bleeding." *Journal of Caring Sciences* 2, no. 3 (2013): 245–54. doi: 10.5681/jcs.2013.030.

71. Solmaz, Soner. "An Overlooked Side Effect of Iron Treatment: Changes in Menstruation." *International Journal of Hematology Research* 2, no. 1 (2016): 120–23. doi: 10.17554/j.issn.2409-3548.2015.01.26.

72. Jewson, Michaela, Prashant Purohit, and Mary Ann Lumsden. "Progesterone and Abnormal Uterine Bleeding/Menstrual Disorders." *Best Practice and Research Clinical Obstetrics and Gynaecology* 69 (2020): 62–73. doi: 10.1016/j.bpobgyn.2020.05.004.

73. "Uterine Fibroids and Polycystic Ovarian Syndrome: Is There a Connection?" Fibroid Treatment Collective. Accessed July 10, 2019. https://fibroids.com/blog/uterine-fibroids-and-polycystic-ovarian-syndrome-is-there-a-connection/.

74. Rajoria et al. "3,3'-Diindolylmethane Modulates Estrogen Metabolism in Patients with Thyroid Proliferative Disease: A Pilot Study."

75. "Calcium-D-Glucarate."

76. Auborn, Karen, Saijun Fan, Eliot Rosen, Leslie Goodwin, Alamelu Chandraskaren, David Williams, DaZhi Chen, and Timothy H. Carter. "Indole-3-Carbinol Is a Negative Regulator of Estrogen." *Journal of Nutrition* 133, no. 7 (2003): 2470S–2475S. doi: 10.1093/jn/133.7.2470s.

77. Lei, Yiming, Lili Yang, Honglian Yang, Min Li, Li Ou, Yang Bai, Taiwei Dong, Feng Gao, and Peifeng Wei. "The Efficacy and Safety of Chinese Herbal Medicine Guizhi Fuling Capsule Combined with Low Dose Mifepristone in the Treatment of Uterine Fibroids: A Systematic Review and Meta-Analysis of 28 Randomized Controlled Trials." *BioMed Central Complementary Medicine and Therapies* 23, no. 54 (2023). doi: 10.1186/s12906-023-03842-y.

78. Briden, Lara. "4 Types of PCOS (a Flowchart)." *The Period Revolutionary*, January 29, 2022. https://www.larabriden.com/4-types-of-pcos-a-flowchart/.

79. Marshall, John C., and Andrea Dunaif. "Should All Women with PCOS Be Treated for Insulin Resistance?" *Fertility and Sterility* 97, no. 1 (2012): 18–22. https://www.ncbi.nlm.nih.gov/pmc/articles/PMC3277302/.

80. Greff, Dorina, Anna E. Juhász, Szilárd Váncsa, Alex Váradi, Zoltán Sipos, Julia Szinte, Sunjune Park, Péter Hegyi, Péter Nyirády, Nándor Ács, Szabolcs Várbíró, and Eszter M. Horváth. "Inositol Is an Effective and Safe Treatment in Polycystic Ovary Syndrome: A Systematic Review and Meta-Analysis of Randomized Controlled Trials." *Reproductive Biology and Endocrinology* 21 (2023): 10. doi: 10.1186/s12958-023-01055-z.

81. Dona, Gabriella, Chiara Sabbadin, Cristina Fiore, Marcantonio Bragadin, Franscesco Giorgino, Eugenio Ragazzi, Giulio Clari, Luciana Bordin, and Decio Armanini. "Inositol Administration Reduces Oxidative Stress in Erythrocytes of Patients with Polycystic Ovary Syndrome." *European Journal of Endocrinology* 166, no. 4 (2012): 703–10. doi: 10.1530/EJE-11-0840.

82. Kalra, Bharti, Sanjay Kalra, and J. B. Sharma. "The Inositols and Polycystic Ovary Syndrome." *Indian Journal of Endocrinology and Metabolism* 20, no. 5 (2016): 720–24. doi: 10.4103/2230-8210.189231.

83. Morais, Jennifer, Juliana Severo, Georgia Alencar, Ana Oliveira, Kyria Cruz, Dilina Marreiro, Betania Freitas, Cecilia Carvalho, Maria Martins, and Karoline Frota. "Effect of Magnesium Supplementation on Insulin Resistance in Humans: A Systematic Review." *Nutrition* 38 (2017): 54–60. doi: 10.1016/j.nut.2017.01.009.

84. Shrivastava, Suyesh, Anamika Sharma, Nishant Saxena, Rashmi Bhamra, and Sandeep Kumar. "Addressing the Preventive and Therapeutic Perspective of Berberine against Diabetes." *Heliyon* 9, no. 11 (2023): e21233. doi: 10.1016/j.heliyon.2023.e21233.

85. Guarano, Alice, Anna Capozzi, Martina Cristodoro, Nicoletta Di Simone, and Stefano Lello. "Alpha Lipoic Acid Efficacy in PCOS Treatment: What Is the Truth?" *Nutrients* 15, no. 14 (2023): 3209. doi: 10.3390/nu15143209.

86. Akbari, Maryam, Vahidreza Ostadmohammadi, Reza Tabrizi, Moein Mobini, Kamran B. Lankarani, Mahmood Moosazadeh, Seyed Taghi Heydari, Maryam Chamani, Fariba Kolahdooz, and Zatollah Asemi. "The Effects of Alpha-Lipoic Acid Supplementation on Inflammatory Markers among Patients with Metabolic Syndrome and Related Disorders: A Systematic Review and Meta-Analysis of Randomized Controlled Trials." *Nutrition and Metabolism* 15, no. 39 (2018): https://doi.org/10.1186/s12986-018-0274-y.

87. Capece, Umberto, Simona Moffa, Ilaria Improta, Gianfranco Di Giuseppe, Enrico Celestino Nista, Chiara M A Cefalo, Francesca Cinti, Alfredo Pontecorvi, Antonio Gasbarrini, Andrea Giaccari, and Teresa Mezza. "Alpha-Lipoic Acid and Glucose Metabolism: A Comprehensive Update on Biochemical and Therapeutic Features." *Nutrients* 15, no. 1 (2022): 18. doi: 10.3390/nu15010018.

88. Foroozanfard, F., M. Jamilian, Z. Jafari, A. Khassaf, A. Hosseini, H. Khorammian, and Z. Asemi. "Effects of Zinc Supplementation on Markers of Insulin Resistance and Lipid Profiles in Women with Polycystic Ovary Syndrome: A Randomized, Double-Blind, Placebo-Controlled Trial." *Experimental and Clinical Endocrinology and Diabetes* 123, no. 4 (2015): 215–20. doi: 10.1055/s-0035-1548790.

89. Rajoria et al. "3,3'-Diindolylmethane Modulates Estrogen Metabolism in Patients with Thyroid Proliferative Disease: A Pilot Study."

90. Lakshmi, Jada Naga, Ankem Narendra Babu, S. S. Mani Kiran, Lakshmi Prasanthi Nori, Nageeb Hassan, Akram Ashames, Richie R Bhandare, and Afzal B. Shaik. "Herbs as a Source for the Treatment of Polycystic Ovarian Syndrome: A Systematic Review." *Biotech* 12, no. 1 (2023): 4. doi: 10.3390/biotech12010004.

91. Greff et al. "Inositol Is an Effective and Safe Treatment in Polycystic Ovary Syndrome."

92. Dona et al. "Inositol Administration Reduces Oxidative Stress in Erythrocytes of Patients with Polycystic Ovary Syndrome."

93. Kalra et al. "The Inositols and Polycystic Ovary Syndrome."

94. Beglaryan, Narine, Gagik Hakobyan, and Eduard Nazaretyan. "Vitamin C Supplementation Alleviates Hypercortisolemia Caused by Chronic Stress." *Stress Health* 40, no. 3 (2024): e3347. doi: 10.1002/smi.3347.

95. Zeng, Ling-Hui, Saba Rana, Liaqat Hussain, Muhammad Asif, Malik Hassan Mehmood, Imran Imran, Anam Younas, Amina Mahdy, Fakhria A. Al-Joufi, and Shaymaa Najm Abed. "Polycystic Ovary Syndrome: A Disorder of Reproductive Age, Its Pathogenesis, and a Discussion on the Emerging Role of Herbal Remedies." *Frontiers in Pharmacology* 13 (2022): 874914. doi: 10.3389/fphar.2022.874914.

96. Mao, Qing-Qiu, Siu-Po Ip, Yan-Fang Xian, Zhen Hu, and Chun-Tao Che. "Anti-Depressant-like Effect of Peony: A Mini-Review." *Pharmaceutical Biology* 50, no. 1 (2012): 72–77. doi: 10.3109/13880209.2011.602696.

97. Kalani, Amir, Gul Bahtiyar, and Alan Sacerdote. "Ashwagandha Root in the Treatment of Non-Classical Adrenal Hyperplasia." *BMJ Case Reports* (2012): doi: 10.1136/bcr-2012-006989.

98. Greff et al. "Inositol Is an Effective and Safe Treatment in Polycystic Ovary Syndrome."

99. Dona et al. "Inositol Administration Reduces Oxidative Stress in Erythrocytes of Patients with Polycystic Ovary Syndrome."

100. Kalra et al. "The Inositols and Polycystic Ovary Syndrome."

101. González, Frank. "Inflammation in Polycystic Ovary Syndrome: Underpinning of Insulin Resistance and Ovarian Dysfunction." *Steroids* 77, no. 4 (2011): 300–305. doi: 10.1016/j.steroids.2011.12.003.

102. Greff et al. "Inositol Is an Effective and Safe Treatment in Polycystic Ovary Syndrome."

103. Dona et al. "Inositol Administration Reduces Oxidative Stress in Erythrocytes of Patients with Polycystic Ovary Syndrome."

104. Kalra et al. "The Inositols and Polycystic Ovary Syndrome."

105. Rezaie et al. "Effects of Curcumin Supplementation on Clinical Features and Inflammation, in Migraine Patients."

106. Guarano et al. "Alpha Lipoic Acid Efficacy in PCOS Treatment: What Is the Truth?"

107. Akbari et al. "The Effects of Alpha-Lipoic Acid Supplementation on Inflammatory Markers among Patients with Metabolic Syndrome and Related Disorders: A Systematic Review and Meta-Analysis of Randomized Controlled Trials."

108. Capece et al. "Alpha-Lipoic Acid and Glucose Metabolism: A Comprehensive Update on Biochemical and Therapeutic Features."

109. Liu, Jiajun, Haodong Su, Xueshan Jin, Lan Wang, and Jieming Huang. "The Effects of N-Acetylcysteine Supplement on Metabolic Parameters in Women with Polycystic Ovary Syndrome: A Systematic Review and Meta-Analysis." *Frontiers in Nutrition* 10 (2023): 1209614. doi: 10.3389/fnut.2023.1209614.

110. Patel, Archan, Deepika Dewani, Arpita Jaiswal, Pallavi Yadav, and Lucky Srivani Reddy. "Exploring Melatonin's Multifaceted Role in Polycystic Ovary Syndrome Management: A Comprehensive Review." *Cureus* 15, no. 11 (2023): e48929. doi: 10.7759/cureus.48929.

111. Smith et al. "Exploring the Efficacy and Safety of a Novel Standardized Ashwagandha (*Withania Somnifera*) Root Extract (Witholytin®) in Adults Experiencing High Stress and Fatigue in a Randomized, Double-Blind, Placebo-Controlled Trial."

112. Kamel, Hany H. "Role of Phyto-Oestrogens in Ovulation Induction in Women with Polycystic Ovarian Syndrome." *European Journal of Obstetrics, Gynecology, and Reproductive Biology* 291 (2013): doi: 10.1016/j.ejogrb.2023.09.027.

113. Meissner, H. O., A. Mscisz, H. Reich-Bilinska, W. Kapczynski, P. Mrozikiewicz, T. Bobkiewicz-Kozlowska, B. Kedzia, A. Lowicka, and I. Barchia. "Hormone-Balancing Effect of Pre-Gelatinized Organic Maca (Lepidium Peruvianum Chacon): (II) Physiological and Symptomatic Responses of Early-Postmenopausal Women to Standardized Doses of Maca in Double Blind, Randomized, Placebo-Controlled, Multi-Centre Clinical Study." *International Journal of Biomedical Science* 2, no. 4 (2006): 360–74. https://www.ncbi.nlm.nih.gov/pmc/articles/PMC3614647/.

114. Zhao, Ting-Tint, Yong-Kang Liu, Jun-Ling Zhou, Hou-Xu Ning, Xiao-Liang Wu, Ya-Fang Song, Jian-Hua Sun, and Li-Xia Pei. "[Effect of Acupuncture on Hypothalamic Functional Connectivity in Patients with Premature OVA-Rian Insufficiency Based on Resting-State Functional Magnetic Resonance Imaging]." *Zhen ci yan jiu* 47, no. 7 (2022): 617–24. doi: 10.13702/j.1000-0607.20210399.

115. Barron, Mary Lee. "Light Exposure, Melatonin Secretion, and Menstrual Cycle Parameters: An Integrative Review." *Biological Research for Nursing* (2007): 49–69. doi: 10.1177/1099800407303337.

116. Zhang, Jianfu, and Bengui Jiang. "Influence of Melatonin Treatment on Emotion, Sleep, and Life Quality in Perimenopausal Women: A Clinical Study." *Journal of Healthcare Engineering* 2023, no. 1 (2023): 2198804. doi: 10.1155/2023/2198804.

117. Rajoria et al. "3,3'-Diindolylmethane Modulates Estrogen Metabolism in Patients with Thyroid Proliferative Disease: A Pilot Study."

118. "Calcium-D-Glucarate."

119. Auborn et al. "Indole-3-Carbinol Is a Negative Regulator of Estrogen."

120. Muto, Michael. "Patient Education: Ovarian Cysts (Beyond the Basics)." *UpToDate*, January 2023. https://www.uptodate.com/contents/ovarian-cysts-beyond-the-basics/print#:~:text=Large%20cysts%20.

121. Inki, P., R. Hurskainen, P. Palo, E. Ekholm, S. Grenman, A. Kivela, E. Kujansuu, J. Teperi, M. Yliskoski, and J. Paavonen. "Comparison of Ovarian Cyst Formation in Women Using the Levonorgestrel-Releasing Intrauterine System vs. Hysterectomy." *Ultrasound in Obstetrics and Gynecology* 20, no. 4 (2002): 381–85. doi: 10.1046/j.1469-0705.2002.00805.x.

122. Pandya, Matangee, Shilpa B. Donga, L. P. Dei, and Anup B. Thakar. "Efficacy of *Virechana*, *Triphaladi* Decoction with Processed *Guggulu* in the Management of Ovarian Cyst: A Pilot Study." *Ayu* 41, no. 3 (2022): 166–72. doi: 10.4103/ayu.AYU_254_19.

123. Wang, Hai-Yan, Xi-Hua Bao, and Jun-Feng Dai. "[Treatment of Ovarian Cyst after Ovulation-Induction with Sanjie Zhentong Capsule]." *Zhongguo Zhong xi yi jie he za zhi Zhongguo Zhongxiyi jiehe zazhi* [Chinese journal of integrated traditional and Western medicine] 28, no. 11 (2008): 1026–28. PMID: 19213349.

124. Hasrat, Nazik H., and Asaad Q. Al-Yassen. "The Relationship between Acne Vulgaris and Insulin Resistance." *Cureus* 15, no. 1 (2023): e34241. doi: 10.7759/cureus.34241.

125. Baldwin, Hilary, and Jerry Tan. "Effects of Diet on Acne and Its Response to Treatment." *American Journal of Clinical Dermatology* 22, no. 1 (2021): 55–65. doi: 10.1007/s40257-020-00542-y.

126. Ugazio, Elena, Vivian Tullio, Arianna Binello, Silvia Tagliapietra, and Franco Dosio. "Ozonated Oils as Antimicrobial Systems in Topical Applications. Their Characterization, Current Applications, and Advances in Improved Delivery Techniques." *Molecules* 25, no. 2 (2020): 334. doi: 10.3390/molecules25020334.

127. Puglia, Lídice Tavares, Jean Lowry, and Gianluca Tamagno. "Vitex Agnus Castus Effects on Hyperprolactinaemia." *Frontiers in Endocrinology* 14 (2023): 1269781. doi: 10.3389/fendo.2023.1269781.

128. Ambrosini et al. "Use of Vitex Agnus-Castus in Migrainous Women with Premenstrual Syndrome: An Open-Label Clinical Observation."

129. Abraham, G. E. "Nutritional Factors in the Etiology of the Premenstrual Tension Syndromes." *Journal of Reproductive Medicine* 28, no. 7 (1983): 446–64. https://pubmed.ncbi.nlm.nih.gov/6684167/.

130. Mumford, Sunni L., Richard W. Browne, Karen C. Schliep, Jonathan Schmelzer, Torie C. Plowden, Kara A. Michels, Lindsey A. Sjaarda, Shvetha M. Zarek, Neil J. Perkins, Lynne C. Messer, Rose G. Radin, Jean Wactawski-Wende, and Enrique F. Schisterman. "Serum Antioxidants Are Associated with Serum Reproductive Hormones and Ovulation among Healthy Women." *Journal of Nutrition* 146, no. 1 (2015): 98–106. doi: 10.3945/jn.115.217620.

BIBLIOGRAPHY

Abbasi, Behnood, Masud Kimiagar, Khosro Sadeghniiat, Minoo M. Shirazi, Mehdi Hedayati, and Bahram Rashidkhani. "The Effect of Magnesium Supplementation on Primary Insomnia in Elderly: A Double-Blind Placebo-Controlled Clinical Trial." *Journal of Research in Medical Sciences* 17, no. 12 (2012): 1161–69. https://www.ncbi.nlm.nih.gov/pmc/articles/PMC3703169/.

Abraham, G. E. "Nutritional Factors in the Etiology of the Premenstrual Tension Syndromes." *Journal of Reproductive Medicine* 28, no. 7 (1983): 446–64. https://pubmed.ncbi.nlm.nih.gov/6684167/.

Adam, Emma K., Meghan E. Quinn, Royette Tavernier, Mollie T. McQuillan, Katie A. Dahlke, and Kirsten E. Gilbert. "Diurnal Cortisol Slopes and Mental and Physical Health Outcomes: A Systematic Review and Meta-Analysis." *Psychoneuroendocrinology* 24, no. 83 (2017): 25–41. https://www.ncbi.nlm.nih.gov/pmc/articles/PMC5568897/#:~:text=Cortisol%20levels%20typically%20follow%20a,1997%3B%20Adam%20and%20Kumari%2C%202009.

Adnane, Mounir, Kieran G. Meade, and Cliona O'Farrelly. "Cervico-Vaginal Mucus (CVM): An Accessible Source of Immunologically Informative Biomolecules." *Veterinary Research Communications* 42, no. 4 (2018): 255–63. https://www.ncbi.nlm.nih.gov/pmc/articles/PMC6244541/.

"Adult Activity: An Overview." *Physical Activity Basics*, December 20, 2023. Centers for Disease Control and Prevention. https://www.cdc.gov/physical-activity-basics/guidelines/adults.html?CDC_AAref_Val=https%3A%2F%2Fwww.cdc.gov%2Fphysicalactivity%2Fbasics%2Fadults%2Findex.htm.

Agbalalah, Tarimoboere, Faith Owabhel Robert, and Emmanuel Amabebe. "Impact of Vitamin B12 on the Reproductive Health of Women with Sickle

Cell Disease: A Narrative Review." *Reproduction & Fertility* 4, no. 3 (2023): e230015. https://www.ncbi.nlm.nih.gov/pmc/articles/PMC10388680/.

Akbari, Maryam, Vahidreza Ostadmohammadi, Reza Tabrizi, Moein Mobini, Kamran B. Lankarani, Mahmood Moosazadeh, Seyed Taghi Heydari, Maryam Chamani, Fariba Kolahdooz, and Zatollah Asemi. "The Effects of Alpha-Lipoic Acid Supplementation on Inflammatory Markers among Patients with Metabolic Syndrome and Related Disorders: A Systematic Review and Meta-Analysis of Randomized Controlled Trials." *Nutrition & Metabolism* 15, no. 39 (2018): https://doi.org/10.1186/s12986-018-0274-y.

"All Birth Control Options: Types of Birth Control: Learn More." *Bedsider*. Accessed June 27, 2024. https://www.bedsider.org/birth-control.

Ambrosini, Anna, Cherubino Di Lorenzo, Gianluca Coppola, and Francesco Pierelli. "Use of Vitex Agnus-Castus in Migrainous Women with Premenstrual Syndrome: An Open-Label Clinical Observation." *Acta Neurologica Belgica* 113, no. 1 (2013): 25–29. https://pubmed.ncbi.nlm.nih.gov/22791378/.

American College of Obstetricians and Gynecologists (ACOG). "Progestin-Only Hormonal Birth Control: Pill and Injection." *Frequently Asked Questions*. ACOG. Accessed June 27, 2024. https://www.acog.org/womens-health/faqs/progestin-only-hormonal-birth-control-pill-and-injection#:~:text=About%204%20in%2010%20women,the%20lining%20of%20the%20uterus.

Aoun, Antoine, Veronique El Khoury, and Roubina Malakieh. "Can Nutrition Help in the Treatment of Infertility?" *Preventive Nutrition and Food Science* 26, no. 2 (2021): 109–20. https://www.ncbi.nlm.nih.gov/pmc/articles/PMC8276703/

Arterburn, Linda, Eileen Hall, and Harry Oken. "Distribution, Interconversion, and Dose Response of N-3 Fatty Acids in Humans." *American Journal of Clinical Nutrition* 83, no. 6 (2006): 1467S–76S. https://pubmed.ncbi.nlm.nih.gov/16841856/.

Asi, Noor, Khaled Mohammed, Qusay Haydour, Michael R. Gionfriddo, Oscar L. Morey Vargas, Larry J. Prokop, Stephanie S. Faubion, and Mohammad Hassan Murad. "Progesterone vs. Synthetic Progestins and the Risk of Breast Cancer: A Systematic Review and Meta-Analysis." *Systematic Reviews* 5, no. 121 (2016): doi: 10.1186/s13643-016-0294-5.

Auborn, Karen, Saijun Fan, Eliot Rosen, Leslie Goodwin, Alamelu Chandraskaren, David Williams, DaZhi Chen, and Timothy H. Carter. "Indole-3-Carbinol Is a Negative Regulator of Estrogen." *Journal of Nutrition* 133, no. 7 (2003): 2470S–75S. doi: 10.1093/jn/133.7.2470s.

Awwad, Johnny, Ghina Ghazeeri, Thomas Toth, Antoine Hannoun, Miche Abou Abdallah, and Chantal Farra. "Fever in Women May Interfere with Follicular Development during Controlled Ovarian Stimulation." *International Journal of Hyperthermia* 28, no. 8 (2012): 742–46. doi: 10.3109/02656736.2012.724516.

Baker, James M., Layla Al-Nakkash, and Melissa Herbst-Kralovets. "Estrogen-Gut Microbiome Axis: Physiological and Clinical Implications." *Maturitas* 103 (2017): 45–53. doi: 10.1016/j.maturitas.2017.06.025.

Baldwin, Hilary, and Jerry Tan. "Effects of Diet on Acne and Its Response to Treatment." *American Journal of Clinical Dermatology* 22, no. 1 (2021): 55–65. doi: 10.1007/s40257-020-00542-y.

Baptiste, Catherine G., Marie-Claude Battista, Andréanne Trottier, and Jean-Patrice Baillargeon. "Insulin and Hyperandrogenism in Women with Polycystic Ovary Syndrome." *Journal of Steroid Biochemistry and Molecular Biology* 122, nos. 1–3 (2009): 42–52. doi: 10.1016/j.jsbmb.2009.12.010.

Barron, Mary Lee. "Light Exposure, Melatonin Secretion, and Menstrual Cycle Parameters: An Integrative Review." *Biological Research for Nursing* (2007): 49–69. doi: 10.1177/1099800407303337.

Bayer Healthcare. Mirena (levonorgestrel-releasing intrauterine system). August 2022. https://labeling.bayerhealthcare.com/html/products/pi/Mirena_PI.pdf.

Beglaryan, Narine, Gagik Hakobyan, and Eduard Nazaretyan. "Vitamin C Supplementation Alleviates Hypercortisolemia Caused by Chronic Stress." *Stress Health* 40, no. 3 (2024): e3347. doi: 10.1002/smi.3347.

Behboodi Moghadam, Zahra, Elham Rezaei, Roghaieh Shirood Gholami, Masomeh Kheirkhah, and Hamid Haghani. "The Effect of Valerian Root Extract on the Severity of Pre-Menstrual Syndrome Symptoms." *Journal of Traditional and Complementary Medicine* 6, no. 3 (2016): 309–15. doi: 10.1016/j.jtcme.2015.09.001.

Bentov, Yaakov, Thomas Hannam, Andrea Jurisicova, Navid Esfandiari, and Robert F. Casper. "Coenzyme Q10 Supplementation and Oocyte Aneuploidy in Women Undergoing IVF-ICSI Treatment." *Clinical Medicine Insights: Reproductive Health* 8 (2014): 31–36. doi: 10.4137/CMRH.S14681.

Berdah, J. "[Pros and Cons of Triphasic Oral Contraception]." *Contraception, fertilite, sexualite* 13, no. 12 (1985): 1205–10. https://pubmed.ncbi.nlm.nih.gov/12267512/.

Berkey, Jennifer. "Staying Active Increases Your Long-Term Happiness." Michigan State University Extension, March 8, 2013. https://www.canr.msu.edu/news/staying_active_increases_your_long-term_happiness#:~:text=Recent%20research%20published%20in%20the,activity%20tend%20to%20be%20unhappier.

Beyer, Kirsten M. M., Aniko Szabo, Kelly Hoormann, and Melinda Stolley. "Time Spent Outdoors, Activity Levels, and Chronic Disease among American Adults." *Journal of Behavioral Medicine* 41, no. 4 (2018): 494–503. doi: 10.1007/s10865-018-9911-1.

Biro, Frank, Suzanne Summer, Bin Huang, Chen Chen, Janie Benoit, and Susan Pinney. "The Impact of Macronutrient Intake on Sex Steroids during Onset of Puberty." *Journal of Adolescent Health* 70, no. 3 (2022): 483–87. doi: 10.1016/j.jadohealth.2021.10.011.

"Birth Control Implant (Nexplanon): Costs, Benefits, and Side Effects." *Bedsider*. Accessed June 26, 2024. https://www.bedsider.org/birth-control/implant.

"Birth Control Shot (Depo-Provera): Costs, Benefits, and Side Effects." *Bedsider*. Accessed June 26, 2024. https://www.bedsider.org/birth-control/the_shot.

"Birth Control Sponges?" Planned Parenthood. Accessed June 27, 2024. https://www.plannedparenthood.org/learn/birth-control/birth-control-sponge.

Bixo, M., M. Johansson, E. Timby, L. Michalski, and T. Bäckström. "Effects of GABA Active Steroids in the Female Brain with a Focus on the Premenstrual Dysphoric Disorder." *Journal of Neuroendocrinology* 30, no. 2 (2018). doi: 10.1111/jne.12553.

Boberg, Julie, Camilla Taxvig, Sofie Christiansen, and Ulla Hass. "Possible Endocrine Disrupting Effects of Parabens and Their Metabolites." *Reproductive Toxicology* 30 no. 2 (2010): 301–12. doi: 10.1016/j.reprotox.2010.03.011.

Bondi, Cara A. M., Julia L. Marks, Lauren B. Wroblewski, Heidi S. Raatikainen, Shannon R. Lenox, and Kay E. Gebhardt. "Human and Environmental Toxicity of Sodium Lauryl Sulfate (SLS): Evidence for Safe Use in Household Cleaning Products." *Environmental Health Insights* 9 (2015): 27–32. doi: 10.4137/EHI.S31765.

Bouma, E. M. C., H. Riese, J. Ormel, F. C. Verhulst, and A. J. Oldehinkl. "Adolescents' Cortisol Responses to Awakening and Social Stress; Effects of Gender, Menstrual Phase and Oral Contraceptives. The TRAILS Study." *Psychoneuroendocrinology* 34, no. 6 (2009): 884–93. https://doi.org/10.1016/j.psyneuen.2009.01.003.

Bowman, Katy. "Thanks for the Mammaries." *Nutritious Movement*, June 1, 2017. https://www.nutritiousmovement.com/thanks-for-the-mammaries/.

"BPA and BPS in Thermal Paper." Minnesota Pollution Control Agency. Accessed June 26, 2024. https://www.pca.state.mn.us/business-with-us/bpa-and-bps-in-thermal-paper#:~:text=Studies%20have%20found%20that%20individual,in%20a%20can%20of%20food.

Bretveld, Reini W., Chris M. G. Thomas, Paul T. J. Scheepers, Gerhard A. Zielhuis, and Nel Roeleveld. "Pesticide Exposure: The Hormonal Function of the Female Reproductive System Disrupted?" *Reproductive Biology and Endocrinology* 4, no. 30 (2006): https://doi.org/10.1186/1477-7827-4-30.

Briden, Lara. "4 Types of PCOS (a Flowchart)." *The Period Revolutionary*, January 29, 2022. https://www.larabriden.com/4-types-of-pcos-a-flowchart/.

Brooks, Nicole, Gisela Wilcox, Karen Walker, John Ashton, Marc Cox, and Lily Stojanovska. "Beneficial Effects of Lepidium Meyenii (MACA) on Psychological Symptoms and Measures of Sexual Dysfunction in Postmenopausal Women Are Not Related to Estrogen or Androgen Content." *Menopause* 15, no. 6 (2008): 1157–62. doi: 10.1097/gme.0b013e3181732953.

Buford, Thomas W., Matthew B. Cooke, Liz L. Redd, Geoffrey M. Hudson, Brian D. Shelmadine, and Darryn S. Willoughby. "Protease Supplementation Improves Muscle Function after Eccentric Exercise." *Medicine and Science in Sports and Exercise* 41, no. 10 (2009): 1908–14. doi: 10.1249/MSS.0b013e3181a518f0.

Bumrungpert, Akkarach, Patcharanee Pavadhgul, Theera Piromsawasdi, and M. R. Mozafari. "Efficacy and Safety of Ferrous Bisglycinate and Folinic Acid in the Control of Iron Deficiency in Pregnant Women: A Randomized, Controlled Trial." *Nutrients* 14, no. 3 (2022): 452. doi: 10.3390/nu14030452.

Butler, Karyn Geralyn. "Relationship between the Cortisol-Estradiol Phase Difference and Affect in Women." *Journal of Circadian Rhythms* 16, no. 3 (2018): article 3. doi: 10.5334/jcr.154.

Cahill, David J., Peter G. Wardle, Christopher R. Harlow, and M. G. R. Hull. "Onset of the Preovulatory Luteinizing Hormone Surge: Diurnal Timing and Critical Follicular Prerequisites." *Fertility and Sterility* 70, no. 1 (1998): 56–59. https://doi.org/10.1016/S0015-0282(98)00113-7.

"Calcium-D-Glucarate." *Alternative Medicine Review: A Journal of Clinical Therapeutic* 7, no. 4 (2002): 336–39. https://pubmed.ncbi.nlm.nih.gov/12197785/.

Canning, Sarah, Mitch Waterman, Nic Orsi, Julie Ayres, Nigel Simpson, and Louise Dye. "The Efficacy of Hypericum Perforatum (St. John's Wort) for the Treatment of Premenstrual Syndrome: A Randomized, Double-Blind, Placebo-Controlled Trial." *CNS Drugs* 24, no. 3 (2010): 207–25. https://pubmed.ncbi.nlm.nih.gov/20155996/.

Capece, Umberto, Simona Moffa, Ilaria Improta, Gianfranco Di Giuseppe, Enrico Celestino Nista, Chiara M. A. Cefalo, Francesca Cinti, Alfredo Pontecorvi, Antonio Gasbarrini, Andrea Giaccari, and Teresa Mezza. "Alpha-Lipoic Acid and Glucose Metabolism: A Comprehensive Update on Biochemical and Therapeutic Features." *Nutrients* 15, no. 1 (2022): 18. doi: 10.3390/nu15010018.

Carlson, Susan E., John Colombo, Byron J. Gajewski, Kathleen M. Gustafson, David Mundy, John Yeast, Michael K. Georgieff, Lisa A. Markley, Elizabeth H. Kerling, and D. Jill Shaddy. "DHA Supplementation and Pregnancy Outcomes." *American Journal of Clinical Nutrition* 97, no. 4 (2013): 808–15. doi: 10.3945/ajcn.112.050021.

Carson, Sandra Ann, and Amanda N. Kallen. "Diagnosis and Management of Infertility: A Review." *Journal of the American Medical Association (JAMA)* 326, no. 1 (2021): 65–76. doi: 10.1001/jama.2021.4788.

Casey, Frances E. "Fertility Awareness-Based Methods of Contraception." *Merck Manual Consumer Version*, August 2023. https://www.merckmanuals.com/home/women-s-health-issues/family-planning/fertility-awareness-based-methods-of-contraception#:~:text=Thus%2C%20of%20the%20fertility%20awareness,she%20gets%20out%20of%20bed.

"Cervical Cap: Birth Control: How It Works and Effectiveness." *Bedsider*. Accessed June 27, 2024. https://www.bedsider.org/birth-control/cervical_cap.

Chandrasekaran, Anita, Bhuvan Molparia, Ehsaan Akhtar, Xiaoyun Wang, James D. Lewis, John T. Chang, Glenn Oliveira, Ali Torkamani, and Gauree Gupta Konijeti. "The Autoimmune Protocol Diet Modifies Intestinal RNA Expression in Inflammatory Bowel Disease." *Crohn's & Colitis* 1, no. 3 (2019): otz016. https://doi.org/10.1093/crocol/otz016.

Chaput, Jean-Philippe, Caroline Dutil, and Hugues Sampasa-Kanyinga. "Sleeping Hours: What Is the Ideal Number and How Does Age Impact This?" *Nature and Science of Sleep* 10 (2018): 421–30. doi: 10.2147/NSS.S163071.

Chen, Li, Rui Chen, Hua Wang, and Fengxia Liang. "Mechanisms Linking Inflammation to Insulin Resistance." *International Journal of Endocrinology* 2015, no. 1 (2015): 50/8409. doi: 10.1155/2015/508409.

Ciarambino, Tiziana, Pietro Crispino, Gloria Guarisco, and Mauro Giordano. "Gender Differences in Insulin Resistance: New Knowledge and Perspectives." *Current Issues in Molecular Biology* 45, no. 10 (2023): 7845–61. https://doi.org/10.3390/cimb45100496.

Cirillo, Michela, Rossella Fucci, Sara Rubini, Maria Elisabetta Coccia, and Cinzia Fatini. "5-Methyltetrahydrofolate and Vitamin B12 Supplementation Is Associated with Clinical Pregnancy and Live Birth in Women Undergoing Assisted Reproductive Technology." *International Journal of Environmental Research and Public Health* 18, no. 23 (2021): 12280. doi: 10.3390/ijerph182312280.

Coad, Felicity, and Charlotte Frise. "Tachycardia in Pregnancy: When to Worry?" *Clinical Medicine* 21, no. 5 (2021): e434–37. doi: 10.7861/clinmed.2021-0495.

Cohen, J. "Clinical Use of Biphasic and Triphasic Pills." *International Planned Parenthood Federation (IPPF) Medical Bulletin* 19, no. 4 (1985): 1–2. PMID: 12280230.

Cole, Laurence A., Jaime M. Sutton-Riley, Sarah A. Khanlian, Marianna Borkovskaya, Brittany B. Rayburn, and William F. Rayburn. "Sensitivity of Over-the-Counter Pregnancy Tests: Comparison of Utility and Marketing Messages." *Journal of the American Pharmacists Association (JAPhA)* 45, no. 5 (2005): 608–15. doi: 10.1331/1544345055001391.

Cooper, Danielle B., and Preeti Patel "Oral Contraceptive Pills." *StatPearls* (online). Treasure Island, FL: StatPearls Publishing, 2024. https://www.ncbi.nlm.nih.gov/books/NBK430882/.

"Copper IUD Contraception." Sexual Health Victoria. Accessed June 26, 2024. https://shvic.org.au/for-you/contraception/iud-intrauterine-device/copper-iud#how-does-the-copper-iud-work.

Cornell. "Progestin-Only Oral Contraceptives (Minipills)." Cornell Health. Accessed June 27, 2024. https://health.cornell.edu/sites/health/files/pdf-library/MiniPills.pdf.

Cropley, Mark, Adrian Banks, and Julia Boyle. "The Effects of Rhodiola Rosea L. Extract on Anxiety, Stress, Cognition, and Other Mood Symptoms." *Phytotherapy Research* 29, no. 12 (2015): 1934–39. doi: 10.1002/ptr.5486.

D'Arrigo, Terri. "Risk of Depression May Increase during First Two Years of Oral Contraceptive Use." *Psychiatric News* 58, no. 9 (2023): https://doi.org/10.1176/appi.pn.2023.09.9.6.

D'souza, Naomi, Rishikesh V. Behere, Bindu Patni, Madhavi Deshpande, Dattatray Bhat, Aboli Bhalerao, Swapnali Sonawane, Rohan Shah, Rasika Ladkat, Pallavi Yajnik, Souvik K. Bandyopadhyay, Kalyanaraman Kumaran, Caroline Fall, and Chittaranjan S. Yajnik. "Pre-Conceptional Maternal Vitamin B12 Supplementation Improves Offspring Neurodevelopment at 2 Years of Age: Priya Trial." *Frontiers in Pediatrics* 9 (2021): 755977. doi: 10.3389/fped.2021.755977

Dasharathy, Sonya S., Sunni L. Mumford, Anna Z. Pollack, Neil J. Perkins, Donald R. Mattison, Jean Wactawski-Wende, and Enrique F. Schisterman. "Menstrual Bleeding Patterns Among Regularly Menstruating Women." *American Journal of Epidemiology* 175, no. 6 (2012): 536–45. doi: 10.1093/aje/kwr356.

Davtyan, Camelia. "Four Generations of Progestins in Oral Contraceptives." *Clinical Vignette*, Proceedings of UCLA Healthcare 16 (2012). https://www.proceedings.med.ucla.edu/wp-content/uploads/2017/01/Four-generations-of.pdf.

Delgado, Benjamin J., and Wilfredo Lopez-Ojeda. "Estrogen." *StatPearls* (online). Treasure Island, FL: StatPearls Publishing, 2023. https://www.ncbi.nlm.nih.gov/books/NBK538260/.

Depo-Provera Contraceptive Injection. "Highlights of Prescribing Information." October 2010. https://www.accessdata.fda.gov/drugsatfda_docs/label/2010/020246s036lbl.pdf.

Dietz, Birgit M., Atieh Hajirahimkhan, Tareisha L. Dunlap, and Judy L. Bolton. "Botanicals and Their Bioactive Phytochemicals for Women's Health." *Pharmacological Reviews* 68, no. 4 (2016): 1026–73. doi: 10.1124/pr.115.010843.

Dona, Gabriella, Chiara Sabbadin, Cristina Fiore, Marcantonio Bragadin, Franscesco Giorgino, Eugenio Ragazzi, Giulio Clari, Luciana Bordin, and Decio Armanini. "Inositol Administration Reduces Oxidative Stress in Erythrocytes of Patients with Polycystic Ovary Syndrome." *European Journal of Endocrinology* 166, no. 4 (2012): 703–10. doi: 10.1530/EJE-11-0840.

Doyle, Brian J., Jonna Frasor, Lauren E. Bellows, Tracie D. Locklear, Alice Perez, Jorge Gomez-Laurito, and Gail B. Mahady. "Estrogenic Effects of Herbal Medicines from Costa Rica Used for the Management of Menopausal Symptoms." *Menopause* 16, no. 4 (2009): 748–55. doi: 10.1097/gme.0b013e3181a4c76a.

"Drug-Nutrient Check." Integrative Therapeutics®. Accessed June 27, 2024. https://integrativepro.com/pages/drug-nutrient-interaction-checker.

Duclos, Martine, and Antoine Tabarin. "Exercise and the Hypothalamo-Pituitary-Adrenal Axis." *Frontiers of Hormone Research* 47 (2016): 12–26. doi: 10.1159/000445149.

Dull, Ana-Maria, Marius Alexandru Moga, Oana Gabriela Dimienescu, Gabriela Sechel, Victoria Burtea, and Costin Vlad Anastasiu. "Therapeutic Approaches of Resveratrol on Endometriosis via Anti-Inflammatory and Anti-Angiogenic Pathways." *Molecules* 24, no. 4 (2019): 667. doi: 10.3390/molecules24040667.

Dunne, F. P., D. G. Barry, J. B. Ferriss, Ginsen Grealy, and D. Murphy. "Changes in Blood Pressure during the Normal Menstrual Cycle." *Clinical Science* 81, no. 4 (1991): 515–18. doi: 10.1042/cs0810515.

Edwards, Michael. "Progestins." *StatPearls* (online). Treasure Island, FL: StatPearls Publishing, 2024. https://www.ncbi.nlm.nih.gov/books/NBK563211/#:~:text=Each%20of%20the%20progestin%20drugs,levonorgestrel%2C%20desogestrel%2C%20norgestimate%2C%20gestodene.

Emet, Mucahit, Halil Ozcan, Lutfu Ozel, Muhammed Yayla, Zekai Halici, and Ahmet Hacimuftuoglu. "A Review of Melatonin, Its Receptors and Drugs." *Eurasian Journal of Medicine* 48, no. 2 (2016): 135–41. https://www.ncbi.nlm.nih.gov/pmc/articles/PMC4970552/.

Eriksson, Olle, Anders Wall, Ulf Olsson, Ina Marteinsdottir, Maria Holstad, Hans Ågren, Per Hartvig, Bengt Långström, and Tord Naessén. "Women with Premenstrual Dysphoria Lack the Seemingly Normal Premenstrual Right-Sided Relative Dominance of 5-HTP-Derived Serotonergic Activity in the Dorsolateral

Prefrontal Cortices: A Possible Cause of Disabling Mood Symptoms." *PloS One* 11, no. 9 (2016): e01595838. doi: 10.1371/journal.pone.0159538.

Eshaghian, Razieh, Mohammad Mazaheri, Mustafa Ghanadian, Safoura Rouholamin, Awat Feizi, and Mahmoud Babaeian. "The Effect of Frankincense (Boswellia Serrata, Oleoresin) and Ginger (Zingiber Officinale, Rhizoma) on Heavy Menstrual Bleeding: A Randomized, Placebo-Controlled, Clinical Trial." *Complementary Therapies in Medicine* 42 (2018): 42–47. https://pubmed.ncbi.nlm.nih.gov/30670277/.

Eske, Jamie. "Period Blood Chart: What Does the Blood Color Mean?" *Medical News Today*, November 23, 2023. https://www.medicalnewstoday.com/articles/324848#black.

Ewert, Alan, and Yun Chang. "Levels of Nature and Stress Response." *Behavioral Sciences* 8, no. 5 (2018): doi: 10.3390/bs8050049.

"EWG Skin Deep®: Your Guide to Safer Personal Care Products." Skin Deep (online database). Accessed June 26, 2024. https://www.ewg.org/skindeep/.

Farwell, Alan, ed. "Volume 7 Issue 1." *Clinical Thyroidology for the Public*, 2014. https://www.thyroid.org/patient-thyroid-information/ct-for-patients/vol-7-issue-1/.

Fehring, Richard J., Donna Lawrence, and Connie Philpot. "Use Effectiveness of the Creighton Model Ovulation Method of Natural Family Planning." *Journal of Obstetric, Gynecologic, and Neonatal Nursing* 23, no. 4 (2015): 303–9. https://doi.org/10.1111/j.1552-6909.1994.tb01881.x.

Fern, M., D. P. Rose, and E. B. Fern. "Effect of Oral Contraceptives on Plasma Androgenic Steroids and Their Precursors." *Obstetrics and Gynecology* 51, no. 5 (1978): 541–44. doi: 10.1097/00006250-197805000-00005.

"Fish: Friend or Foe?" *The Nutrition Source*. Harvard T.H. Chan School of Public Health, May 9, 2024. https://nutritionsource.hsph.harvard.edu/fish/.

Foroozanfard, F., M. Jamilian, Z. Jafari, A. Khassaf, A. Hosseini, H. Khorammian, and Z. Asemi. "Effects of Zinc Supplementation on Markers of Insulin Resistance and Lipid Profiles in Women with Polycystic Ovary Syndrome: A Randomized, Double-Blind, Placebo-Controlled Trial." *Experimental and Clinical Endocrinology and Diabetes* 123, no. 4 (2015): 215–20. doi: 10.1055/s-0035-1548790.

Garner, Tyler, James Malcolm Hester, Allison Carothers, and Francisco J. Diaz. "Role of Zinc in Female Reproduction." *Biology of Reproduction* 104, no. 5 (2021): 976–94. doi: 10.1093/biolre/ioab023.

Ginsen, ed. "Period Colour Meaning According to Chinese Medicine." *TCM Blog*, August 16, 2023. https://tcmblog.co.uk/what-can-we-learn-from-period-colour/#:~:text=If%20the%20blood%20is%20slimy,fever%20and%20other%20inflammatory%20conditions.

Glasier, A., and A. Gebbie. "Spermicide." *International Encyclopedia of Public Health*. Cambridge, MA: Academic Press, 2008. https://www.sciencedirect.com/topics/agricultural-and-biological-sciences/spermicide#:~:text=Use%20of%20a%20spermicide%20more,urinary%20tract%20infections%20to%20thrive.

González, Frank. "Inflammation in Polycystic Ovary Syndrome: Underpinning of Insulin Resistance and Ovarian Dysfunction." *Steroids* 77, no. 4 (2011): 300–305. doi: 10.1016/j.steroids.2011.12.003.

Goshtasebi, Azita, Ziba Mazari, Samira Behboudi Gandevani, and Mohsen Naseri. "Anti-Hemorrhagic Activity of Punica Granatum L. Flower (Persian Golnar) against Heavy Menstrual Bleeding of Endometrial Origin: A Double-Blind, Randomized Controlled Trial." *Medical Journal of the Islamic Republic of Iran* 29 (2015): 199. https://www.ncbi.nlm.nih.gov/pmc/articles/PMC4476216/.

Goyal, Madhav, Sonal Singh, Erica M S Sibinga, Neda F Gould, Anastasia Rowland-Seymour, Ritu Sharma, Zackary Berger, et al. "Meditation Programs for Psychological Stress and Well-Being: A Systematic Review and Meta-Analysis." *JAMA Internal Medicine* 174, no. 3 (2014): 357–68. doi: 10.1001/jamainternmed.2013.13018.

Granda, Dominika, Maria Karolina Szmidt, and Joanna Kaluza. "Is Premenstrual Syndrome Associated with Inflammation, Oxidative Stress and Antioxidant Status? A Systematic Review of Case-Control and Cross-Sectional Studies." *Antioxidants* 10, no. 4 (2021): 604. doi: 10.3390/antiox10040604.

Graydon, James S., Karla Claudio, Seth Baker, Mohan Kocherla, Mark Ferreira, Abiel Roche-Lima, Jovaniel Rodríguez-Maldonado, Jorge Duconge, and Gualberto Ruaño. "Ethnogeographic Prevalence and Implications of the 677C>T and 1298A>C *MTHFR* Polymorphisms in US Primary Care Populations." *Biomarkers in Medicine* 13, no. 8 (2019): 649–61. doi: 10.2217/bmm-2018-0392.

Greff, Dorina, Anna E. Juhász, Szilárd Váncsa, Alex Váradi, Zoltán Sipos, Julia Szinte, Sunjune Park, Péter Hegyi, Péter Nyirády, Nándor Ács, Szabolcs Várbíró, and Eszter M. Horváth. "Inositol Is an Effective and Safe Treatment in Polycystic Ovary Syndrome: A Systematic Review and Meta-Analysis of Randomized Controlled Trials." *Reproductive Biology and Endocrinology* 21 (2023): 10. doi: 10.1186/s12958-023-01055-z.

Grieger, Jessica A., and Robert J. Norman. "Menstrual Cycle Length and Patterns in a Global Cohort of Women Using a Mobile Phone App: Retrospective Cohort Study." *Journal of Medical Internet Research* 22, no. 6 (2020): e17109. doi: 10.2196/17109.

Gross, Rachel E. "The Clitoris, Uncovered: An Intimate History." *Scientific American*, March 4, 2020. https://www.scientificamerican.com/article/the-clitoris-uncovered-an-intimate-history/.

Guarano, Alice, Anna Capozzi, Martina Cristodoro, Nicoletta Di Simone, and Stefano Lello. "Alpha Lipoic Acid Efficacy in PCOS Treatment: What Is the Truth?" *Nutrients* 15, no. 14 (2023): 3209. doi: 10.3390/nu15143209.

Gupta, K., and M. K. Rana. "Brussels Sprout." *Encyclopedia of Food Sciences and Nutrition*. Cambridge, MA: Academic Press, 2003. https://www.sciencedirect.com/topics/pharmacology-toxicology-and-pharmaceutical-science/brussels-sprout.

Hajizadeh, Khadije, Sakineh Mohammad Alizadeh Charandabi, Robab Hazanzade, and Mojgan Mirghafourvand. "Effect of Vitamin E on Severity and Duration of Cyclic Mastalgia: A Systematic Review and Meta-Analysis." *Complementary Therapies in Medicine* 44 (2019): 1–8. doi: 10.1016/j.ctim.2019.03.014.

Hall, Marianna, Magdalena Walicka, and Iwona Traczyk. "[Reactive Hypoglycemia: An Interdisciplinary Approach of the Disease of XXI Century]." *Wiadomosci lekarskie* 73, no. 2 (2020): 384–89. Polish. PMID: 32248180.

Halmos, Gabor, and Andrew Schally. "Thyrotropin Release." In *Hormonal Signaling in Biology and Medicine*, edited by Gerald Litwack, 43–68. Cambridge, MA: Academic Press, 2020. doi: 10.1016/B978-0-12-813814-4.00003-1.

Han, Joan, and Nazia Sadiq. "Anatomy, Abdomen and Pelvis: Fallopian Tube." *StatPearls* (online). Treasure Island, FL: StatPearls Publishing, 2023. https://www.ncbi.nlm.nih.gov/books/NBK547660/.

Hapangama, Dharani K., and Judith N. Bulmer. "Pathophysiology of Heavy Menstrual Bleeding." *Women's Health* 12, no. 1 (2016): 3–13. doi: 10.2217/whe.15.81.

Hartley, Sarah, Sylvie Royant-Parola, Ayla Zayoud, Isabelle Gremy, and Bobette Matulonga. "Do Both Timing and Duration of Screen Use Affect Sleep Patterns in Adolescents?" *PloS One* 17, no. 10 (2022): e0276226. doi: 10.1371/journal.pone.0276226.

Hasrat, Nazik H., and Asaad Q. Al-Yassen. "The Relationship between Acne Vulgaris and Insulin Resistance." *Cureus* 15, no. 1 (2023): e34241. doi: 10.7759/cureus.34241.

"Headaches." Headaches & Migraines, Menopause Information & Articles | The North American Menopause Society, NAMS. Accessed June 29, 2024. https://www.menopause.org/for-women/menopauseflashes/women's-health-and-menopause/headaches#:~:text=The%20fluctuation%20in%20estrogen%20levels,to%20have%20headaches%20after%20menopause.

"Healthy Habits Can Lengthen Life." National Institutes of Health (NIH), May 7, 2018. https://www.nih.gov/news-events/nih-research-matters/healthy-habits-can-lengthen-life.

Heitmann, Ryan, Kelly Langan, Raywin Huang, Gregory Chow, and Richard Burney. "Premenstrual Spotting of ≥2 Days Is Strongly Associated with Histologically Confirmed Endometriosis in Women with Infertility." *American Journal of Obstetrics and Gynecology* 211, no. 4 (2014): 358.e–6. doi: 10.1016/j.ajog.2014.04.041.

Hemmatzadeh, Shahla, Sakineh Mohammad Alizadeh Charandabi, Afsaneh Veisy, and Mojgan Mirghafourvand. "Evening Primrose Oil for Cervical Ripening in Term Pregnancies: A Systematic Review and Meta-Analysis." *Journal of Complementary and Integrative Medicine* 20, no. 2 (2021): 328–37. doi: 10.1515/jcim-2020-0314.

Hermann, Anne, Anne Nafziger, Jennifer Victory, Robert Kulaway, Mario Rocci, and Joseph Bertino. "Over-the-Counter Progesterone Cream Produces Significant Drug Exposure Compared to a Food and Drug Administration-Approved Oral Progesterone Product." *Journal of Clinical Pharmacology* 45, no. 6 (2005): 614–19. https://doi.org/10.1177/0091270005276621.

Hertel, Johannes, Johanna König, Georg Homuth, Sandra Van der Auwera, Katharina Wittfeld, Maik Pietzner, Tim Kacprowski, et al. "Evidence for Stress-like Alterations in the Hpa-Axis in Women Taking Oral Contraceptives." *Scientific Reports* 7 (2017): 14111. doi: 10.1038/s41598-017-13927-7.

Hill, Sarah. "What Does the Pill's Effect on the Human Stress Response Mean?" Sarah E. Hill, March 31, 2021. https://www.sarahehill.com/pill_and_stress/.

Hilton, Robin. "The History of the Clitoris." University of Regina Students Union, October 1, 2021. https://ursu.ca/the-history-of-the-clitoris/.

Hlisníková, Henrieta, Ida Petrovičová, Branislav Kolena, Miroslava Šidlovská, and Alexander Sirotkin. "Effects and Mechanisms of Phthalates' Action on Reproductive Processes and Reproductive Health: A Literature Review." *International Journal of Environmental Research and Public Health* 17, no. 18 (2020): 6811. doi: 10.3390/ijerph17186811.

Hodges, Romilly E., and Deanna M. Minich. "Modulation of Metabolic Detoxification Pathways Using Foods and Food-Derived Components: A Scientific Review with Clinical Application." *Journal of Nutrition and Metabolism* 1 (2015): doi: 10.1155/2015/760689.

"How Effective Is Pulling Out?" Planned Parenthood. Accessed June 27, 2024. https://www.plannedparenthood.org/learn/birth-control/withdrawal-pull-out-method/how-effective-is-withdrawal-method-pulling-out#:~:text=What%20we%20do%20know%20is,or%20not%20you're%20ovulating.

"How to Take a Basal Body Temperature." Pedagogy Education. Accessed June 26, 2024. https://pedagogyeducation.com/getmedia/f6b6c1a6-d4ca-40ca-b119-a4b06cfbc3a2/Basal-Temperature.pdf.

Inki, P., R. Hurskainen, P. Palo, E. Ekholm, S. Grenman, A. Kivela, E. Kujansuu, J. Teperi, M. Yliskoski, and J. Paavonen. "Comparison of Ovarian Cyst Formation in Women Using the Levonorgestrel-Releasing Intrauterine System vs. Hysterectomy." *Ultrasound in Obstetrics and Gynecology* 20, no. 4 (2002): 381–85. doi: 10.1046/j.1469-0705.2002.00805.x.

"Intercourse Timing and Frequency." Fertility Friend. Accessed June 28, 2024. https://www.fertilityfriend.com/Faqs/Intercourse-Timing-and-Frequency.html.

"Internal Condoms: How to Use an Internal Condom (Insertion and Removal)." *Bedsider*. Accessed June 27, 2024. https://www.bedsider.org/birth-control/internal_condom.

Jacobson, Amanda, Sara Vesely, Terah Koch, Janis Campbell, and Sarah O'Brien. "Patterns of von Willebrand Disease Screening in Girls and Adolescents with Heavy Menstrual Bleeding." *Obstetrics & Gynecology* 131, no. 6 (2018): 1121–29. doi: 10.1097/AOG.0000000000002620.

Jacobson, Melanie H., Penelope P. Howards, James S. Kesner, Juliana W. Meadows, Celia E. Dominguez, Jessica B. Spencer, Lyndsey A. Darrow, Metrecia L. Terrell, and Michele Marcus. "Hormonal Profiles of Menstrual Bleeding Patterns during the Luteal-Follicular Transition." *Journal of Clinical Endocrinology and Metabolism* 105, no. 5 (2020): e2024–31. doi: 10.1210/clinem/dgaa099.

Jamilian, Mehri, Fatemeh Foroozanfard, Fereshteh Bahmani, Rezvan Talee, Mahshid Monavari, and Zatollah Asemi. "Effects of Zinc Supplementation on Endocrine Outcomes in Women with Polycystic Ovary Syndrome: A Randomized, Double-Blind, Placebo-Controlled Trial." *Biological Trace Element Research* 170, no. 2 (2015): 271–78. doi: 10.1007/s12011-015-0480-7.

Jewson, Michaela, Prashant Purohit, and Mary Ann Lumsden. "Progesterone and Abnormal Uterine Bleeding/Menstrual Disorders." *Best Practice and Research Clinical Obstetrics and Gynaecology* 69 (2020): 62–73. doi: 10.1016/j.bpobgyn.2020.05.004.

Johnson, Sarah, Lorrae Marriott, and Michael Zinaman. "Increased Likelihood of Pregnancy from Sex on the Two Days Before Ovulation." *Obstetrics & Gynecology* 131 (2018): 20S. doi: 10.1097/01.AOG.0000532907.57204.dd.

Jurczewska, Justyna, and Dorota Szostak-Węgierek. "The Influence of Diet on Ovulation Disorders in Women-A Narrative Review." *Nutrients* 14, no. 8 (2022):1556. doi: 10.3390/nu14081556.

Kalani, Amir, Gul Bahtiyar, and Alan Sacerdote. "Ashwagandha Root in the Treatment of Non-Classical Adrenal Hyperplasia." *BMJ Case Reports* (2012): doi: 10.1136/bcr-2012-006989.

Kalra, Bharti, Sanjay Kalra, and J. B. Sharma. "The Inositols and Polycystic Ovary Syndrome." *Indian Journal of Endocrinology and Metabolism* 20, no. 5 (2016): 720–24. doi: 10.4103/2230-8210.189231.

Kamel, Hany H. "Role of Phyto-Oestrogens in Ovulation Induction in Women with Polycystic Ovarian Syndrome." *European Journal of Obstetrics, Gynecology, and Reproductive Biology* 291 (2013): doi: 10.1016/j.ejogrb.2023.09.027.

Kazemi, Farideh, Seyedeh Zahra Masoumi, Arezoo Shayan, and Khodayar Oshvandi. "The Effect of Evening Primrose Oil Capsule on Hot Flashes and Night Sweats in Postmenopausal Women: A Single-Blind Randomized Controlled Trial." *Journal of Menopausal Medicine* 27, no. 1 (2021): 8–14. doi: 10.6118/jmm.20033.

Keefe, Catherine E., Renee Mirkes, and Patrick Yeung. "The Evaluation and Treatment of Cervical Factor Infertility a Medical-Moral Analysis." *Linacre Quarterly* 79, no. 4 (2012): 409–25. doi: 10.1179/002436312804827127.

Kerin, J. "Ovulation Detection in the Human." *Clinical Reproduction and Fertility* 1, no. 1 (1982): 27–54. PMID: 6821195.

Kessler, Jack. "The Effect of Supraphysiologic Levels of Iodine on Patients with Cyclic Mastalgia." *Breast Journal* 10, no. 4 (2004): 328–36. https://onlinelibrary.wiley.com/.

Kikuchi, K., H. Tagami, R. Akaraphanth, and S. Aiba. "Functional Analyses of the Skin Surface of the Areola Mammae: Comparison between Healthy Adult Male and Female Subjects and between Healthy Individuals and Patients with Atopic Dermatitis." *British Journal of Dermatology* 164, no. 1 (2011): 97–102. doi: 10.1111/j.1365-2133.2010.10076.x.

Ko, Jade Heejae, and Seung-Nam Kim. "A Literature Review of Women's Sex Hormone Changes by Acupuncture Treatment: Analysis of Human and Animal

Studies." *Evidence-Based Complementary and Alternative Medicine*, no. 1 (2018): doi: 10.1155/2018/3752723.

Kohama, Takafumi, Kotaro Herai, and Masaki Inoue. "Effect of French Maritime Pine Bark Extract on Endometriosis as Compared with Leuprorelin Acetate." *Journal of Reproductive Medicine* 52, no. 8 (2007): 703–8. doi: 10.1155/2018/3752723.

Komori, Teruhisa. "The Effects of Phosphatidylserine and Omega-3 Fatty Acid–Containing Supplement on Late Life Depression." *Mental Illness* 7, no. 1 (2015): 5647. doi: 10.4081/mi.2015.5647.

Korsmo, Hunter W., Xinyin Jiang, and Marie A. Caudill. "Choline: Exploring the Growing Science on Its Benefits for Moms and Babies." *Nutrients* 11, no. 8 (2019): https://www.ncbi.nlm.nih.gov/pmc/articles/PMC6722688/.

Kozimor, Amanda, Hui Chang, and Jamie Cooper. "Effects of Dietary Fatty Acid Composition from a High Fat Meal on Satiety." *Appetite* 69 (2013): 39–45. doi: 10.1016/j.appet.2013.05.006.

"Label: Liletta—Levonorgestrel Intrauterine Device." DailyMed (online database). US National Library of Medicine. Last updated June 9, 2023. https://dailymed.nlm.nih.gov/dailymed/lookup.cfm?setid=aaf0eb2a-f88a-4f26-a445-0fd30176c326.

Lakshmi, Jada Naga, Ankem Narendra Babu, S. S. Mani Kiran, Lakshmi Prasanthi Nori, Nageeb Hassan, Akram Ashames, Richie R. Bhandare, and Afzal B. Shaik. "Herbs as a Source for the Treatment of Polycystic Ovarian Syndrome: A Systematic Review." *Biotech* 12, no. 1 (2023): 4. doi: 10.3390/biotech12010004.

Lambert, Charles P. "Saturated Fat Ingestion Regulates Androgen Concentrations and May Influence Lean Body Mass Accrual." *Journals of Gerontology* 63, no. 11 (2008): 1260–61. https://doi.org/10.1093/gerona/63.11.1260.

Lanfranchi, Angela. "A Scientific Basis for Humanae Vitae and Natural Law: The Role of Human Pheromones on Human Sexual Behavior Preferences by Oral Contraceptives and the Abortifacient Effects of Oral Contraceptives." *Linacre Quarterly* 85, no. 2 (2018): 148–54. doi: 10.1177/0024363918756191.

Langsjoen, Peter, and Alena Langsjoen. "Comparison Study of Plasma Coenzyme Q10 Levels in Healthy Subjects Supplemented with Ubiquinol Versus Ubiquinone." *Clinical Pharmacology in Drug Development* 3, no. 1 (2014): 13–17. doi: 10.1002/cpdd.73.

Leblanc, Erin S., and Ami Laws. "Benefits and Risks of Third-Generation Oral Contraceptives." *Journal of General Internal Medicine* 14, no. 10 (1999): 625–32. doi: 10.1046/j.1525-1497.1999.08108.x.

Lei, Yiming, Lili Yang, Honglian Yang, Min Li, Li Ou, Yang Bai, Taiwei Dong, Feng Gao, and Peifeng Wei. "The Efficacy and Safety of Chinese Herbal Medicine Guizhi Fuling Capsule Combined with Low Dose Mifepristone in the Treatment of Uterine Fibroids: A Systematic Review and Meta-Analysis of 28 Randomized Controlled Trials." *BioMed Central Complementary Medicine and Therapies* 23, no. 54 (2023): https://doi.org/10.1186/s12906-023-03842-y.

"Levonorgestrel IUDs: Mirena, Kyleena, and Skyla." University Health Services (clinical handout), January 2023. https://uhs.berkeley.edu/sites/default/files/iud_hormonal.pdf.

LeWine, Howard. "How Much Protein Do You Need Every Day?" *Harvard Health*, June 22, 2023. https://www.health.harvard.edu/blog/how-much-protein-do-you-need-every-day-201506188096.

Lewis, Radha, Deshawn Taylor, Melissa Natavio, Alexander Melamed, Juan Felix, and Daniel Mishell. "Effects of the Levonorgestrel-Releasing Intrauterine System on Cervical Mucus Quality and Sperm Penetrability." *Contraception* 82, no. 6 (2010): 491–96. doi: 10.1016/j.contraception.2010.06.006.

Li, De-Kun, Liyan Liu, and Roxana Odouli. "Exposure to Non-Steroidal Anti-Inflammatory Drugs during Pregnancy and Risk of Miscarriage: Population Based Cohort Study." *BMJ (British Medical Journal)* 327, no. 7411 (2003): 368. doi: 10.1136/bmj.327.7411.368.

Li, Quan-Zhen, David R. Karp, Jiexia Quan, Valerie K. Branch, Jinchun Zhou, Yun Lian, Benjamin F. Chong, Edward K. Wakeland, and Nancy J. Olsen. "Risk Factors for Ana Positivity in Healthy Persons." *Arthritis Research and Therapy* 13, no. 2 (2011): R38. doi: 10.1186/ar3271.

Liang Ooi, Soo, Stephanie Watts, Rhett McClean, and Sok Cheon Pak. "Vitex Agnus-Castus for the Treatment of Cyclic Mastalgia: A Systematic Review and Meta-Analysis." *Journal of Women's Health* 29, no. 2 (2020): 262–78. doi: 10.1089/jwh.2019.7770.

Lim, Meng Thiam, Bernice Jiaqi Pan, Darel Wee Kiat Toh, Clarinda Nataria Sutanto, and Jung Eun Kim. "Animal Protein versus Plant Protein in Supporting Lean Mass and Muscle Strength: A Systematic Review and Meta-Analysis of Randomized Controlled Trials." *Nutrients* 13, no. 2 (2021): 661. doi: 10.3390/nu13020661.

Liu, Jiajun, Haodong Su, Xueshan Jin, Lan Wang, and Jieming Huang. "The Effects of N-Acetylcysteine Supplement on Metabolic Parameters in Women with Polycystic Ovary Syndrome: A Systematic Review and Meta-Analysis." *Frontiers in Nutrition* 10 (2023): 1209614. doi: 10.3389/fnut.2023.1209614.

Liu, Zhan-Wen, Jin Shu, Jia-Ying Tu, Cui-Hong Zhang, and Jue Hong. "Liver in the Chinese and Western Medicine." *Integrative Medicine International* 4, nos. 1–2 (2017): 39–45. doi: 10.1159/000466694.

Loeffelholz, Christian von, and Andreas L. Birkenfeld. "Non-Exercise Activity Thermogenesis in Human Energy Homeostasis." In *Endotext* (online) edited by Kenneth R. Feingold et al. South Dartmouth, MA: MDText.com, Inc., 2000 November 25, 2022. https://www.ncbi.nlm.nih.gov/books/NBK279077/.

Loukas, Marios, Michael Hanna, Nada Alsaiegh, Mohammadali Shoja, and Shane Tubbs. "Clinical Anatomy as Practiced by Ancient Egyptians." *Clinical Anatomy* 24, no. 4 (2011): 409–15. doi: 10.1002/ca.21155.

"Low Blood Glucose (Hypoglycemia)." National Institute of Diabetes and Digestive and Kidney Diseases (NIH). Accessed June 25, 2024. https://www.niddk.nih.gov/health-information/diabetes/overview/preventing-problems/

low-blood-glucose-hypoglycemia#:~:text=Although%20you%20may%20not%20wake,blood%20glucose%20during%20the%20day.
Madore, Kevin P., and Anthony D. Wagner. "Multicosts of Multitasking." *Cerebrum* (2019): cer-04-19. https://www.ncbi.nlm.nih.gov/pmc/articles/PMC7075496/.
Maffei, Massimo E. "5-Hydroxytryptophan (5-HTP): Natural Occurrence, Analysis, Biosynthesis, Biotechnology, Physiology and Toxicology." *International Journal of Molecular Sciences* 22, no. 1 (2020): 181. doi: 10.3390/ijms22010181.
Malanchuk, Larysa, Mariia Riabokon, Artem Malanchuk, Svitlana Riabokon, Serhiy Malanchuk, Viktoriia Martyniuk, Tetiana Grabchak, and Inna Pitsyk. "Relationship between Pathological Menstrual Symptoms and the Development of Extragenital Forms of Local Inflammation." *Wiadomosci lekarskie* 74, no. 1 (2021): 64–67. PMID: 33851589.
Malherbe, Kathryn. "Fibrocystic Breast Disease." *StatPearls* (online). Treasure Island, FL: StatsPearls Publishing, 2023. https://www.ncbi.nlm.nih.gov/books/NBK551609/.
Malik, Mokerrum, Henry Adekola, William Porter, and Janet Poulik. "Passage of Decidual Cast Following Poor Compliance with Oral Contraceptive Pill." *Fetal and Pediatric Pathology* 34, no. 2 (2014): 103–7. doi: 10.3109/15513815.2014.970263.
Manley, Hannah, James Sprinks, and Phillip Breedon. "Menstrual Blood-Derived Mesenchymal Stem Cells: Women's Attitudes, Willingness, and Barriers to Donation of Menstrual Blood." *Journal of Women's Health* 28, no. 12 (2019): https://doi.org/10.1089/jwh.2019.7745.
Manthou, Eirini, Maria Kanaki, Kalliopi Georgakouli, Chariklia K. Deli, Dimitrios Kouretas, Yiannis Koutedakis, and Athanasios Z. Jamurtas. "Glycemic Response of a Carbohydrate-Protein Bar with Ewe-Goat Whey." *Nutrients* 6, no. 6 (2014): 2240–50. doi: 10.3390/nu6062240.
Mao, Qing-Qiu, Siu-Po Ip, Yan-Fang Xian, Zhen Hu, and Chun-Tao Che. "Anti-Depressant-like Effect of Peony: A Mini-Review." *Pharmaceutical Biology* 50, no. 1 (2012): 72–77. doi: 10.3109/13880209.2011.602696.
Marshall, John C., and Andrea Dunaif. "Should All Women with PCOS Be Treated for Insulin Resistance?" *Fertility and Sterility* 97, no. 1 (2012): 18–22. https://www.ncbi.nlm.nih.gov/pmc/articles/PMC3277302/.
Martinez, LaQuita. "Cell Division" *MedlinePlus Medical Encyclopedia* (video). August 23, 2023. https://medlineplus.gov/ency/anatomyvideos/000025.htm#:~:text=For%20the%20first%2012%20hours,made%20up%20of%2016%20cells.
Mauvais-Jarvis, Franck, Deborah J. Clegg, and Andrea L. Hevener. "The Role of Estrogens in Control of Energy Balance and Glucose Homeostasis." *Endocrine Reviews* 34, no. 3 (2013): 309–38. doi: 10.1210/er.2012-1055.
Mayo Clinic Staff. "Period Irregularities to Get Checked Out." Mayo Clinic, April 22, 2023. https://www.mayoclinic.org/healthy-lifestyle/womens-health/in-depth/menstrual-cycle/art-20047186.
McDonald, Daniel, et al. "American Gut: An Open Platform for Citizen Science Microbiome Research" *mSystems*, May 15, 2018. https://doi.org/10.1128/msystems.00031-18.

McEvedy, Samantha, Gillian Sullivan-Mort, Sian McLean, and Michaela Pascoe. "Ineffectiveness of Commercial Weight-Loss Programs for Achieving Modest but Meaningful Weight Loss: Systematic Review and Meta-Analysis." *Journal of Health Psychology* 22, no. 12 (2017): 1614–27. doi: 10.1177/1359105317705983.

Mckellar, Kerry, and Elizabeth Sillence. "Menstrual Cycle." In *Teenagers, Sexual Health Information and the Digital Age*. Cambridge, MA: Academic Press, 2020. https://doi.org/10.1016/C2018-0-01310-9.9.

McKinley, Paula S., Arlene R. King, Peter A. Shapiro, Iordan Slavov, Yixin Fang, Ivy S. Chen, Larry D. Jamner, and Richard P. Sloan. "The Impact of Menstrual Cycle Phase on Cardiac Autonomic Regulation." *Psychophysiology* 46, no. 4 (2009): 904–11. doi: 10.1111/j.1469-8986.2009.00811.x.

McLaughlin, Jessica E. "Menstrual Cycle." *Merck Manual Consumer Version*, September 2022. https://www.merckmanuals.com/home/women-s-health-issues/biology-of-the-female-reproductive-system/menstrual-cycle.

Meissner, H. O., A. Mscisz, H. Reich-Bilinska, W. Kapczynski, P. Mrozikiewicz, T. Bobkiewicz-Kozlowska, B. Kedzia, A. Lowicka, and I. Barchia. "Hormone-Balancing Effect of Pre-Gelatinized Organic Maca (Lepidium Peruvianum Chacon): (II) Physiological and Symptomatic Responses of Early-Postmenopausal Women to Standardized Doses of Maca in Double Blind, Randomized, Placebo-Controlled, Multi-Centre Clinical Study." *International Journal of Biomedical Science* 2, no. 4 (2006): 360–74. https://www.ncbi.nlm.nih.gov/pmc/articles/PMC3614647/.

Mergenthaler, Philipp, Ute Lindauer, Gerald A. Dienel, and Andreas Meisel. "Sugar for the Brain: The Role of Glucose in Physiological and Pathological Brain Function." *Trends in Neurosciences* 36, no. 10 (2013): 587–97. doi: 10.1016/j.tins.2013.07.001.

Mihm, M., S. Gangooly, and S. Muttukrishna. "The Normal Menstrual Cycle in Women." *Animal Reproduction Science* 124, no. 3–4 (2011): 229–36. doi: 10.1016/j.anireprosci.2010.08.030.

Mindell, Jodi, and Ariel Williamson. "Benefits of a Bedtime Routine in Young Children: Sleep, Development, and Beyond." *Sleep Medicine Reviews* 40 (2018): 93–108. doi: 10.1016/j.smrv.2017.10.007.

Mirabi, Parvaneh, Seideh Hanieh Alamolhoda, Seddigheh Esmaeilzadeh, and Faraz Mojab. "Effect of Medicinal Herbs on Primary Dysmenorrhoea: A Systematic Review." *Iranian Journal of Pharmaceutical Research* 13, no. 3 (2014): 757–67. https://www.ncbi.nlm.nih.gov/pmc/articles/PMC4177637/.

Mitchell, Jon-Benay, Sarentha Chetty, and Fatima Kathrada. "Progestins in the Symptomatic Management of Endometriosis: A Meta-Analysis on Their Effectiveness and Safety." *BioMed Central Women's Health* 22 (2022): 526. doi: 10.1186/s12905-022-02122-0.

Mohammadi, Mohammad, Nahid Nayeri, Monireh Mashhadi, and Shokoh Varei. "Effect of Omega-3 Fatty Acids on Premenstrual Syndrome: A Systematic Review and Meta-Analysis." *Journal of Obstetrics and Gynaecology Research* 48, no. 6 (2022): 1293–305. doi: 10.1111/jog.15217.

Mokra, Katarzyna. "Endocrine Disruptor Potential of Short- and Long-Chain Perfluoroalkyl Substances (PFASs)—a Synthesis of Current Knowledge with Proposal of Molecular Mechanism." *International Journal of Molecular Sciences* 22, no. 4 (2021): 2148. doi: 10.3390/ijms22042148.

Morais, Jennifer, Juliana Severo, Georgia Alencar, Ana Oliveira, Kyria Cruz, Dilina Marreiro, Betania Freitas, Cecilia Carvalho, Maria Martins, and Karoline Frota. "Effect of Magnesium Supplementation on Insulin Resistance in Humans: A Systematic Review." *Nutrition* 38 (2017): 54–60. doi: 10.1016/j.nut.2017.01.009.

Mounsey, Anne, and Rita M. Lahlou. "Heavy Menstrual Bleeding in Premenopausal Patients and the Role of NSAIDs." *American Family Physician* 102, no. 3 (2020): 147–48. https://www.aafp.org/pubs/afp/issues/2020/0801/p147.html.

Mumford, Sunni L., Richard W. Browne, Karen C. Schliep, Jonathan Schmelzer, Torie C. Plowden, Kara A. Michels, Lindsey A. Sjaarda, Shvetha M. Zarek, Neil J. Perkins, Lynne C. Messer, Rose G. Radin, Jean Wactawski-Wende, and Enrique F. Schisterman. "Serum Antioxidants Are Associated with Serum Reproductive Hormones and Ovulation among Healthy Women." *Journal of Nutrition* 146, no. 1 (2015): 98–106. doi: 10.3945/jn.115.217620.

Munro, Malcom, Hillary Critchley, and Ian Fraser. "The Figo Classification of Causes of Abnormal Uterine Bleeding in the Reproductive Years." *Fertility and Sterility* 95, no. 7 (2011): 2024–8. doi: 10.1016/j.fertnstert.2011.03.079.

Muto, Michael. "Patient Education: Ovarian Cysts (Beyond the Basics)." *UpToDate*, January 2023. https://www.uptodate.com/contents/ovarian-cysts-beyond-the-basics/print#:~:text=Large%20cysts%20.

Najmabadi, Shahpar, Karen C. Schliep, Sara E. Simonsen, Christina A. Porucznik, Marlene J. Egger, and Joseph B. Stanford. "Cervical Mucus Patterns and the Fertile Window in Women without Known Subfertility: A Pooled Analysis of Three Cohorts." *Human Reproduction* 36, no. 7 (2021): 1784–95. doi: 10.1093/humrep/deab049.

Nasiadek, Marzenna, Joanna Stragierowicz, Michał Klimczak, and Anna Kilanowicz. "The Role of Zinc in Selected Female Reproductive System Disorders." *Nutrients* 12, no. 8 (2020): 2464. doi: 10.3390/nu12082464.

National Health Service. (NHS). "How Well Contraception Works at Preventing Pregnancy." Last updated January 31, 2024. https://www.nhs.uk/contraception/choosing-contraception/how-well-it-works-at-preventing-pregnancy/#:~:text=Contraceptive%20pill&text=than%2099%25%20effective.-,Fewer%20than%201%20in%20100%20women%20will%20get%20pregnant%20in,get%20pregnant%20in%20a%20year.

Nguyen, John D. "Anatomy, Abdomen and Pelvis: Female External Genitalia." StatPearls (online). Treasure Island, FL: StatPearls Publishing, 2023. https://www.ncbi.nlm.nih.gov/books/NBK547703/.

"Nexplanon (Etonogestrel Implant): Side Effects, Uses, Dosage, Interactions, Warnings." RxList. Last updated October 17, 2023. https://www.rxlist.com/nexplanon-drug.htm.

"NIH Study Shows How Insulin Stimulates Fat Cells to Take in Glucose." News Releases. National Institutes of Health (NIH). September 7, 2010. https://www

.nih.gov/news-events/news-releases/nih-study-shows-how-insulin-stimulates-fat-cells-take-glucose#:~:text=September%207%2C%202010-,NIH%20study%20shows%20how%20insulin%20stimulates%20fat%20cells%20to%20take,glucose%20in%20a%20rat%20model.

Ogunrinola, Grace A., John O. Oyewale, Oyewumi O. Oshamika, and Grace I. Olasehinde. "The Human Microbiome and Its Impacts on Health." *International Journal of Microbiology* (2020): 8045646. doi: 10.1155/2020/8045646.

"Omega-3 Fatty Acids: Fact Sheet for Health Professionals." National Institutes of Health, Office of Dietary Supplements. Accessed June 26, 2024. https://ods.od.nih.gov/factsheets/Omega3FattyAcids-HealthProfessional/.

Omidvar, Shabnam, Sedighe Esmailzadeh, Mahmood Baradaran, and Zahra Basirat. "Effect of Fennel on Pain Intensity in Dysmenorrhoea: A Placebo-Controlled Trial." *Ayu* 33, no. 2 (2012): 311–13. doi: 10.4103/0974-8520.105259.

Ong, Hooi-Theng, Hayati Samsudin, and Herlinda Soto-Valdez. "Migration of Endocrine-Disrupting Chemicals into Food from Plastic Packaging Materials: An Overview of Chemical Risk Assessment, Techniques to Monitor Migration, and International Regulations." *Critical Reviews in Food Science and Nutrition* 62, no. 4 (2022): 957–79. doi: 10.1080/10408398.2020.1830747.

Oriji, P. C., D. O. Allagoa, A. E. Ubom, and V. K. Oriji. "A 5-Year Review of Incidence, Presentation and Management of Bartholin Gland Cysts and Abscesses in a Tertiary Hospital, Yenagoa, South-South Nigeria." *medRxiv* (2022). doi: 10.1101/2022.05.01.22274551.

Ośko, Justyna, Wiktoria Pierlejewska, and Małgorzata Grembecka. "Comparison of the Potential Relative Bioaccessibility of Zinc Supplements-in Vitro Studies." *Nutrients* 15, no. 12 (2023): 2813. doi: 10.3390/nu15122813.

"Overview: Heavy Periods." InformedHealth.org. Last updated June 17, 2021. https://www.ncbi.nlm.nih.gov/books/NBK279294/#:~:text=Although%20it%20can%20feel%20like,pad%20to%20become%20fully%20soaked.

Pacyga, Diana C., Catheryne Chiang, Zhong Li, Rita S. Strakovsky, and Ayelet Ziv-Gal. "Parabens and Menopause-Related Health Outcomes in Midlife Women: A Pilot Study." *Journal of Women's Health* 31, no. 11 (2022): 1645–54. doi: 10.1089/jwh.2022.0004.

Palacios, S., C. Mustata, J. M. Rizo, and P. A. Regidor. "Improvement in Menopausal Symptoms with a Nutritional Product Containing Evening Primrose Oil, Hop Extract, Saffron, Tryptophan, Vitamins B6, D3, K2, B12, and B9." *European Review for Medical and Pharmacological Sciences* 27, no. 17 (2023): 8180–89. doi: 10.26355/eurrev_202309_33578.

Pandya, Matangee, Shilpa B. Donga, L. P. Dei, and Anup B. Thakar. "Efficacy of *Virechana*, *Triphaladi* Decoction with Processed *Guggulu* in the Management of Ovarian Cyst: A Pilot Study." *Ayu* 41, no. 3 (2022): 166–72. doi: 10.4103/ayu.AYU_254_19.

Parazzini, Fabio, Mirella Martino, and Paolo Pellegrino. "Magnesium in the Gynecological Practice: A Literature Review." *Magnesium Research* 30, no. 1 (2017): 1–7. doi: 10.1684/mrh.2017.0419.

Pareek, Anil, Manish Suthar, Garvendra S. Rathore, and Vijay Bansal. "Feverfew (Tanacetum Parthenium L.): A Systematic Review." *Pharmacognosy Reviews* 5, no. 9 (2011): 103–10. doi: 10.4103/0973-7847.79105.

Patel, Archan, Deepika Dewani, Arpita Jaiswal, Pallavi Yadav, and Lucky Srivani Reddy. "Exploring Melatonin's Multifaceted Role in Polycystic Ovary Syndrome Management: A Comprehensive Review." *Cureus* 15, no. 11 (2023): e48929. doi: 10.7759/cureus.48929.

Patel, Palak S., and Mia T. Minen. "Complementary and Integrative Health Treatments for Migraine." *Journal of Neuroophthalmology* 39, no. 3 (2019): 360–69. doi: 10.1097/WNO.0000000000000841.

Patel, S. "Fragrance Compounds: The Wolves in Sheep's Clothings." *Medical Hypotheses* 102 (2017): 106–11. doi: 10.1016/j.mehy.2017.03.025.

Pistollato, Francesca, Sandra Sumalla Cano, Iñaki Elio, Manuel Masias Vergara, Francesca Giampieri, and Maurizio Battino. "Associations between Sleep, Cortisol Regulation, and Diet: Possible Implications for the Risk of Alzheimer Disease." *Advances in Nutrition* 7, no. 4 (2016): 679–89. doi: 10.3945/an.115.011775.

"Pre-Seed™ Fertility Lubricant." First Response™. Accessed June 27, 2024. https://www.firstresponse.com/en/product-listings/fertility-lubricant.

Priyanto, Bambang, Rohadi Rosyidi, Andi Islam, Agus Turchan, and Tusra Pintaningrum. "The Effect of Progesteron for Expression Delta (δ) Opioid Receptor Spinal Cord through Peripheral Nerve Injury." *Annals of Medicine and Surgery* 75 (2022): 103376. doi: 10.1016/j.amsu.2022.103376.

Pruthi, Sandhya, Dietlind Wahner-Roedler, Carolyn Torkelson, Stephen Cha, Lori Thicke, Jennifer Hazelton, and Brent Bauer. "Vitamin E and Evening Primrose Oil for Management of Cyclical Mastalgia: A Randomized Pilot Study." *Alternative Medicine Review* 15, no. 1 (2010): 59–67. https://pubmed.ncbi.nlm.nih.gov/20359269/.

Puglia, Lídice Tavares, Jean Lowry, and Gianluca Tamagno. "Vitex Agnus Castus Effects on Hyperprolactinaemia." *Frontiers in Endocrinology* 14 (2023): 1269781. doi: 10.3389/fendo.2023.1269781.

Qu, Jingwen, Huiru Hu, Haoyuan Niu, Xiaomei Sun, and Yongjun Li. "Melatonin Restores the Declining Maturation Quality and Early Embryonic Development of Oocytes in Aged Mice." *Theriogenology* 210 (2023): 110–18. doi: 10.1016/j.theriogenology.2023.07.021.

Rafieian-Kopaei, Mahmoud, and Mino Movahedi. "Systematic Review of Premenstrual, Postmenstrual and Infertility Disorders of Vitex Agnus Castus." *Electronic Physician* 9, no. 1 (2017): 3685–89. doi: 10.19082/3685.

Rajoria, Shilpi, Robert Suriano, Perminder Singh Parmar, Yushan Lisa Wilson, Uchechukwu Megwalu, Augustine Moscatello, H. Leon Bradlow, Daniel W. Sepkovic, Jan Geliebter, Stimson P. Schantz, and Raj K. Tiwari. "3,3'-Diindolylmethane Modulates Estrogen Metabolism in Patients with Thyroid Proliferative Disease: A Pilot Study." *Thyroid* 21 no. 3 (2011): 299–304. doi: 10.1089/thy.2010.0245.

Reiter, R. J., J. R. Calvo, M. Karbownik, W. Qi, and X. Tan. "Melatonin and Its Relation to the Immune System and Inflammation." *Annals of the New York Academy of Sciences* 917 (2000): 376–86. https://pubmed.ncbi.nlm.nih.gov/11268363/.

Reyes-Hernández, Octavio Daniel, Gabriela Figueroa-González, Laura Itzel Quintas-Granados, Stephany Celeste Gutiérrez-Ruíz, Hector Hernández-Parra, Alejandra Romero-Montero, María Luisa Del Prado-Audelo, Sergio Alberto Bernal-Chavez, Hernán Cortés, Sheila I. Peña-Corona, Lashyn Kiyekbayeva, Dilek Arslan Atessahin, Tamar Goloshvili, Gerardo Leyva-Gómez, and Javad Sharifi-Rad. "3,3'-Diindolylmethane and Indole-3-Carbinol: Potential Therapeutic Molecules for Cancer Chemoprevention and Treatment via Regulating Cellular Signaling Pathways." *Cancer Cell International* 23 (2023): 180. doi: 10.1186/s12935-023-03031-4.

Rezaie, Sheyda, Gholamreza Askari, Fariborz Khorvash, Mohammad Javad Tarrahi, and Reza Amani. "Effects of Curcumin Supplementation on Clinical Features and Inflammation, in Migraine Patients: A Double-Blind Controlled, Placebo Randomized Clinical Trial." *International Journal of Preventive Medicine* 12 (2021): 161. doi: 10.4103/ijpvm.IJPVM_405_20.

Rhyu, Mee-Ra, Jian Lu, Donna E. Webster, Daniel S. Fabricant, Norman R. Farnsworth, and Z. Jim Wang. "Black Cohosh (Actaea Racemosa, CIMICIFUGA Racemosa) Behaves as a Mixed Competitive Ligand and Partial Agonist at the Human MU Opiate Receptor." *Journal of Agricultural and Food Chemistry* 54, no. 26 (2006): 9852–57. doi: 10.1021/jf062808u.

Rivard, Allyson B., Laura Galarza-Paez, and Diana C. Peterson. "Anatomy, Thorax, Breast." *StatPearls* (online). Treasure Island, FL: StatPearls Publishing, 2023.

Robinson, Janet, Melanie Wakelin, and Jayne Ellis. "Increased Pregnancy Rate with Use of the Clearblue Easy Fertility Monitor." *Fertility and Sterility* 87, no. 2 (2007): 329–34. doi: 10.1016/j.fertnstert.2006.05.054.

Rodríguez-Varela, Cristina, and Elena Labarta. "Does Coenzyme Q10 Supplementation Improve Human Oocyte Quality?" *International Journal of Molecular Sciences* 22, no. 17 (2021): 9541. doi: 10.3390/ijms22179541.

Rösner, Harald, Wolfgang Möller, Sabine Groebner, and Pompilio Torremante. "Antiproliferative/Cytotoxic Effects of Molecular Iodine, Povidone-Iodine and Lugol's Solution in Different Human Carcinoma Cell Lines." *Oncology Letters* 12, no. 3 (2016): 2159–62. doi: 10.3892/ol.2016.4811.

Ryterska, Karina, Agnieszka Kordek, and Patrycja Załęska. "Has Menstruation Disappeared? Functional Hypothalamic Amenorrhea—What Is This Story About?" *Nutrients* 13, no. 8 (2021): 2827. doi: 10.3390/nu13082827.

Rytz, Andreas, Dorothée Adeline, Kim-Anne Lê, Denise Tan, Lisa Lamothe, Olivier Roger, and Katherine Macé. "Predicting Glycemic Index and Glycemic Load from Macronutrients to Accelerate Development of Foods and Beverages with Lower Glucose Responses." *Nutrients* 11, no. 5 (2019): 1172. doi: 10.3390/nu11051172.

Samuels, Michelle. "When Does Fertility Return after Stopping Contraceptive Use?" *Birth Control*, November 16, 2020. https://www.bu.edu/sph/news/

articles/2020/when-does-fertility-return-after-stopping-contraceptive-use/#:~:text=Earlier%20research%20has%20focused%20mainly,after%20women%20stopped%20taking%20them.

Sergin, Selin, Vijayashree Jambunathan, Esha Garg, Jason E. Rowntree, and Jenifer I. Fenton. "Fatty Acid and Antioxidant Profile of Eggs from Pasture-Raised Hens Fed a Corn- and Soy-Free Diet and Supplemented with Grass-Fed Beef Suet and Liver." *Foods* 11, no. 21 (2022): 3404. doi: 10.3390/foods11213404.

Sharma, Alok, and Pratap Kumar. "Understanding Implantation Window, a Crucial Phenomenon." *Journal of Human Reproductive Sciences* 5, no. 1 (2012): 2–6. doi: 10.4103/0974-1208.97777.

Sharma, Anup, Patricia Gerbarg, Teodoro Bottiglieri, Lila Massoumi, Linda L. Carpenter, Helen Lavretsky, Philip R. Muskin, Richard P. Brown, David Mischoulon, and Work Group of the American Psychiatric Association Council on Research. "S-Adenosylmethionine (Same) for Neuropsychiatric Disorders: A Clinician-Oriented Review of Research." *Journal of Clinical Psychiatry* 78, no. 6 (2017): e656–67. doi: 10.4088/JCP.16r11113.

Sharma, Medhavi. "Ovulation Induction Techniques." *StatPearls* (online). Treasure Island, FL: StatPearls Publishing, 2023. https://www.ncbi.nlm.nih.gov/books/NBK574564/.

Sharts-Hopko, N. C. "Depo–Provera." *American Journal of Maternal/Child Nursing (MCN)* 18, no. 2 (1993): 128. doi: 10.1097/00005721-199303000-00015.

Shaw, Sarah, Katrina Wyatt, John Campbell, Edzard Ernst, and Joanna Thompson-Coon. "Vitex Agnus Castus for Premenstrual Syndrome." *Cochrane Database of Systematic Reviews* 2018, no. 3 (2018): CD004632. doi: 10.1002/14651858.CD004632.pub2.

Shoupe, Donna. "The Progestin Revolution 2: Progestins Are Now a Dominant Player in the Tight Interlink between Contraceptive Protection and Bleeding Control-plus More: Contraception and Reproductive Medicine." *Contraceptive and Reproductive Medicine* 8, no. 48 (2023). doi: 10.1186/s40834-023-00249-5.

Shrivastava, Suyesh, Anamika Sharma, Nishant Saxena, Rashmi Bhamra, and Sandeep Kumar. "Addressing the Preventive and Therapeutic Perspective of Berberine against Diabetes." *Heliyon* 9, no. 11 (2023): e21233. doi: 10.1016/j.heliyon.2023.e21233.

"Side Effects of NEXPLANON." Risks and Side Effects of NEXPLANON® (etonogestrel implant) 68 mg Radiopaque. Organon. Accessed June 26, 2024. https://www.nexplanon.com/side-effects/.

Singla, Rajiv, Yashdeep Gupta, Manju Khemani, and Sameer Aggarwal. "Thyroid Disorders and Polycystic Ovary Syndrome: An Emerging Relationship." *Indian Journal of Endocrinology and Metabolism* 19, no. 1 (2015): 25–29. doi: 10.4103/2230-8210.146860.

Smith, R. L., K. L. Vernon, D. E. Kelley, J. R. Gibbons, and C. J. Mortensen. "Impact of Moderate Exercise on Ovarian Blood Flow and Early Embryonic Outcomes in Mares." *Journal of Animal Science* 90, no. 11 (2012): 3770–77. doi: 10.2527/jas.2011-4713.

Smith, Stephen J., Adrian L. Lopresti, and Timothy J. Fairchild. "Exploring the Efficacy and Safety of a Novel Standardized Ashwagandha (*Withania Somnifera*) Root Extract (Witholytin®) in Adults Experiencing High Stress and Fatigue in a Randomized, Double-Blind, Placebo-Controlled Trial." *Journal of Psychopharmacology* 37, no. 11 (2023): 1091–1104. doi: 10.1177/02698811231200023.

Sohrabi, Nahid, Maryam Kashanian, Sima Ghafoori, and Seyed Malakouti. "Evaluation of the Effect of Omega-3 Fatty Acids in the Treatment of Premenstrual Syndrome: 'A Pilot Trial.'" *Complementary Therapies in Medicine* 21, no. 3 (2013): 141–46. doi: 10.1016/j.ctim.2012.12.008.

Solmaz, Soner. "An Overlooked Side Effect of Iron Treatment: Changes in Menstruation." *International Journal of Hematology Research* 2, no. 1 (2016): 120–23. doi: 10.17554/j.issn.2409-3548.2015.01.26.

Stanhiser, J., A. M. Z. Jukic, D. R. McConnaughey, and A. Z. Steiner. "Omega-3 Fatty Acid Supplementation and Fecundability." *Human Reproduction* 37, no. 5 (2022): 1037–46. doi: 10.1093/humrep/deac027.

"Sterilization as Birth Control: Types, Cost, Side Effects & Benefits." *Bedsider*. Accessed June 26, 2024. https://www.bedsider.org/birth-control/sterilization.

Sun, Jiayi, Xin Shen, Hui Liu, Siying Lu, Jing Peng, and Haibin Kuang. "Caloric Restriction in Female Reproduction: Is It Beneficial or Detrimental?" *Reproductive Biology and Endocrinology* 19, no. 1 (2021): 1. doi: 10.1186/s12958-020-00681-1.

Suzuki, Nobutaka, Kazuo Uebaba, Takafumi Kohama, Nobuhiko Moniwa, Naohiro Kanayama, and Koji Koike. "French Maritime Pine Bark Extract Significantly Lowers the Requirement for Analgesic Medication in Dysmenorrhea: A Multicenter, Randomized, Double-Blind, Placebo-Controlled Study." *Journal of Reproductive Medicine* 53, no. 5 (2008): 338–46. PMID: 18567279.

"Sympto-Thermal Method." Fertility Appreciation Collaborative to Teach the Science (FACTS), 2014. https://www.factsaboutfertility.org/wp-content/uploads/2014/09/SymptoThermalPEH.pdf.

Taran, F. A., E. A. Stewart, and S. Brucker. "Adenomyosis: Epidemiology, Risk Factors, Clinical Phenotype and Surgical and Interventional Alternatives to Hysterectomy." *Geburtshilfe und Frauenheilkunde* 73, no. 9 (2013): 924–31. doi: 10.1055/s-0033-1350840.

Taşkaldıran, Işılay, Emre Vuraloğlu, Yusuf Bozkuş, Özlem Turhan İyidir, Aslı Nar, and Neslihan Başçıl Tütüncü. "Menstrual Changes after COVID-19 Infection and COVID-19 Vaccination." *International Journal of Clinical Practice* (2022): 3199758. doi: 10.1155/2022/3199758.

Taylor, Alison. "ABC of Subfertility: Extent of the Problem." *British Medical Journal (BMJ)* 327, no. 7412 (2003): 434–36. doi: 10.1136/bmj.327.7412.434.

Teicholz, Nina. "A Short History of Saturated Fat: The Making and Unmaking of a Scientific Consensus." *Current Opinion in Endocrinology, Diabetes, and Obesity* 30, no. 1 (2022): 65–71. doi: 10.1097/MED.0000000000000791.

Thiyagarajan, Dhanalakshmi K. "Physiology, Menstrual Cycle." *StatPearls* (online). Treasure Island, FL: StatPearls Publishing, 2023. https://www.ncbi.nlm.nih.gov/books/NBK500020/.

Torre F., A. E. Calogero, R. A. Condorelli, R. Cannarella, A. Aversa, and S. La Vignera. "Effects of Oral Contraceptives on Thyroid Function and Vice Versa." *Journal of Endocrinological Investigation* 43, no. 9 (2020): 1181–88. doi: 10.1007/s40618-020-01230-8.

Travis, Ruth C., and Timothy J. Key. "Oestrogen Exposure and Breast Cancer Risk." *Breast Cancer Research (BCR)* 5, no. 5 (2003): 239–47. doi: 10.1186/bcr628.

Ugazio, Elena, Vivian Tullio, Arianna Binello, Silvia Tagliapietra, and Franco Dosio. "Ozonated Oils as Antimicrobial Systems in Topical Applications. Their Characterization, Current Applications, and Advances in Improved Delivery Techniques." *Molecules* 25, no. 2 (2020): 334. doi: 10.3390/molecules25020334.

Ułamek-Kozioł, Marzena, Stanisław J. Czuczwar, Sławomir Januszewski, and Ryszard Pluta. "Ketogenic Diet and Epilepsy." *Nutrients* 11, no. 10 (2019): 2510. doi: 10.3390/nu11102510.

Underwood, E. Ashworth, and Robert Richardson. "History of Medicine." *Encyclopædia Britannica*, last updated December 13, 2024. https://www.britannica.com/science/history-of-medicine.

"Uterine Fibroids and Polycystic Ovarian Syndrome: Is There a Connection?" Fibroid Treatment Collective. Accessed July 10, 2019. https://fibroids.com/blog/uterine-fibroids-and-polycystic-ovarian-syndrome-is-there-a-connection/.

Van Vliet, H., D. A. Grimes, F. M. Helmerhorst, and K. F. Schulz. "Biphasic versus Monophasic Oral Contraceptives for Contraception." *Cochrane Database of Systematic Reviews* 2006, no. 3 (2006): CD0022032. doi: 10.1002/14651858.CD002032.pub2.

Van Vliet, Hubertus, and Kenneth Schulz. "Triphasic Contraceptive Agent." *Contraception* 65, no. 5 (2002): 321–24. doi: 10.1016/S0010-7824(01)00314-6.

Vekemans, M. "Postpartum Contraception: The Lactational Amenorrhea Method." *European Journal of Contraception and Reproductive Health Care* 2, no. 2 (1997): 105–11. doi: 10.3109/13625189709167463.

Venkatasamy, Vighnesh Vetrivel, Sandeep Pericherla, Sachin Manthuruthil, Shikha Mishra, and Ram Hanno. "Effect of Physical Activity on Insulin Resistance, Inflammation and Oxidative Stress in Diabetes Mellitus." *Journal of Clinical and Diagnostic Research (JCDR)* 7, no. 8 (2013): 1764–66. doi: 10.7860/JCDR/2013/6518.3306.

Verhaeghe, J., R. Gheysen, and P. Enzlin. "Pheromones and Their Effect on Women's Mood and Sexuality." *Facts, Views, and Vision in ObGyn* 5, no. 3 (2013): 189–95. https://pubmed.ncbi.nlm.nih.gov/24753944/.

"Vitamin B12: Fact Sheet for Health Professionals." National Institutes of Health, Office of Dietary Supplements. Accessed June 27, 2024. https://ods.od.nih.gov/factsheets/VitaminB12-HealthProfessional/#:~:text=Even%20at%20large%20doses%2C%20vitamin,does%20not%20store%20excess%20amounts.

Vliet, Hubertus van, and Kenneth Schultz. "Triphasic Contraceptive Agent." Triphasic Contraceptive Agent—an overview. ScienceDirect Topics, 2002. https://www.sciencedirect.com/topics/medicine-and-dentistry/triphasic-contraceptive-agent.

Vom Saal, Frederick S., and Laura N. Vandenberg. "Update on the Health Effects of Bisphenol A: Overwhelming Evidence of Harm." *Endocrinology* 162, no. 3 (2020): bqaa171. doi: 10.7860/JCDR/2013/6518.3306.

Walker, Matthew H., and Kyle Tobler. "Female Infertility." *StatPearls* (online). Treasure Island, FL: StatPearls Publishing, 2023. https://www.ncbi.nlm.nih.gov/books/NBK556033/#:~:text=Ovulatory%20disorders%20make%20up%2025,opportunity%20for%20fertilization%20and%20pregnancy.

Wang, Hai-Yan, Xi-Hua Bao, and Jun-Feng Dai. "[Treatment of Ovarian Cyst after Ovulation-Induction with Sanjie Zhentong Capsule]." *Zhongguo Zhong xi yi jie he za zhi* [Chinese journal of integrated traditional and Western medicine] 28, no. 11 (2008): 1026–28. PMID: 19213349.

Wang, Ruohan, Ying Feng, Jiahe Chen, Yingjiao Chen, and Fang Ma. "Association between Polyunsaturated Fatty Acid Intake and Infertility among American Women Aged 20–44 Years." *Frontiers in Public Health* 10 (2022): 938343. doi: 10.3389/fpubh.2022.938343.

Wang, Xiaoxia, Tongzhang Xian, Xiaofan Jia, Lina Zhang, Li Liu, Fuli Man, Xianbo Zhang, Jie Zhang, Qi Pan, and Lixin Guo. "A Cross-Sectional Study on the Associations of Insulin Resistance with Sex Hormone, Abnormal Lipid Metabolism in T2DM and IGT Patients." *Medicine* 96, no. 26 (2017): doi: 10.1097/MD.0000000000007378.

Wartella, E. A., A. H. Lichenstein, and C. S. Boon, eds. "History of Nutrition Labeling." In *Front-of-Package Nutrition Rating Systems and Symbols: Phase I Report*. Washington, DC: National Academies Press, 2010. https://www.ncbi.nlm.nih.gov/books/NBK209859/.

Weisz, George, and Loes Knaapen. "Diagnosing and Treating Premenstrual Syndrome in Five Western Nations." *Social Science & Medicine* 68, no. 8 (2009): 1498–1505. doi: 10.1016/j.socscimed.2009.01.036.

"What Is Implantation Bleeding?" American Pregnancy Association, September 20, 2023. https://americanpregnancy.org/pregnancy-symptoms/what-is-implantation-bleeding/#:~:text=Generally%2C%20around%20a%20third%20of,is%20lighter%20than%20menstrual%20bleeding.

"When Can I Expect a Positive HPT If I Am Pregnant?" Fertility Friend. Accessed June 28, 2024. https://www.fertilityfriend.com/Faqs/When-can-I-expect-a-positive-HPT-if-I-am-pregnant.html.

Whitehead, Brenda R., and C. S. Bergeman. "Daily Religious Coping Buffers the Stress-Affect Relationship and Benefits Overall Metabolic Health in Older Adults." *Psychology of Religion and Spirituality* 12, no. 4 (2019): 393–99. doi: 10.1037/rel0000251.

Wilcox, A. J., D. D. Baird, and C. R. Weinberg. "Time of Implantation of the Conceptus and Loss of Pregnancy." *New England Journal of Medicine* 340, no. 23 (1999): 1796–99. doi: 10.1056/NEJM199906103402304.

Wise, Amber, Kacie O'Brien, and Tracey Woodruff. "Are Oral Contraceptives a Significant Contributor to the Estrogenicity of Drinking Water?" *Environmental Science and Technology* 45, no. 1 (2011): 51–60. doi: 10.1021/es1014482.

Wise, Lauren A., Amelia K. Wesselink, Katherine L. Tucker, Shilpa Saklani, Ellen M. Mikkelsen, Heidi Cueto, Anders H. Riis, Ellen Trolle, Craig J. McKinnon, Kristen A. Hahn, Kenneth J. Rothman, Henrik Toft Sørensen, and Elizabeth E. Hatch. "Dietary Fat Intake and Fecundability in 2 Preconception Cohort Studies." *American Journal of Epidemiology* 187, no. 1 (2018): 60–74. doi: 10.1093/aje/kwx204.

Woo, Hye Lin, Hae Ri Ji, Yeon Kyoung Pak, Hojung Lee, Su Jeong Heo, Jin Moo Lee, and Kyoung Sun Park. "The Efficacy and Safety of Acupuncture in Women with Primary Dysmenorrhea: A Systematic Review and Meta-Analysis." *Medicine* 97, no 23 (2018): e11007. https://www.ncbi.nlm.nih.gov/pmc/articles/PMC5999465/.

Wooltorton, Eric. "The Evra (Ethinyl Estradiol/Norelgestromin) Contraceptive Patch: Estrogen Exposure Concerns." *Canadian Medical Association Journal (CMAJ)* 174, no. 2 (2006): 164–65. doi: 10.1503/cmaj.051623.

Wu, Guoyao. "Dietary Protein Intake and Human Health." *Food & Function* 7, no. 3 (2016): 1251–65. doi: 10.1039/c5fo01530h.

Wyatt, K. M., P. W. Dimmock, P. W. Jones, and P. M. Shaughn O'Brien. "Efficacy of Vitamin B-6 in the Treatment of Premenstrual Syndrome: Systematic Review." *British Medical Journal (BMJ)* 318, no. 7195 (1999): 1375–81. doi: 10.1136/bmj.318.7195.1375.

Xiao, Bryan, Tianna Zeng, S. Wu, H. Sun, and N. Xiao. "Effect of Levonorgestrel-Releasing Intrauterine Device on Hormonal Profile and Menstrual Pattern after Long-Term Use." *Contraception* 51, no. 6 (1995): 359–65. doi: 10.1016/0010-7824(95)00102-g.

Xiao, Keyi, Akiko Furutani, Hiroyuki Sasaki, Masaki Takahashi, and Shigenobu Shibata. "Effect of a High Protein Diet at Breakfast on Postprandial Glucose Level at Dinner Time in Healthy Adults." *Nutrients* 15, no. 1 (2022): 85. doi: 10.3390/nu15010085.

Xiping, Liu, W. U. Xiaqiu, Bao Lirong, Peng Jin, and Ka-Kit Hui. "Menstrual Cycle Characteristics as an Indicator of Fertility Outcomes: Evidence from Prospective Birth Cohort Study in China." *Journal of Traditional Chinese Medicine* 42, no. 2 (2022): 272–78. doi: 10.19852/j.cnki.jtcm.2022.02.010.

"XULANE-Norelgestromin and Ethinyl Estradiol Patch." Xulane. Accessed June 27, 2024. https://dailymed.nlm.nih.gov/dailymed/fda/fdaDrugXsl.cfm?setid=f7848550-086a-43d8-8ae5-047f4b9e4382&type=display.

Yan, Han, Yi Chen, Hong Zhu, Wei-Hua Huang, Xin-He Cai, Dan Li, Ya-Juan Lv, Si-Zhao, Hong-Hao Zhou, Fan-Yan Luo, Wei Zhang, and Xi Li. "The Relationship among Intestinal Bacteria, Vitamin K and Response of Vitamin K Antagonist: A Review of Evidence and Potential Mechanism." *Frontiers in Medicine* 9 (2022): 829304. doi: 10.3389/fmed.2022.829304.

Yavarikia, Parisa, Mahnaz Shahnazi, Samira Hadavand Mirzaie, Yousef Javadzadeh, and Razieh Lutfi. "Comparing the Effect of Mefenamic Acid and Vitex Agnus on Intrauterine Device Induced Bleeding." *Journal of Caring Sciences* 2, no. 3 (2013): 245–54. doi: 10.5681/jcs.2013.030.

"Yaz (drospirenone and ethinyl estradiol) Tablets." Accessed June 25, 2024. https://www.accessdata.fda.gov/drugsatfda_docs/label/2010/021676s009lbl.pdf.

Yoon, Seonmin, Jung-Ick Byun, and Won Chul Shin. "Efficacy and Safety of Low-Dose Gamma-Aminobutyric Acid from Unpolished Rice Germ as a Health Functional Food for Promoting Sleep: A Randomized, Double-Blind, Placebo-Controlled Trial." *Journal of Clinical Neurology* 18, no. 4 (2022): 478–80. doi: 10.3988/jcn.2022.18.4.478.

Zabin, L. S., P. W. Scher, R. H. DuRant, J. D. Forrest, S. K. Henshaw, and S. J. Emans. "Contraceptive Compliance with a Triphasic and a Monophasic Norethindrone-Containing Oral Contraceptive Pill in a Private Adolescent Practice." *Adolescent and Pediatric Gynecology* 7, no. 1 (1994). https://www.sciencedirect.com/science/article/abs/pii/S0932861012801757.

Zaccaro, Andrea, Andrea Piarulli, Marco Laurino, Erika Garbella, Danilo Menicucci, Bruno Neri, and Angelo Gemignani. "How Breath-Control Can Change Your Life: A Systematic Review on Psycho-Physiological Correlates of Slow Breathing." *Frontiers in Human Neuroscience* 12 (2018): 353. doi: 10.3389/fnhum.2018.00353.

Zduńska, Anna, Joanna Cegielska, and Izabela Domitrz. "The Pathogenetic Role of Melatonin in Migraine and Its Theoretic Implications for Pharmacotherapy: A Brief Overview of the Research." *Nutrients* 14, no. 16 (2022): 3335. doi: 10.3390/nu14163335.

Zeng, Ling-Hui, Saba Rana, Liaqat Hussain, Muhammad Asif, Malik Hassan Mehmood, Imran Imran, Anam Younas, Amina Mahdy, Fakhria A. Al-Joufi, and Shaymaa Najm Abed. "Polycystic Ovary Syndrome: A Disorder of Reproductive Age, Its Pathogenesis, and a Discussion on the Emerging Role of Herbal Remedies." *Frontiers in Pharmacology* 13 (2022): 874914. doi: 10.3389/fphar.2022.874914.

Zhan, Xiaoshu, Lauren Fletcher, Serena Dingle, Enzo Baracuhy, Bingyun Wang, Lee-Anne Huber, and Julang Li. "Choline Supplementation Influences Ovarian Follicular Development." *Frontiers in Bioscience* 26, no. 12 (2021): 1525–36. doi: 10.52586/5046.

Zhang, Jianfu, and Bengui Jiang. "Influence of Melatonin Treatment on Emotion, Sleep, and Life Quality in Perimenopausal Women: A Clinical Study." *Journal of Healthcare Engineering* 2023, no. 1 (2023): 2198804. doi: 10.1155/2023/2198804.

Zhao, Ting-Tint, Yong-Kang Liu, Jun-Ling Zhou, Hou-Xu Ning, Xiao-Liang Wu, Ya-Fang Song, Jian-Hua Sun, and Li-Xia Pei. "[Effect of Acupuncture on Hypothalamic Functional Connectivity in Patients with Premature OVA-Rian Insufficiency Based on Resting-State Functional Magnetic Resonance Imaging]." *Zhen ci yan jiu* 47, no. 7 (2022): 617–24. doi: 10.13702/j.1000-0607.20210399.

Zhu, Zhanhui, Yang Lei, and Zheng Lin. "Effects of Crohn's Disease Exclusion Diet on Remission: A Systematic Review." *Therapeutic Advances in Gastroenterology* 16 (2023): doi: 10.1177/17562848231184056.

Zucca-Matthes, Gustavo, Cícero Urban, and André Vallejo. "Anatomy of the Nipple and Breast Ducts." *Gland Surgery* 5, no. 1 (2016): 32–36. doi: 10.3978/j.issn.2227-684X.2015.05.10.

INDEX

Note: Page numbers in *"italics"* represents figures in the text.

5-Hydroxytryptophan (5-HTP), 203
150-minute rule, 75

A1 β-casein, 82
A2 β-casein, 82
abnormal bleeding (spotting), 214, 217, 227
acupuncture, 92, 95, 207, 225
adenomyosis, 41, 208–10
adrenal dysfunction, 198, 221, 247
adrenal fatigue a.ka. "Burnout Syndrome," 247
adrenal hormone imbalances: adrenal dysfunction, 198, 221, 247; adrenal fatigue a.ka. "Burnout Syndrome," 247; chronic stress response, 246
alpha lipoic acid (ALA), 219, 223
amenorrhea, 4–6, 87, 147; hypothalamic amenorrhea (HA), 224–25; lactational amenorrhea, 165–66

American Academy of Sleep Medicine, 72
American Gut Project, 92
American Journal of Endocrinology, 63
anemia, 21–22, 63, 133, 195, 196, 213
Angelou, Maya, 11
animal protein, 82, 86–87
anxiety, 2, 7, 77, 81, 84, 135, 141, 154, 176, 199, 200–204
ashwagandha *(Withania somnifera),* 201, 202, 221, 225
autoimmune diseases, 21
average-cycle-minus-fourteen rule, 112

Bartholin's glands, 35
basal body temperature (BBT), 137, 179; average basal body temperature, 113; charting, 111, 115–17, *117;* definition, 111; limitations, 117–18; measuring

steps, 114–15; *vs.* resting heart rate (RHR), 119; thermometer, 114
BBT. *See* basal body temperature (BBT)
berberine, 219
bicornuate uterus, 41, *42*
binding globulin availability hypothyroidism, 242
birth control. *See also* birth control pills; contraceptives
birth control pills, 2–10, 76; combined pills, 152; estrogen-containing pills, 152; first-generation progestins/estranes, 153; fourth-generation progestin, 154; high-risk contraceptives, 8; hormonal fluctuations, 56, *57*; Lo Loestrin Fe, 152; monophasic combined pills, 154–55; multiphasic combined pills, 155; multiphasic pills, 152; negative side effects, 172; placebo pills, 151; progestin-only pills, 152, 156; risks and complications, 4, 7–9; second-generation progestins/gonanes, 153; synthetic estrogen compounds, 7; third-generation progestins, 153–54; ulipristal, 163; Yaz, 5–7; *See also* contraceptives
black cohosh *(Cimicifuga racemosa)*, 192, 201, 225
blastocyst, 181
Blood sugar balance, 83–85
Borrelia burgdorferi, 20
Bowman, Katy, 38
breast anatomy: anatomical diagram, 37; areola, 38, 39; fascia, 37; glandular tissue, 38; muscle of Meyerholz, 39; muscle of Sappey, 39; supernumerary nipples, 36; suspensory ligaments, 37
breast movement, 38
breast self-examination, 39

breast tenderness, 9, 39, 59, 112, 132, 190; caused by estrogen dominance, 195; caused by fibrocystic breast disease, 194; pharmacological treatment, 193–94

calcium-D-glucarate (CDG), 209–10, 216, 228
calories, 81
carbohydrates, 4, 82–88, 91, 138
celiac disease, 22
Centers for Disease Control and Prevention (CDC), 75
cervical checking, 42
cervical fluid tracking, 120–23
cervical mucus, 55, 66, 67, *67,* 121, 123, 126, 150, 156, 158, 179–82
chaste tree *(Vitex agnus-castus),* 192, 201, 203, 214, 232
chronic infections, 20–21, 42
chronic stress response, 246
Cipro, 6
clean eating, 96
clitoris *(Corpus cavernosum),* 34–35
common period-tracking app, 60
condoms, 11; female/internal condoms, 160–61; male/external condoms, 159–60
congenital adrenal hyperplasia, 221
contraceptives, 2, 188; cervical cap, 161–62; condoms, 11, 159–61; diaphragm, 161–62; emergency contraception, 163–64; ethinylestradiol, 143, 144; fertility awareness methods (FAM), 166–67; intrauterine devices (IUDs). *See* intrauterine devices (IUDs); lactational amenorrhea, 165–66; levonorgestrel (LNG), 146; patch, 157–58; ring, 158; sponge, 162–63; sterilization techniques, 144; tubal ligation/removal, 145–46; vasectomy, 144–45; ways to support

your body, 173–74; withdrawal method, 11, 164–65; *See also* birth control pills
copper IUD, 148–49, 163
corpus luteum, 53, 55, 110, 117, 135, 137, 138, 181
COVID-19 pandemic, 19
Creighton Model Method, 122
cycle syncing method, 129, 130
cyclic therapy, 226

Dalton, Katharina, 68
day-twenty-one progesterone tests, 110
dehydroepiandrosterone (DHEA), 24, 26, 46, 55, 76, 218
Depo-Provera, 150–51
dietary fat: animal fats, 90; deficiency of, 88; diet-heart hypothesis, 90; fat-restricted diet, 88–91; ill-gotten reputation, 89; omega-3 fatty acids, 89, 90; saturated, 88, 91; unsaturated, 88–89
diindolylmethane (DIM), 201, 209, 214–16, 220, 228
The Dirty Dozen, 101
Dong quai *(Angelica sinensis)*, 210
dysmenorrhea, 4, 205

eating disorders, 80–81
emergency contraception, 163–64
endometriosis, 41, 170, 210–12
environmental contaminants, 101
Environmental Working Group's (EWG's): *Guide to Healthy Cleaning*, 104; *Skin Deep* website, 103
Epstein Barr Virus, 20
estrobolome, 173–74
estrogen, 53–56, 66–68, 88, 92, 100, 103, 111, 113, 119–23, 132–38, 140, 152, 153, 166, 181, 188, 190, 192–95, 203, 209, 210, 225, 227–28; artificial estrogen, 155, 224; binding, 173; deficiency, 23, 25, 63, 200–201; dominance, 24, 25, 200–202, 243, 244; estrogen-containing contraceptives, 156, 173, 191; estrogen-dominant conditions, 41, 211, 213, 215, 221; estrogen-gut microbiome axis, 23; estrogenic acne, 230; metabolism, 214, 216, 220; migraines, 191; pills, 152, 154, 191; synthetic estrogen, 154
Evening primrose oil (EPO), 123
exercises, 3, 4, 34, 74–76, 80, 89, 97, 98, 134, 136, 138, 140–42, 224, 225
external genital anatomy. *See* vulva

family planning, 2, 169–71; after coming off of hormonal contraceptives, 173–74; preconception support, 174–76; prenatal vitamins, 176–78; return to fertility, 171; trying to conceive (TTC), 178–80; two-week-wait, 180–85
fatigue, 64, 66, 76, 84, 130, 221; caused by HPA axis dysfunction, 198; caused by inflammation, 198–99; caused by iron deficiency, 196–97; pharmacological treatment, 196
feedback loops, 51
female reproductive hormones. *See* estrogen; progesterone
fennel *(Foeniculum vulgare)*, 206
fertile window, 170
fertility awareness methods (FAM), 166–67
Fertility Friend app, 116
Feverfew *(Tanacetum parthenium)*, 191, 192
fiber, 83, 84, 91–92, 133, 173
fibrocystic breast disease, 194
fibroids, 41, 63, 163, 213, 215–16

first response early result (FRER) test, 183–84
Five Elements theory, 93–95, *94,* 98–99
follicle-stimulating hormone (FSH), 51, 54, 132, 133, 224–26, 231
follicular phase, 54, 113, 116, 121, 124; days, 131; emotional health, 133; energy and sleep, 132–33; exercise, 134; hormonal review, 132; nutrition, 133–34; sexuality, 134; TCM perspective, 132
Food and Drug Administration (FDA), 177
food-borne illnesses, 20
Frankincense *(Olibanum),* 214

GABA, 204
Galen, Claudius, 31
gastrointestinal (GI) disorders, 22
ginger *(Zinziber officinale),* 206, 214
gonadotropin-releasing hormone (GnRH), 51
Guide to Healthy Cleaning, 104
Gui Zhi Fu Ling Wan, 216

Hashimoto's hypothyroidism, 240–41
health-o-meter, 18–20
heavy periods, 212–15
high androgens, 26
high-intensity interval training (HIIT) workouts, 134
Hill, Sarah, 57
hormonal acne, 230–31
hormonal birth control, 57, 214, 229
hormone receptor competition hypothyroidism, 241–42
Hornsby, Paige Perry, 62
human chorionic gonadotrophin (hCG), 181
hyperprolactinemia, 171, 231–32
hyperthyroidism, 28

hypothalamic amenorrhea (HA), 224–25
hypothalamic hypothyroidism, 240
hypothalamicpituitary-adrenal axis (HPA axis), 51
hypothalamic-pituitary-adrenal-thyroid-gonadal-axis (HPATG) axis, 27, 49–51, *50,* 55, 76, 87, 117, 118, 137
hypothalamic-pituitary-gonadal axis (HPG axis), 51–52, 132
hypothalamic-pituitary-thyroid axis (HPT) axis, 51
hypothyroidism, 5, 27, 28, 63, 114, 187, 205, 213; binding globulin availability hypothyroidism, 242; Hashimoto's hypothyroidism, 240–41; hormone receptor competition hypothyroidism, 241–42; hypothalamic hypothyroidism, 240; nutrient deficiency hypothyroidism, 242–43; peripheral conversion defect hypothyroidism, 241; primary hypothyroidism, 239

Indole-3-carbinol (I3C), 216, 228
infertility, 21, 42, 49, 63, 90, 170
inflammation, 19, 20, 22, 28, 35, 40, 45, 63, 64, 66, 71, 76, 82, 83, 90, 100, 132, 139, 192–95, 198–200, 203, 204, 207, 209–11, 222, 223
inositol, 219, 221–23
insulin resistance, 83
intermittent fasting, 84
internal genital anatomy. *See* uterus
International Federation of Gynecology and Obstetrics (FIGO), 63
intrauterine devices (IUDs), 8, 171; advantages, 147; copper IUD, 148–49, 163; drawbacks, 147–48; Kyleena IUD, 146; levonorgestrel (LNG), 146; Liletta IUD, 147; Mirena IUD, 147; nonhormonal

IUD option, 148–51; Skyla IUD, 146; T-shaped device, 146
in vitro fertilization (IVF) egg retrieval cycles, 110
irregular periods, 217
irritability and/or anxiety, 2, 7, 77, 81, 84, 135, 141, 154, 176, 199, 200–204; caused by estrogen deficiency, 200–201; caused by estrogen dominance, 201; caused by HPA axis dysfunction, 202
IUDs. *See* intrauterine devices (IUDs)

Journal of Behavioral Medicine, 79

Kabat-Zinn, Jon, 77
Kegels, 34
ketogenic diet, 79
Kyleena IUD, 146

lactational amenorrhea, 165–66
Lady's mantle *(Alchemilla vulgaris)*, 210
L-arginine, 123
levonorgestrel (LNG), 146
Liletta IUD, 147
Listeria monocytogenes, 20
liver detox, 173
Lo Loestrin Fe, 152
Loperamide, 6
low androgens, 26–28
lubricants, 179–80
luteal phase, 53, 66, 111, 112, 116, 121–22, 124, 131; days, 136; defect (luteal phase deficiency), 232–33; emotional health, 137; energy and sleep, 137; exercise, 138; hormonal review, 137; nutrition, 137–38; sexuality, 138; TCM review, 137
luteinizing hormone (LH), 51, 72, 132; strips, 116, 124–25, 179; surge, 55

maca *(Lepidium meyenii)*, 200–202, 225
MacKillop, Alexandra, 15

macronutrients, 81–83, 85
magnesium glycinate, 192–93, 206, 219
male fertility, 170
male reproductive hormones. *See* DHEA; testosterone
Mayo Clinic, 60
melatonin, 74, 193, 223, 226
membranous dysmenorrhea, 64
menstrual cycle, 51; anovulatory cycle, 56; blood color, 63–64; breast changes, 68; cervical mucus, 66–67, *67*; cramps and pain, 66; cycle length, 60, 62; cycle syncing method, 129, 130, 142; flow, 65; follicle (egg) maturation process, 54; follicular phase, 54, 113, 116, 121, 124, 131–34; foundational habits, 130; frequency, 60, 62; hormonal fluctuations, 56, *57*; hormonal signaling, 54, *54*; late follicular phase, 121; length of cycles, 53; luteal phase, 53, 66, 111, 112, 116, 121–22, 124, 131, 136–38; menstrual blood measurement, 65, *65*; menstrual phase, 53, 121, 124, 131, 140–42; midcycle bleeding, 63; mood changes, 67–68; normal period characteristics, 60, *61*; ovulatory/fertile phase, 53, 121, 124, 131, 134–36; pale pink bleeding, 64; period length, 62; pregnancy, 124; premenstrual phase, 131, 138–40; spotting, 62, 63; texture, 64–65; twenty-eight-day cycle, 53, 59, 112
Menstrual Disorders Committee (MDC), 63
menstrual irregularities, 12
menstrual phase, 53, 121, 124, 131, 140–42
menstrual products, 207–8
mental and emotional disorders, 2

Merck Manual, 60
microbiome, 22–24, 27
Mirena IUD, 147
monophasic combined pills, 154–55
Montgomery's tubercles, 38
mood changes: depression, 202–3; irritability and/or anxiety, 200–202; pharmacological treatment, 199–200; premenstrual dysphoric disorder (PMDD), 204
multiphasic combined pills, 155
muscle of Meyerholz, 39

N-acetyl-cysteine (NAC), 223
National Library of Medicine, 60
natural progesterone, 233
Nexplanon, 149–50
nonhormonal IUD option: copper IUD, 148–49; Depo-Provera, 150–51; Nexplanon, 149–50; Paragard, 148–49
normal period characteristics, 60, *61*
nutrient deficiency hypothyroidism, 242–43
nutrition, 133–34; A1 β-casein, 82; A2 β-casein, 82; animal protein, 86–87; blood sugar balance, 83–85; calories, 81; carbohydrates, 87–88; dietary fat, 88–91; dietary intervention, 79; eating disorders, 80–81; fiber, 91–92; ketogenic diet, 79; macronutrients, 81–83, 85; omega-3 fatty acids, 174; protein, 85–86; therapeutic dietary modifications, 79
Nutrition Labeling and Education Act, 81

O'Connell, Helen, 34
oil-based cleanser, 231
omega-3 fatty acids (docosahexaenoic acid (DHA)), 89, 90, 141, 174, 176, 198–99, 201, 203, 206, 210, 212
omega-6 fatty acids, 89, 90
oocyte quality, 174
ovarian cysts, 228–30
ovulation, 25, 43, 44, 52–56, 60, 66, 68, 109, 130, 134–38, 144, 146, 149–52, 157, 158, 163–66, 170, 178–82, 189–91, 219, 223, 224, 227, 230, 231; average-cycle-minus-fourteen rule, 112; basal body temperature (BBT), 111–18; cervical fluid tracking, 120–23; cervical position, 123–24; cycle tracking, 126–27, *127*; Fertility Friend app, 116; 5 + 2 rule, 113; luteinizing hormone test strips, 116, 124–25; predicting and confirming, 110–25; resting heart rate (RHR), 118–20, *120*; symptothermal method, 116; tracking app, 111–12; women chart, 113
ovulatory disorders, 170–71
ovulatory/fertile phase, 53, 121, 124, 131; days, 134; emotional health, 136; energy and sleep, 135; exercise, 136; hormonal review, 135; nutrition, 136; sexuality, 136; TCM review, 135
ozonated oil, 231

painful periods: acupuncture, 207; causes, 208; degree of pelvic tenderness, 204; dysmenorrhea, 205; fennel *(Foeniculum vulgare)*, 206; ginger *(Zinziber officinale)*, 206; inflammation, 204; magnesium glycinate, 206; omega-3 fatty acids, 206; pharmacological treatment, 205; pycnogenol (French pine bark), 206–7; turmeric *(Curcuma cyminum)*, 206
Paragard, 148–49
partial mastectomy, 36

PCOS. *See* polycystic ovarian syndrome (PCOS)
pelvic adhesions, 170–71
perimenopause, 225–26
peripheral conversion defect hypothyroidism, 241
pesticides, 100–101
pheromones, 33
PMS. *See* premenstrual syndrome (PMS)
polycystic ovarian syndrome (PCOS), 43, 71, 117, 153, 217–23, 245; *post-pill PCOS,* 222–23
polyps, 63, 213, 215–16
polysorbate-60, 103
pomegranate flower (*Punica granatum,* Persian Golnar), 214
post birth-control syndrome/post-pill syndrome, 172
preconception support: choline (phosphatidylcholine), 176; CoEnzyme Q10 (ubiquinol), 175; nutrient-dense diet, 174; omega-3 fatty acids (docosahexaenoic acid (DHA)), 174, 176; vitamin B12 (Methylcobalamin), 175–76; zinc bisglycinate, 175
premenstrual dysphoric disorder (PMDD), 204
premenstrual headaches: causes, 190; migraines caused by estrogen withdrawal, 191–92; migraines caused by inflammation, 192–93; pharmacological treatment, 190–91
premenstrual phase: days, 138; emotional health, 139; energy and sleep, 139; exercise, 140; hormonal review, 138–39; nutrition, 139–40; sexuality, 140; TCM review, 139
premenstrual spotting, 62, 63
premenstrual syndrome (PMS), 12, 22, 39, 68–69, 76; abnormal bleeding (spotting), 227; adenomyosis, 208–10; breast tenderness, 193–96; endometriosis, 210–12; estrogen dominance (excess estrogen), 228; estrogen dominance (low progesterone), 227–28; fatigue, 195–99; fibroids, 215–16; heavy periods, 212–15; hormonal acne, 230–31; hyperprolactinemia, 231–32; hypothalamic amenorrhea, 224–25; irregular periods, 217; luteal phase defect (luteal phase deficiency), 232–33; mood changes, 199–204; ovarian cysts, 228–30; painful periods, 204–8; perimenopause, 225–26; polycystic ovarian syndrome (PCOS), 217–23; polyps, 215–16; premenstrual headaches, 190–93; symptoms, 190
prenatal vitamins: choline, 177; folate, 176; iron, 177–78; vitamin A, 177; vitamin B12, 176; vitamin D, 177
PreSeed™ Fertility Lubricant, 179, 180
primary hypothyroidism, 239
progesterone, 24, 26, 53, 55, 56, 67, 76, 109, 111, 116, 144; cream, 188–89, 192, 210, 212; day-twenty-one progesterone tests, 110; deficiency, 25, 66, 112; measurement, 110
progestin-only pills, 156
pro-inflammatory chemicals, 66
prolactin, 165, 231, 232
prostaglandins, 20, 53, 66, 183, 192, 194, 204, 206
protein, 46, 82–87, 138
proteolytic enzymes, 209, 211–12
pycnogenol (French pine bark), 206–7, 212

Qi, 95

reactive hypoglycemia, 84

remote reproductive organs. *See* thyroid gland
reproductive hormones, 51
resting heart rate (RHR), 118–20, *120*
resveratrol, 212
rhodiola *(Rhodiola rosea),* 202

S-adenosylmethionine (SAMe), 203
Sanjie zhentong, 229–30
septate uterus, 41, *42*
sex education ("sex ed"), 1, 10–11, 169
sex hormone imbalances, 23–24; estrogen excess (estrogen dominance), 243; low androgens, 245; other estrogen dominance, 244; polycystic ovarian syndrome (PCOS). *See* polycystic ovarian syndrome (PCOS); progesterone deficiency (estrogen dominance), 244; sex hormone deficiency, 246
sex hormone receptors, 3
sexually transmitted infections (STIs), 11
Skene's glands, 35
Skin Deep website, 103
Skyla IUD, 146
sleep: bedtime routines, 73; daily schedule, 72; difficulty sleeping, 72–73; diurnal, 72; hormones reset, 72; medications, 73; quality improvement, 73; sleep-wake cycle, 72; supplements to support sleep, 73–74
spearmint tea, 220
spotting, 62, 63; abnormal bleeding (spotting), 214, 217, 227; premenstrual spotting, 62, 63
St. John's wort *(Hypericum perforatum),* 204
stress: 4-7-8 breathing, 77; allostatic load, 76; clear your schedule, 78; cultivating a spiritual practice, 77; ditch multitasking, 77–78; get outside, 78–79; hormones, 19, 28–29; impacts, 76; meditation, 77; mindfulness, 77; mitigation techniques, 77–79; wellness techniques, 77–79
supernumerary nipple, 36
supplements to support sleep, 73–74
symptothermal method, 116

tampons, 5, 13, 43, 64, 65, 207, 208
TCM. *See* Traditional Chinese Medicine (TCM)
testosterone, 26, 27, 55, 67, 83, 153, 219, 220, 224
thyroid gland, *45,* 45–47
thyroid imbalances, 28; binding globulin availability hypothyroidism, 242; Hashimoto's hypothyroidism, 240–41; hormone receptor competition hypothyroidism, 241–42; hypothalamic hypothyroidism, 240; nutrient deficiency hypothyroidism, 242–43; peripheral conversion defect hypothyroidism, 241; primary hypothyroidism, 239
time-restricted eating, 84
toxins: cleaning products, 104–5; clothing, 105; cookware, 101–2; do-it-yourself (DIY) projects, 106–7; environmental exposures, 105–7; in food, 100–102; footwear, 105–6; furniture products, 105–6; grocery receipts, 105; personal care products, 102–3; pesticides, 100–101; plastic compound bisphenol A (BPA), 100; plastic packaging, 101; surfactant chemicals, 100; in water, 102
Traditional Chinese Medicine (TCM), 64, 99, 129, 131–33, 207; acupuncture, 92; benefits, 93; Five Elements theory, 93–95, *94,* 98–99;

lifestyle changes, 92; Qi, 95; yin-yang theory, 93, 96–98
triphaladi kayasha, 229
"triple protection plan," 11
trying to conceive (TTC): antihistamines (allergy medications), 180; cervical mucus, 179; lubricants, 179–80; non-steroidal anti-inflammatory drugs (NSAIDs), 180; timing of intercourse, 178–79
T-shaped device, 146
TTC. *See* trying to conceive (TTC)
tubal blockages, 171
tubal/uterine abnormalities, 171
turmeric *(Curcuma cyminum)*, 206
turmeric *(Curcuma longa)*, 193, 199, 212, 223
two-week wait: cervical mucus, 181–82; cervical position, 181; implantation bleeding, 182–83; implantation cramping, 183; implantation dip, 182; increased resting heart rate (RHR), 183; sustained high temperatures, 182; triphasic chart, 182; urine tests, 183–84

ulipristal, 163
uterus: anatomical diagram, 40, *41*; anterior fornix, 43; bicornuate uterus, 41, *42*; body, 41; cervical checking, 42; cervix, 41–43; endometrium, 40, 41; fallopian tubes, 43, 44; fundus, 41; isthmus, 41; myometrium, 40; ovaries, 43; posterior fornix, 43; septate uterus, 41, *42*

valerian root, 202
vasectomy, 144–45
vestibular bulbs, 34
vitality, 14, 17, 19, 88
vitamin B6, 123, 203, 233
vitamin C (ascorbic acid), 221, 233
vitamin K, 23
vulva: anatomical diagram, 32, *33*; Bartholin's glands, 35; clitoris *(Corpus cavernosum)*, 34–35; labia majora (outer lips), 34; labia minora (inner lips), 34; mons pubis, 33; Skene's glands, 35; urethra, 35; vaginal opening, 35; vestibular bulbs, 34; vulva vestibule, 35

Wherever You Go, There You Are (Kabat-Zinn), 77
white peony *(Paeonia lactiflora)*, 221
withdrawal method, 11, 164–65

Yaz, 5–7
yin-yang theory, 93; activity, 97–98; exchange of ideas, 98; light and darkness, 97; mental and physical load, 98; sound, 98; temperature and humidity, 97
Yuka app, 103

ABOUT THE AUTHOR

Dr. Alexandra MacKillop is a fertility-focused functional medicine physician, acupuncturist, food scientist, and women's health advocate. Passionate about supporting the natural design of women's bodies, she seeks to change the cultural conversations surrounding female health through her writing. She is also the author of *Fulfilled*, a non-diet nutrition self-help book, as well as several journaling guides related to women's health topics. In addition to her books, Dr. MacKillop's work can be found online at AlexandraMacKillop.com

   Clinically, Dr. MacKillop treats women suffering from infertility, premenstrual syndrome, painful periods, PCOS, and other cycle-related problems. She sees patients in person and through telemedicine near Chicago, Illinois.